The War Injured Child

Ghassan Soleiman Abu-Sittah
Jamal J. Hoballah

Editors

The War Injured Child

From Point of Injury Treatment Through
Management and Continuum of Care

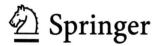 Springer

Editors
Ghassan Soleiman Abu-Sittah
Department of Plastic and
Reconstructive Surgery
American University of Beirut
Beirut, Lebanon

Jamal J. Hoballah
Department of Surgery
American University of Beirut
Medical Center
Beirut, Lebanon

ISBN 978-3-031-28612-4   ISBN 978-3-031-28613-1   (eBook)
https://doi.org/10.1007/978-3-031-28613-1

This Springer imprint is published by the registered company Springer Nature Switzerland AG
The registered company address is: Gewerbestrasse 11, 6330 Cham, Switzerland

To the war injured child…tomorrow is a better day

Acknowledgments

This book represents an attempt to capture the wealth of expertise that has developed over the years within the American University of Beirut Medical Center in the treatment of children with war related and weapons inflicted injuries. My thanks go to everyone within that institution, which is the Middle East's primary academic medical institution and the world's leading civilian academic institution with such unique experience and expertise.

I would like to acknowledge the support given to this project by the Global Health Institute at the American University of Beirut, which is leading the way in undertaking and disseminating research on the clinical burden of war injuries. My gratitude also goes to the Center for Blast Injury Studies at Imperial College which supports collaborative research on war injuries through the ProTect project consortium and to the National Institute for Health Research (UK) which has been funding these international research partnerships looking at the complex relationship between protracted conflict and health. I am grateful to the UK charity Save The Children which was the first to highlight the need for more clinical data on pediatric war injuries and launched the Pediatric Blast Injury Network that continues to work on improving outcome in pediatric war injuries.

The partnership forged between the Department of Surgery at the AUBMC and the charity the International Network for Aid Relief and Assistance (INARA) and the United Nations Children's Fund (UNICEF) to set up the Pediatric War Injuries Program at the Division of Plastic and Reconstructive Surgery was a critical step towards developing a multidisciplinary approach to the treatment of these injuries.

My personal gratitude goes to Dean Mohammed Sayegh (Raja N. Khuri Dean of the Faculty of Medicine and Executive Vice President of Medicine and Global Strategy at the American University of Beirut (AUB) from 2009 to 2020) for his support and encouragement in developing the field of Conflict Medicine at the AUBMC and to my friend and colleague Dr. Imad Kaddoura who was my strongest supporter and ally in developing these projects and partnerships. Most of all my heartfelt thanks and enduring gratitude to Professor Jamal Hoballah, Head of the Department of Surgery at the AUBMC for agreeing to co-edit this book but most importantly for spearheading the initiative to develop the AUBMC into an academic center of excellence in the management of war injuries and in particular in children.

My deep appreciation goes out to all the books' contributors for their hard work and patience. It also goes out to Dr. Ismael Soboh and Dr. Theresa Farahat who helped me edit this book.

But most of all, I will be forever grateful to and in awe of the children whom I have treated over the past 25 years in wars not only in Lebanon, but also in Palestine (Gaza Strip), Iraq, Syria, and Yemen. They continue to inspire me in both my work and my daily life.

Ghassan Soleiman Abu-Sittah MBcHB FRCS(Plast)

Associate Professor of Surgery

Plastic, Reconstructive and Aesthetic Surgeon

Honorary Senior Lecturer, Center for Blast Injury Studies, Imperial College London University

Visiting Senior Lecturer, Conflict & Health Research Group, Faculty of Life Sciences and Medicine, King's College London University

Director, Conflict Medicine Program, Global Health Institute, American University of Beirut

Clinical Lead, Trauma Advisory & Operational Team, WHO-EMRO

Contents

Part I

Introduction

The Epidemiology of the Pediatric War Injuries

1

Ismail Soboh and Ghassan Soleiman Abu-Sittah

1.1   Introduction

"Every war is a war against children," said Eglantynne Jebb over 100 years ago [1]. According to the "Save the Children" reports, more than 357 million children live in conflict zones and are at risk of grave violations [1].

It is significantly important to know that children injured in a war setting need special treatment considerations that differ from adults. Even trained medical staff such as surgeons, nurses, and therapists may lack the expertise and training they need to treat injured children in conflict zones [1]. Such experts are supposed to make complex decisions in the terrible situations of war, like whether to amputate a child's leg or how best to help a child with a life-changing injury reintegrate back into society [1].

This book was written to address the necessity of having a backbone for the treatment and management of pediatric war injuries especially due to the very little information available in this regard. In fact, pediatric war injuries require specific considerations of early and late management that are way different from adults.

Readers of this manual are going to be mainly surgeons who are not really exposed to the practice of pediatric war injuries and its literature. Even general pediatricians can benefit from the information provided. This chapter on the epidemiology of pediatric war wounds introduces a specific approach to the factors influencing war injured child treatments and outcomes.

I. Soboh
Division of Plastic Surgery, Department of Surgery, American University of Beirut Medical Center, Beirut, Lebanon

G. S. Abu-Sittah (✉)
Conflict Medicine Program, Global Health Institute, American University of Beirut, Beirut, Lebanon
e-mail: ga60@aub.edu.lb

© Springer Nature Switzerland AG 2023
G. S. Abu-Sittah, J. J. Hoballah (eds.), *The War Injured Child*,
https://doi.org/10.1007/978-3-031-28613-1_1

1.2   Public Health Consequences of Armed Conflict on Children

More than 1 in every 6 children is affected by armed conflicts globally in 2016 [2]. This number has increased by 30 million to reach 420 million in 2017 [3]. Children living in conflict zones are subjected to several forms of not only physical injuries but also physiological and mental health problems. During the past several decades, health facilities, health workers, and schools have become direct targets, increasing the impact of war on children [4]. The pediatric population that is affected whether directly or indirectly from war conflicts suffers from mild to severe effects that might persist throughout the life course.

The direct effects of war on children range from physical injury, medical illness, and psychological trauma to death [3]. In addition, a complex set of political, economic, environmental, and social factors have an indirect impact on child health in areas of combat [4]. Therefore, it is extremely challenging for the medical and public health systems to function normally after the destruction of their infrastructure, limiting both the access and the quality of care provided.

1.2.1   Geographical Spread of Children Living in Conflict Zones

During the period 1946–2016, there were 280 distinct armed conflicts around the world [5]. Of these conflicts, 165 took place in the last 30 years [4]. Although there is a lack of data regarding child health in most of the past conflicts, the number of children living in conflict zones has increased drastically. It has increased by 75 percent from the early 1990s when it was about 200 million to reach around 357 million in 2016 and 420 million in 2017 according to "Save the Children" reports [1, 3] (Fig. 1.1).

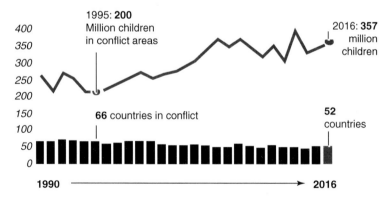

Fig. 1.1   The Chart shows the number of children living in conflict zones and the number of countries in conflict between 1990 and 2016 [1]. Source: War on Children

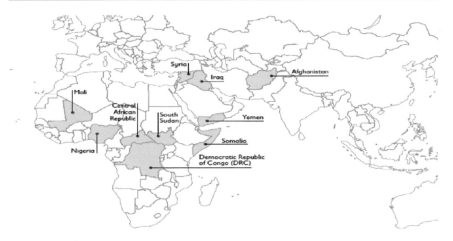

Fig. 1.2 Map showing the 10 worst conflict-affected countries for children to live in. Source: Stop the war on Children

According to the UN's provided Data and PRIO's Research, the "Save the children" institute identified the 10 worst conflict-affected countries for children in their report referring to several indicators such as conflict intensity, number of grave violations, prevalence of children living in conflict zones, etc. [3]. The worst 10 countries can be identified in Fig. 1.2.

1.2.2   Historical Overview

It is commonly known that war conflict leads to a greater percentage of civilian victims rather than military and that children have a big share in this. In all main combats over the last 100 years, with some exceptions, civilians have become a direct target and accounted for around two-thirds of the casualties [6]. Therefore, the heavy burden on the public health of children in contemporary conflicts is not new and children had, throughout history, paid the cost of wars that others start and end. Indeed, in certain conflicts, the destabilization of political, social, and economic infrastructures, the destruction of cultural institutions, and the psychological terrorizing of civilians, especially children, have led to 2–15 times more civilian deaths than direct injuries [6].

1.2.3   The Public Health Effects of Social Disruption

One of the most dangerous effects of war conflicts is social disruption. This includes the displacement of the population whether internally or externally from their homeland, the breakdown of nutrition and Sanitary conditions, pauperization, polluted drinking water, and the disruption of the whole medical system [6]. Nevertheless, there is no doubt regarding the tremendous effects—whether direct or indirect—of political violence on health services and the health system in general (Table 1.1).

Table 1.1 Effects of political violence on health and health systems [7]

Direct effects	Indirect effects
Death	Reduced food distribution and production
Disability	Economic pressures and disruption
Injury	Environmental disruption
Destruction of health system	Internal displacement and refugees
Disruption of the health programs	Family disruption
Psychological stress	Impact on housing, water supply, and sewage disposal

Source: Toward an epidemiology of political violence in the third world

Thousands of children have been dying all over the globe because of violence at war every year [8]. They become direct targets whether citizens or recruited worriers on the battlefield or die for ethnic reasons [8]. Preventable diseases are epidemic during the war due to the lack of proper vaccination in addition to a significant increase in infant mortality when compared to peacetime or in comparison with peaceful parts of the same country [4]. Furthermore, children in conflict zones suffer from various types of injuries and mutilation. There is a wide range of injuries affecting all organs of the body and they are broadly classified as crush injuries, blunt trauma, penetrating injuries, and burns [4]. They are all attributed to gunshots, explosions, Motor Vehicle Accidents (MVAs), buildings destruction, and shelling [4]. The most important heritage of war is the fact that children are mainly affected by landmines. Mine explosions have a higher incidence of injury and a greater mortality rate among children than adults leading to foot and lower limb injuries, genital injuries, blindness, and deafness [8].

Nevertheless, damage to the health system in the areas of conflict extremely affects children's health. They will be exposed to several types of infectious diseases that are easily transmitted in camps and refugee gatherings. This is the result of the lack of proper health facilities, lack of immunizations, contaminated water, malnutrition, and exposure to vectors. Moreover, the adverse effects of population displacement, destruction of social infrastructure, economic sanctions, and environmental damage may compromise children's access to basic needs such as food, health care, and education, for decades [9]. Similarly, schools have been direct targets in any raising armed conflict, and children are being targeted in their way whether to or back from school. What is worst is the fact that schools in many conflicts are being used as shields and bases for combatants or governments in the recruitment of children into war [9]. Therefore, children living in areas of conflict suffer from various terrible consequences—direct or indirect—on public health as the result of social disruption ranging from injury and malnutrition to death.

1.2.4 The Burden of War Wounded Children

Pediatric war injuries have been always a major cause of morbidity, mortality, and disability all over the globe; especially in Low and Middle-Income Countries (LMICs) [10]. These injuries are a growing global concern, which falls disproportionately on developing countries where the public health system and the health facilities are initially not well prepared [11]. That is also because the consequences of injury do not fall only on the injured child but also place a substantial burden on family members, institutions, and society in general provoking poverty and social disability. According to the World Health Organization (WHO), around 15% of the burden of diseases worldwide in the 1990s was due to war injuries [12].

1.2.5   Six Grave Violations

Since the official council of the Special Representative for Children and Armed Conflicts was established in 1996, the United Nations (UN) general assembly has been trying to promote data gathering in terms of children, who are the victims of armed conflicts, in order to raise awareness globally and ensure international cooperation to strengthen protection of these children [13]. As a result, a Monitoring and Reporting Mechanism (MRM) was created to track grave violations against children in 2005 by UN Security Council [3]. These criteria serve as the basis to report and gather information on violations affecting children all over the globe [13].

Killing and maiming are one of these violations that are being practiced against children in conflict zones. According to the "save the children" report, around 73,000 children have been killed or maimed across 25 conflicts between 2005 and 2016 [1] (Fig. 1.3). In some reports of Children and Armed Conflicts (CAAC), it was stated that children are being directly targeted in order to create maximum

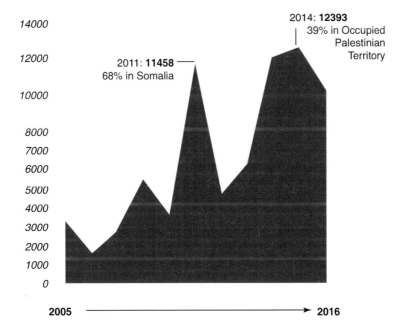

Fig. 1.3   Killing and maiming of children. Source: War on children

emotional damage or to get rid of the next generations of certain ethnic or religious groups [14].

Recruitment of children into conflicts is also one of the major grave violations breaching children's rights. Around 49,650 verified cases of both sexes were recruited by armed forces between 2005 and 2016, according to the UN CAAC annual report [1]. Being used or recruited by combatants in armed groups may leave behind a significant negative life-long impact on the recruited or used children, for those who survived the experience [1]. The traumatic aspect of the brutality they have witnessed and experienced can have tremendous psychological effects that will accompany them into adulthood [1].

Nevertheless, **sexual violence** is a hugely under-reported facet of conflicts and outside the conflicts too [1]. The Sexual Violence in Armed Conflict (SVAC) database, which includes "sexual slavery, forced prostitution, rape, forced pregnancy, forced sterilization/abortion, sexual mutilation, and sexual torture shows that globally 35% of conflicts involved some sort of sexual violence against children between 1998 and 2009" [1]. Moreover, Children can also be **abducted** or **seized** during conflicts which can take many forms ranging from conscription to kidnapping. Other Violations include **attacks on hospitals and schools** along with **humanitarian access denial** which is also considered of major importance in reflecting the present and future of children in conflict.

1.3 Global Epidemiology of War Injured Children

Children are resilient and they represent a high-risk population for injuries worldwide. One of the major direct ramifications of wars and combats on children is being—whether intentionally or unintentionally—targeted and injured. Injuries in this case can take several forms and each requires special considerations regarding the treatment options. However, these injuries fluctuate between blunt injuries, which the child might face in a collapsed building, for example, to penetrating wounds, landmine injuries, and explosive blast injuries.

1.3.1 Blunt Injuries and Penetrating GSWs

Blunt trauma represents a separate category of injury that has several characteristics that overlap with blast injury [15]. This is because sometimes, and due to blast explosion, the victims might be thrown over hard solid objects or be under the threat of a collapsed building resulting in blunt injury.

Penetrating wounds of pediatric populations mainly due to gunshot wounds (GSWs), in war settings, are under-reported in most of the studies done. This is because GSWs in the pediatric population occur mainly in high-income countries and places where weapons are easily accessible as per law. In the USA, for example, guns are ubiquitous and it is estimated that over 90 million firearms are present in civilian homes [16]. That is why firearm-related deaths are the third leading cause of death among US children aged 1–17 years and it is the second leading cause of death-related injuries after car crashes [17]. Although relatively rare compared to adolescents and adults, deaths occurring in young children represent a particularly tragic subcategory of firearms-related fatalities [18]. Nearly 33,636 firearm-related deaths were reported in the USA in 2013 [18]. According to the NVSS and NEISS*, 1300 children died and 5790 were injured and treated in the USA each year as a result of firearm-related injury [19]. Fifty-three percent of those who died were homicides, 38% were suicides, and 6% were unintentional firearm deaths; the remaining 3% were due to legal intervention and deaths of undetermined intent [19].

1.3.2 Blast and Landmine Injuries

Although explosions might be the result of civilian actions such as industrial accidents or fireworks, most of them globally stem from terror or conflict-related attacks [20]. More than 90% of death-related injuries occur in LMICs, where these countries are under-resourced in terms of treatment and prevention [21]. It is worth mentioning that the pathophysiology of blast injuries differs significantly from other forms of injuries and traumas resulting in a multiple and scattered numbers of distinctly patterned injuries [22]. That is why, blast and landmine injuries resulted in three-quarters of all child casualties in the five deadliest conflicts (Afghanistan, Yemen, Syria, Nigeria, and Iraq) for children in 2017, according to the Save the Children analysis of the UN data [23] (Table 1.2). It is estimated that 7364 children were killed or maimed in conflicts in 2017 through which 5322 were linked to blast explosions [23]. Nevertheless, the unexploded ordnance along with landmines injuries constitutes a major risk for injury to children living in conflict areas. A review of surveillance data done between 1997 and 2002 in Afghanistan showed that 6114 injuries were due to unexploded ordnance and landmines, in which 54% of those injured were children under the age of 18 years [24]. It also indicated that children who were mostly affected by unexploded ordnance were playing or tampering with these explosives because of its higher visibility, whereas the adults sustained their

Table 1.2 The number of total child casualties and those linked to blasts in the five deadliest conflicts for children in 2017 [23]

Country	Total child casualties (2017)	Child casualties linked to blast n (%) (2017)
Afghanistan	3,179 (251 girls)	2,216 (70%)
Yemen	1,316 (369 girls)	814 (62%)
Syria	1,271	1,058 (83%)
Nigeria	881	672 (76%)
Iraq	717 (227 girls)	562 (78%)
Total	7,364	5,322 (72%)

Source: SAVE THE CHILDREN (BLAST INJURIES)

injuries mainly while traveling or performing activities of economic necessity by landmines [24, 25]. This was also confirmed by another surveillance study, done in the same country between 2002 and 2006, showing that 92% of the victims were civilians through which children less than 18 years constitute 47% [25]. A higher percentage of children sustained upper limb amputation as compared to adults, whereas more adults sustained lower limb amputations when compared to children [25]. Among Children, the study showed that 65% of the injuries were related to unexploded ordnance whereas 56% of adults' injuries were related to landmines [25]. Therefore, any area contaminated with unexploded ordnance should be cleared in order to decrease the incidence of injured children in areas of conflict. This should also be associated with risk awareness training campaigns and programs for children addressing the danger of unexploded ordnance and the risky behavior by children such as tampering in these special circumstances [25].

Explosive charges can be divided into High-order explosives (HE) and low-order explosives which will lead to either primary, secondary, tertiary, and/or quaternary blast injuries [26] (Refer to Chap. 2).

Nearly 83% of children and only 12% of the combatants of the people killed in Syria's conflict were killed by blasts (Table 1.2) [23]. Indeed, children killed by blast injuries are 7 times more likely to be the victims of blast injuries than combatants involved in the fighting. Similarly in Afghanistan, approximately a third of all casualties in 2017 were children (Table 1.2) [23]. According to the Action on Armed Violence (AOAV), around 42,000 deaths and injuries in 2017 resulted from explosive violence, which is 38% more than the year before [27]. The continuous use of explosive blasts in areas inhabited by civilians will result in a greater number of child casualties when compared to adults and combatants living in the same conflict zone.

1.4 Anatomic Distribution

The epidemiological study of the anatomic distribution of war-related pediatric injuries facilitates the proper identification of the etiology related to the injury and the expectations of the treatment plans and outcomes.

Approximately 70% of pediatric blast injury patients have multiple body regions affected, with burns and penetrating injuries to the extremities present in around 70–80% of the injured pediatric population, according to the pediatric blast injury review [28]. Penetrating injuries to the head, neck, upper limb, and trunk affect over 80% of the children injured by blast explosions when compared to adults in which 31% were affected [28].

Children are subjected to an extremely high-energy burden following exposure to a blast, which is measured through a widely used consensus called Injury Severity Score (ISS) [20]. However, the ideal scoring system for injury is still unknown [29]. According to a literature review done on the Impact of Blast Injuries on Children, 20–36% of children experience severe injury with an ISS score of more than 15, while 8–16% are critically injured with an ISS of more than 25 [20]. This can also be classified according to the age group affected by the injuries. Children older than

9 years have been shown to have a greater ISS score with a greater number of surgical interventions needed following blast injuries [20].

1.4.1 Thermal Injuries

Thermal burns are relatively common injuries following blast exposure in the pediatric population, with a prevalence of around 60–70% regardless of the age group of the child [30]. They result in multi-systemic insults affecting not only the dermis, but the pulmonary, cardiovascular, inflammatory, and metabolic systems [31]. The severity of the burn has been used as a prognostic factor to expect the mortality of the injured child, with severe burns exceeding 30% of the total body surface area (TBSA) in children under 15 years old being the major cause of death [30]. When compared to adults, for example, a burn to the face and scalp constitutes only 9% of the TBSA through which no fluid resuscitation is needed in this case, whereas the same injury in a pediatric patient represents 19% of the TBSA and necessitates IV fluid management [32]. It is also worth mentioning that children less than 2 years of age have a relatively smaller subcutaneous layer and skin thickness when compared to younger children or adults [20]. Thus, clinical assessment according to burn depth in such cases is not accurate as thermal burns in such cases result in greater protein, fluid, and heat loss at a lower energy level [33]. Through impairment of wound healing, increased risk of infection, and nutritional deficiencies associated with burn injuries, pediatric victims are at increased risk of hospitalization, mortality, and morbidity long after the initial insult [34]. Therefore, a thorough examination and specific considerations should be taken in terms of management and rehabilitation for children who suffered from thermal injuries due to blast explosions.

1.4.2 Head and Spinal Injuries

The prevalence of pediatric head injuries following blast varies significantly between 15 and 60% [30, 35]. Studies have shown that the younger the child is, the more he is at risk of having a head injury. Victims under 7 years of age are almost twice as likely to present with head injuries when compared to older children [30]. For patients under the age of 3 years, neurosurgical decompression is the most common surgical intervention done overall following a blast [36]. This is mainly due to anatomical immaturity in skull compositions because of the incomplete ossification along with the thin structure it constitutes [37]. Thus, blast-induced traumatic brain injuries (bTBI) are more common in victims under the age of 10 years when compared to adolescents and adults [35]. It has also been shown that head and cervical spine injury was the second most common cause of mortality in pediatrics post-blast exposure regardless of age [30].

Spinal injury in pediatrics represents a much lower percentage than head injury following a blast (1–3%) [38, 39]. This type of injury is mostly associated with a concurrent head injury [30]. Cervical spine injuries characterize 60–80% of total pediatric injuries, as compared to adults (15–45%) [40, 41].

1.4.3   Torso Injuries

Chest and abdominal Trauma is common following blast injuries, with incidence fluctuating between 32–50% and a peak in the 5–10 years age group of children [35, 39]. Primary Blast lung injury (PBLI) is the most common fatal injury following exposure to overpressure waves [31]. However, pediatric-specific data on PBLI is lacking with documented incidents coming only from case series or reports [42, 43]. Furthermore, injuries to the abdomen following blast explosions can be life-threatening resulting in severe hemorrhage, mucosal layer separation, and infarction [44]. Vascular injuries following penetrating trauma in pediatric blast victims result in significant morbidity and mortality (4%) when compared to injuries in civilian trauma (0.3%) [45]. Approximately 71% of children undergoing vascular penetrating injuries post-blast die during surgery [45].

1.4.4   Extremity Injuries

Extremity injuries in children have been shown to be age dependent. Around 11% of infants and 20% of children less than 7 years of age experience extremity injuries as compared to 50% of older children [46]. Younger children also are subjected more to upper limb injuries whereas adolescents suffer more from lower limb injuries [28]. The incidence of long bone fractures is around 45% in blast pediatric victims, and it is more commonly present in the upper limbs [47]. Traumatic amputations following blasts in pediatrics range from 11 to 31% and they occur mostly in the lower limbs [36].

1.4.5   Ophthalmologic and Otology Injuries

Despite its small surface area, the eye is sensitive to injury following blast explosions with an incidence of greater than 60% of victims performing mine clearance operations [38]. It is important to know more about pediatric eye injuries during conflict because of the significant impact that vision loss would have on the child over the long term.

One of the major primary blast injuries persisting for a long period after the initial insult is hearing loss [48]. Children suffering from hearing impairment are going to suffer from social and academic underachievement along with a negative impact on their future employment and psychological well-being.

1.5   Conclusion

1.5.1   Lessons to Be Gained from the Study of Epidemiology

As a result of this brief Overview of the epidemiology of pediatric war injuries, several conclusions can be drawn out.

1. For the pediatric population living in conflict zones, the impact of war on public health is considered more dangerous than the effect of trauma resulting from direct targeting. However, the destruction of the health system, malnutrition, and social and environmental disruption all carry a huge burden in terms of increased prevalence of mortality and morbidity along war injured children.

2. Children living in conflict zones are subjected to killing or maiming, sexual violence, recruitment for war, abduction, and seizing. Their schools and even hospitals might be directly targeted by the combatants. These all are considered as GRAVE VIOLATIONS that serve as the basis for information gathering and reporting.

3. GSWs, especially in high-income countries, are nowadays ubiquitous and present in many civilian homes. Firearm-related deaths, in the USA, for example, are one of the leading causes of death among children aged 1–17 years.

4. Most of the explosions worldwide are either conflict-related or due to terror attacks. Blast and landmine injuries constitute more than 75% of all child casualties in the five deadliest conflicts for children in 2017.

5. Children are mainly subjected to upper limb injuries while tampering or playing with unexploded ordnance which necessitates educational campaigns to decrease the incidence of child casualties in conflict areas.

6. Around 70% of pediatric blast injury patients have multiple body regions affected, with burns and penetrating injuries to the extremities presenting in around 70–80% of the injured pediatric population.

7. Thermal burns are relatively common injuries following blast exposure in the pediatric population. They result in multisystemic insults affecting not only the dermis but also the pulmonary, cardiovascular, inflammatory, and metabolic systems.

8. It has been shown that head and cervical spine injury was the second most common cause of mortality in pediatrics post-blast exposure regardless of age.

9. Primary Blast lung injury (PBLI) is the most common fatal injury following exposure to overpressure waves.

References

1. Save the Children. The war on children. Save the children; 2018 5–40.
2. Wessells M. Children and armed conflict: interventions for supporting war-affected children. Peace Confl: J Peace Psychol. 2017;23(1):4–13.
3. Graham G, Kirollos M, Fylkesnes G, Salarkia K, Wong N. Stop the war on children. Genevae. 2017:4–60.
4. Kadir A, Shenoda S, Goldhagen J. Effects of armed conflict on child health and development: a systematic review. PLoS One. 2019;14(1):e0210071.
5. (PRIO) P. Trends in Armed Conflict, 1946–2016 [Internet]. Prio.org. 2020 [cited 12 May 2020]. Available from: https://www.prio.org/Publications/Publication/?x=10599
6. Giannou C, Baldan M. War surgery. Geneva: ICRC; 2010. p. 50–120.
7. Zwi A, Ugalde A. Towards an epidemiology of political violence in the third world. Soc Sci Med. 1989;28(7):633–42.
8. Çelik N, Özpınar S. Children and health effects of war being a war child. Cumhuriyet Med J. 2017:639–43.

9. Kadir A, Shenoda S, Goldhagen J, Pitterman S. The effects of armed conflicts on children. Pediatrics. 2018;142(6).
10. Mosleh M, Dalal K, Aljeesh Y, Svanström L. The burden of war-injury in the Palestinian health care sector in Gaza Strip. BMC Int Health Hum Rights. 2018;18:1.
11. Hyder A, Wali S, Fishman S, Schenk E. The burden of unintentional injuries among the under-five population in South Asia. Acta Paediatr. 2008;97(3):267–75.
12. World Health Organization (WHO). The global burden of disease. Geneva: WHO; 2004. update. p. 2008.
13. The Six Grave Violations - United Nations Office of the Special Representative of the Secretary-General for Children and Armed Conflict | To promote and protect the rights of all children affected by armed conflict [Internet]. United Nations Office of the Special Representative of the Secretary-General for Children and Armed Conflict [cited 12 May 2020]. https://childrenandarmedconflict.un.org/six-grave-violations/
14. Hall DM. The future of child protection. J R Soc Med. 2006;99(1):6–9.
15. Miller D, Mansour K. Blunt Traumatic Lung Injuries. Thorac Surg Clin. 2007;17(1):57–61.
16. Newton G, and Zimring F. Firearms and violence in American Life, pp. 1–71. National Commission on the Causes and Prevention of Violence. U.S. Government Printing Office, Washington, D. C., 1968.
17. Lilyea J. Hand-wringing about gun violence [Internet]. This ain't Hell, but you can see it from here. 2020 [cited 12 May 2020]. https://valorguardians.com/blog/?p=72848
18. Prahlow J. Fatal gunshot wounds in young children. Acad Forensic Pathol. 2016;6(4):691–702.
19. Fowler K. Childhood firearm injuries in the United States [internet]. Res Gate. 2017; [cited 12 May 2020]. https://pediatrics.aappublications.org/content/pediatrics/early/2017/06/15/peds.2016-3486.full.pdf
20. [Internet]. Imperial.ac.uk. 2020 [cited 12 May 2020]. https://www.imperial.ac.uk/media/imperial-college/research-centres-and-groups/centre-for-blast-injury-studies/Literature-Review-on-paediatric-blast-injury.pdf
21. Wesson HK, Boikhutso N, Bachani AM, Hofman KJ, Hyder AA. The cost of injury and trauma care in low- and middle-income countries: a review of economic evidence. Health Policy Plan. 2014;29:795–808.
22. Quintana D, Jordan F, Tuggle D, Mantor P, Tunell W. The spectrum of pediatric injuries after a bomb blast. J Pediatr Surg. 1997;32(2):307–11.
23. Denselow J, Salarkia K, Edwards J. [Internet]. Savethechildren.org.uk. 2018 [cited 12 May 2020]. https://www.savethechildren.org.uk/content/dam/gb/reports/blast_injuries.pdf
24. Bilukha O, Brennan M. Injuries and deaths caused by unexploded ordnance in Afghanistan: review of surveillance data, 1997-2002. BMJ. 2005;330(7483):127–8.
25. Bilukha O, Brennan M, Anderson M. The lasting legacy of war: epidemiology of injuries from landmines and unexploded ordnance in Afghanistan, 2002–2006. Prehosp Disaster Med. 2008;23(6):493–9.
26. Hamele M. Disaster preparedness, pediatric considerations in primary blast injury, chemical, and biological terrorism. World J Crit Care Med. 2014;3(1):15.
27. Action on Armed Violence | AOAV [Internet]. AOAV. 2020 [cited 12 May 2020]. https://aoav.org.uk/
28. Bendinelli C, 2009. 'Effects of land mines and unexploded ordnance on the pediatric population and comparison with adults in rural Cambodia'. World J Surg. In Hargrave, M., 2019. The Impact of Blast Injury on Children: A multidisciplinary literature review. Centre for Blast Injuries Study, Imperial College London.
29. Stevenson M. An overview of the injury severity score and the new injury severity score. Inj Prev. 2001;7(1):10–3.
30. Edwards MJ, Lustik M, Eichelberger MR, Elster E, Azarow K, Coppola C. Blast injury in children: an analysis from Afghanistan and Iraq, 2002-2010. J Trauma Acute Care Surg. 2012;73(5):1278–83.
31. Wolf SJ, Bebarta VS, Bonnett CJ, Pons PT, Cantrill SV. Blast injuries. Lancet. 2009;374(9687):405–15.

32. Allison K, Porter K. Consensus on the pre-hospital approach to burns patient management. Injury. 2004:734–8.
33. Wang XQ, Mill J, Kravchuk O, Kimble RM. Ultrasound assessed thickness of burn scars in association with laser Doppler imaging determined depth of burns in paediatric patients. Burns. 2010;36(8):1254–62.
34. Jeschke MG, Gauglitz GG, Kulp GA, Finnerty CC, Williams FN, Kraft R, et al. Long-term persistance of the pathophysiologic response to severe burn injury. PLoS One. 2011;6:7.
35. Jaffe DH, Peleg K. Terror explosive injuries. Ann Surg. 2010;251(1):138–43.
36. Edwards MJ, Lustik M, Carlson T, Tabak B, Farmer D, Edwards K, et al. Surgical interventions for pediatric blast injury: an analysis from Afghanistan and Iraq 2002 to 2010. J Trauma Acute Care Surg. 2014;76(3):854–8.
37. Chafi MS, Karami G, Ziejewski M. Biomechanical assessment of brain dynamic responses due to blast pressure waves. Ann Biomed Eng. 2010;38(2):490–504.
38. Creamer KM, Edwards MJ, Shields CH, Thompson MW, Yu CE, Adelman W. Pediatric wartime admissions to US Military Combat Support Hospitals in Afghanistan and Iraq: learning from the first 2,000 admissions. Trauma. 2009;67(4):762–9.
39. Waisman Y, Aharonson-Daniel L, Mor M, Amir L, Peleg K. The impact of terrorism on children: a two-year experience. Prehosp Disaster Med. 2003;18(3):242–8.
40. Hasler RM, Exadaktylos AK, Bouamra O, Benneker LM, Clancy M, Sieber R, et al. Epidemiology and predictors of spinal injury in adult major trauma patients: European cohort study. Eur Spine J. 2011;20(12):2174–80.
41. Stephan K, Huber S, Häberle S, Kanz K-G, Bühren V, van Griensven M, et al. Spinal cord injury—incidence, prognosis, and outcome: an analysis of the Trauma Register DGU. Spine J. 2015;15(9):1994–2001.
42. Anwar M, Akhtar J, Khatoon R, Ali R. Blast injuries in children and adolescents. J Surg Pak. 2015;20:1.
43. Ratto J, Johnson BK, Condra CS, Knapp JF. Pediatric blast lung injury from a fireworks-related explosion. Pediatr Emerg Care. 2012;28(6):573–6.
44. Crabtree J. Terrorist homicide bombings: a primer for preparation. J Burn Care Res. 2006;27(5):576–88.
45. Villamaria CY, Morrison JJ, Fitzpatrick CM, Cannon JW, Rasmussen TE. Wartime vascular injuries in the pediatric population of Iraq and Afghanistan: 2002-2011. J Pediatr Surg. 2014;49(3):428–32.
46. Bendinelli C. Effects of land mines and unexploded ordnance on the pediatric population and comparison with adults in rural Cambodia. World J Surg. 2009;33(5):1070–4.
47. Quintana DA, Jordan FB, Tuggle DW, Mantor PC, Tunell WP. The spectrum of pediatric injuries after a bomb blast. J Pediatr Surg. 1997;32(2):307–11.
48. Fausti SA, Wilmington DJ, Gallun FJ, Myers PJ, Henry JA. Auditory and vestibular dysfunction associated with blast-related traumatic brain injury. J Rehabil Res Dev. 2009;46(6):797–810.

Biodynamics of Blast Injury

2

Seif Emseih and Ghassan Soleiman Abu-Sittah

2.1   Introduction

Children are not spared from the horrific injuries inflicted by explosives. While exposure can occur in civilian settings such as fireworks or industrial accidents, the majority stem from conflict or terror-related attacks across the globe [1, 2]. Despite increasing recognition of the complex and unique injury patterns sustained following blast exposure in the adult population [3], the physical and psychological impact on the pediatric population is less well understood.

For the purposes of this review, we define children as any person under the age of 18 years (as specified by the United Nations Convention on the Rights of the Child). The heterogeneity of this group is acknowledged, and most studies will further subdivide this population. These classifications vary and are somewhat arbitrary but can be approximated by the following: infants (under 1 year old), young children (1–8 years old), older children (9–15 years old), and adolescents (16–18 years old).

It is essential to understand the epidemiology of blast injuries within this population to demonstrate the effect of explosive weapons on children and the ensuing burden on both domestic and global health systems. Furthermore, insight into the mechanism of childhood blast insults will further efforts to prevent, mitigate, and effectively treat these injuries [3, 4]. This chapter aims to provide an overview of the fundamentals of blast physics and injuries and review how the injury patterns and biomechanical features of explosive blasts may differ between pediatric and adult

S. Emseih
Division of Plastic Surgery, Department of Surgery, American University of Beirut Medical Center, Beirut, Lebanon

G. S. Abu-Sittah (✉)
Conflict Medicine Program, Global Health Institute, American University of Beirut, Beirut, Lebanon
e-mail: ga60@aub.edu.lb

© Springer Nature Switzerland AG 2023

G. S. Abu-Sittah, J. J. Hoballah (eds.), *The War Injured Child*,
https://doi.org/10.1007/978-3-031-28613-1_2

populations. This will aid in defining future research needs for protection, mitigation, acute medical treatment, and rehabilitation. This work is by definition interdisciplinary and as such, covers material that relates to both the biomedical sciences and engineering domains.

2.2   Explosive Blasts

An explosive is a material capable of producing an explosion using its own stored energy [5]. To understand the impact of blast injury on the human body, an examination of these materials' chemical and physical properties is necessary. The injury potential of explosive munitions is dictated by its properties and the physical changes the material and its surroundings undergo. Based on chemical composition and properties, explosives are classified as high or low [6].

Low explosives undergo deflagration, which is the subsonic combustion of the surface chemicals, comparable to a household fire [5]. This chemical phenomenon is seen in gunpowder propellants, smokeless powder, and fireworks. However, these materials may detonate when confined and used in conjunction with another more powerful explosive [5]. Conversely, high explosives detonate without confinement and are subject to a self-sustaining reaction [6] which is propagated by the high-pressure shockwave traveling through the material. These include PETN, HMX, RDX, and nitroglycerine. They have higher wounding potential due in part to the powerful shock waves that can fracture bone and cause soft tissue trauma [6]. Trauma from low explosives is more commonly confined to soft tissues as these do not produce shock waves [5].

When a high or low explosive detonates, it produces a rapid shift from potential to kinetic energy in roughly 1/1000th of a second. This results in the release of a significant amount of heat and gaseous products that are transmitted as a blast (shock) wave. The shock wave propagates out from the center of the blast by the expansion of gases generated by the reaction, with a pressure pulse a few millimeters thick traveling at supersonic speeds [7]. The spherical outer edge of this blast wave yields a disruptive increase in pressure, density, and temperature, known as a shock front, which exercises severe crushing, shattering, and shearing, as well as partially elucidated effects on cells and various tissues, such as the brain, heart muscle, and lungs [7]. As the superheated detonation products rapidly expand, surrounding cool air is compressed (the blast wave) in front of the expanding gas volume, which contains most of the explosive's energy. This leads to the formation of a subatmospheric pressure phase that sucks in the air behind the blast wave. The resulting turbulence aligns any debris into literal projectiles, whether particulate matter from the explosive itself or matter picked up from the environment as the wave progresses [5]. The air molecules are compressed to such a density that the pressure wave itself (a thin layer of compressed air) acts like a solid object propagating spherically in all directions from the explosion's epicenter. This particularly destructive layer of air is also known as the shock front and is capable of striking soft tissues with enormous force [7].

The variations in air pressure with time at a fixed point in space (the Friedlander relationship) describe the physical properties of a blast wave [5, 8]. The blast shock wave has three different physical properties that are responsible for the pathophysiological effects on biological tissue. These are the amplitude of the peak pressure, the impulse (defined as the time integral of pressure), and the duration of the positive phase overpressure. It has also been proposed that the dynamic overpressure of the detonation products (blast wind) and thermal energy released in the explosion contribute to blast injury.

The first event is the high positive pressure phase occurring immediately after the blast, which is the longest portion of a shock wave and causes a rise in ambient air pressure. It is followed by a negative (subatmospheric) pressure phase. This can be represented graphically as an idealized curve (Fig. 2.1) representing the Friedlander equation which is the variation in blast wave pressure with time, at a fixed point in space (the Friedlander relationship) [5, 8]. The curve shows a rapid increase in ambient air pressure following an explosive event over a short period of time. The negative pressure phase is also visualized by the curve reaching a minimum point that is below the ambient air temperature.

Accompanying the positive and negative pressure phases is the blast wind, a mass movement of air caused by the explosion that lags behind the blast wave (a combination of positive and negative phases of the explosion). The expansion of gaseous byproducts of the explosion accelerates molecules of air into a high-speed wind. This phenomenon is potentiated by a countermovement of ambient air filling the vacuum created by the negative phase. This secondary wave is capable of propelling objects and can be as damaging as the original explosion. Once the blast wind resolves, a return to ambient air pressure occurs. These three components (positive and negative pressure phases followed by the blast wind), determined by the physical properties of the explosive and the surrounding environment,

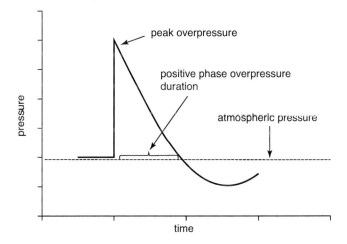

Fig. 2.1 Simplified Friedlander waveform showing pressure changes over time in a free field explosion [5, 8]

collectively form the basis of the injuring processes that act on the human body, which is further explained when considering the human body's response to these rapid changes.

The injuries caused by explosions, whether incurred from blast waves or blast winds, represent a variety of complex traumatic wounds. Various factors such as proximity to the blast determine the complexity and intensity of sustained injuries. The blast wave, for instance, dissipates energy inversely proportionate to the third power of the distance from the detonation point. In CLOSE proximity, injuries are caused directly by the displaced explosive material and its container, rather than the blast wave itself, which is a more common cause of injury further from the epicenter. Because the intensity of the blast (the peak overpressure) decreases rapidly with distance from the detonation point, victims must be in close proximity to sustain primary blast injuries [7]. Context is another important consideration when analyzing trauma from blasts. Many factors need to be considered for a full skeletal assessment such as explosive type, differential survival rates, improved protection (in combat situations), and confined vs. open surroundings.

Blast waves occurring in enclosed spaces behave differently from their open-space counterparts, as waves multiply when they bounce off solid objects such as walls. This produces an erratic network of interfering waves and can intensify the effects on biological systems, making injuries more severe. The medium where the blast wave propagates also alters its effect. Immersion blasts, or shock waves produced in water, create waves of higher intensity and longer duration than atmospheric blasts. Intraabdominal injuries are prominent in such cases: laparotomy findings include sub-serosal hemorrhage and tears in the bowel wall [9].

In summary, shock waves have a number of properties that help explain their effects on tissues [8]).

- They generate highly localized forces with small, but rapid distortions. Pathophysiological effects are at the microvascular level; gross lacerations are not typical.
- They affect organs with marked differences in physical properties (acoustic impedance) particularly hollow gas-containing organs.
- Stress concentration: when a stress wave encounters an interface between two media of different physical properties such as bowel wall tissues and gas-filled lumens, a component of the compressive stress wave is reflected back at the interface as a tension wave. Most materials are weaker under tension to compression, disruption at the interface (tissue damage) may result, and this phenomenon can affect organs far from the site of impact. Stress waves through the thoracic and abdominal walls are responsible for blast lung and primary blast injury of the small bowel, respectively.
- Pressure differentials across delicate structures such as alveolar septa or bowels: compression of a segment (implosion) and SDA subsequent expansion damages the wall of the structure.

2.3   Blast Injury Mechanisms

Blasts produce a unique spectrum of devastating injuries classically divided into primary, secondary, tertiary, and quaternary blast injuries [10]. While this classification is useful for its simplicity and mirrors the principal injury mechanisms, it is based on Second World War data of open field bare explosives [11], a model that does not account for modern variations, i.e., explosive types (Mine, IED, Suicide vest) or environmental factors (open air, confined, buried). Furthermore, multiple mechanisms often overlap, leading to complex injury types in the polytraumatized child [12]. Nevertheless, it constitutes a widely accepted theoretical model for understanding blast injuries [5, 13].

2.3.1   Primary Blast Injury

Primary blast damage is largely a function of the character, magnitude, and rate of pressure fluctuations, and the duration of the pressure pulse [14]. Primary blast injuries are caused by the interaction of the blast wave and its components with the body and are therefore a type of non-penetrating trauma that is estimated to constitute 86% of fatal blast injuries [6, 8].

The effect of blast waves is most profound at air and fluid-filled interfaces in the body which are most sensitive to rapid pressure fluctuations as the blast wave propagates [6]. The brain, ears, spinal cord, gastrointestinal tract, lungs, and cardiovascular system are especially susceptible to damage from the primary blast wave [15].

Damage to human tissues is incurred mainly by four mechanisms: spalling, implosion, acceleration/deceleration, and pressure differentials [15].

1. Spalling occurs when particles from a denser fluid are forcibly pushed through a less dense fluid at the interface of two different media.
2. Implosion implies a contraction of gas pockets that occurs as a blast wave propagates through tissue. The expansion follows rapidly, causing injury from multiple miniature internal disruptions.
3. Acceleration/deceleration injury occurs when the body or its internal organs are accelerated in one direction from contact with the blast wave front, followed by an abrupt change in momentum. This can occur when a reflected blast wave collides with the body from a different direction or when meeting a solid object or wall.
4. Pressure differentials between the outer surface of the body and the internal organs during a blast wave can cause internal injury.

Some studies have shown that survivors of explosive blasts were found to have elevations in plasma arachidonic acid metabolites, thromboxane A, prostacyclin, and sulfidopeptide leukotrienes, suggesting that blast waves can cause extensive, measurable pathophysiologic alterations. Traumatic limb amputation from primary blast waves occurs at a blast wave-induced fracture site rather than joints. Other primary blast wave injuries include traumatic brain injury, tympanic membrane rupture, perforation of the globe of the eye, abdominal hemorrhage, and pulmonary barotraumas. Primary blast injuries in open air tend to be confined to victims in close proximity to the epicenter and are less common than ballistic (secondary) injuries [8]. A casualty close enough to an explosion to sustain serious primary injuries will commonly have lethal secondary and tertiary injuries.

A higher incidence of serious primary blast injury can be observed in the following circumstances:

- Enclosed spaces (vehicles or buildings) where the reflection of the blast wave augments the total blast load.
- Close proximity to the explosion.
- In individuals wearing body armor which confers protection against projectiles but not the blast wave.
- Large-scale explosions.
- Fuel-air explosives and other types of enhanced blast munitions.

2.3.2 Secondary Blast Injury

Secondary blast injury is the most common form encountered in blast-related injuries and is a far greater contributor to mortality in blast victims that survive the primary blast [6, 16]. The mechanism of secondary blast injury is tied to blast winds which lag behind the negative pressure wave that follows the primary blast wave. As the pressure drops below atmospheric levels, the vacuum generates winds that can propel objects in the vicinity of the explosion with considerable destructive force, on par with the blast wave of the initial explosion [15]. The musculoskeletal system is most commonly involved in the form of severe tissue injuries and amputations [15].

Fragmentation is the most common mechanism of secondary blast injuries, capable of damage over large distances. Projectiles, i.e., materials that have been added to the explosive device or built into it by design (fragmentation grenades), are propelled by the blast wave or blast winds [16]. They can travel with varying velocities (up to 2700 feet per second) and emulate ballistic patterns, causing penetrating or blunt ballistic trauma. In addition, blast fragments can carry environmental debris into the wound, seeding wounds with pathogens and impeding proper wound healing [15]. Injury patterns created by penetrating fragments reflect their shape and velocity and are categorized based on their resemblance to ballistic materials (i.e., ball bearings) or irregularly shaped projectiles [6]. The lethality of fragmentation injuries is dependent on the degree of vital structures' penetration. Fragmentation dispersion is chaotic and indiscriminate; the likelihood of penetrating vital organs is increased at shorter distances from the blast epicenter [17]. Small standing individuals such as children will have their vital regions (chest, head, and neck) closer to the epicenter of a buried explosive (mine, IED), increasing their fragmentation exposure. This explains the increased incidence of thoracic, head, and neck injuries in pediatric victims compared to adults [18], and the increased requirement for operative procedures for these body zones [19]. The introduction of enhanced body armor to adult combatants provides partial protection from direct fragmentation strikes on the thorax, head, and neck [20, 21]. Unfortunately, children are unlikely to benefit from this form of protection.

2.3.3 Tertiary Blast Injury

Tertiary blast injuries are defined as the spectrum of injuries sustained through bodily displacement followed by rapid deceleration of the body or its parts, and impact upon the ground, walls, or objects. Additionally, the damage incurred from collapsing structures such as crush injuries is also considered part of this category. Bodily displacement is caused by an acceleration induced by blast winds or expanding gases in violent explosions. Fractures, crush injuries, traumatic limb amputations, severe soft tissue lacerations, and contusions can result [6, 8, 15]. Blunt head injuries and fractures are the most common types sustained, similar to non-combat or conflict-related trauma, although with greater severity [17]. In fact, head injuries are the second most significant cause of mortality following blasts in the pediatric population [12]. The relatively small body mass of pediatric patients increases their predisposition to bodily displacement and resultant blunt traumatic injuries [3]. In addition to differences in size and shape, pediatric tissues have different biophysical properties than their adult counterparts; the biomechanical response to blast loading and impact may differ. Pediatric bone has been shown to be less mineralized than adult bone. Reduced bone ash content leads to a lower modulus of elasticity and lower bending strength; a child's bone will bend more easily when subjected to the same force [24]. The tendency of pediatric bone to absorb energy, bend more, and deform plastically leads to the phenomenon of "greenstick" fractures. These are characterized by bending and unilateral fracture of the bone; this is in contrast to the adult bone which fails and fractures completely when subjected to a lesser degree of bending [25].

2.3.4 Quaternary Blast Injuries

Quaternary blast injuries encompass the wide spectrum of injuries not addressed by the previous three classifications [17]. These include psychological trauma, burns, asphyxia following inhalation of toxic fumes or burned materials, and mucosal edema (oral, nasal, pharyngeal) from high temperatures generated by secondary fires (flammable devices, structures, pavement, vehicles) [16]. Burns are the leading cause of death in children under 15 years old, and alongside head trauma, are the greatest predictor of death in all age groups [26, 27]. Psychological trauma is a complex and underreported issue that often follows a pediatric blast injury.

2.4   Blast Injury Characteristics in the Pediatric Population

While acknowledging that blasts produce a heterogeneous injury pattern within both adult and pediatric populations, epidemiological studies demonstrate certain injury patterns are more common in children. In pediatric populations, multiple body regions are involved in 65–70% of cases [12, 28], with burns and penetrating injuries to the extremities observed in 70–80% of blast victims [12, 18, 22, 27]. Penetrating injuries to the face, head, neck, upper limb, and trunk affects 80% of pediatric patients, significantly higher than the 31% of adult victims [22, 23] (Fig. 2.2). Children experience a high injury burden from blast trauma, as assessed by the injury severity score (ISS—a widely used consensus-based measure of injury severity) [29]. Around 20–36% experience "severe" injury (ISS > 15), while 8-18% are considered "critically injured" (ISS > 25) [10, 18, 19, 30]. Older children have a greater ISS and undergo a higher number of surgical interventions when compared to younger children (<9 years old). Of these, wound debridement and closure are most commonly performed [31], followed by vascular surgeries and exploratory laparotomies. These statistics reflect the prevalence of penetrating trauma as a major mechanism of injury [32].

Pediatric blast victims constitute a disproportionately large resource burden on treatment facilities [32–38], with approximately 56% requiring surgery [19], or twice the requirement of non-blast-related pediatric trauma [35]. Special structural

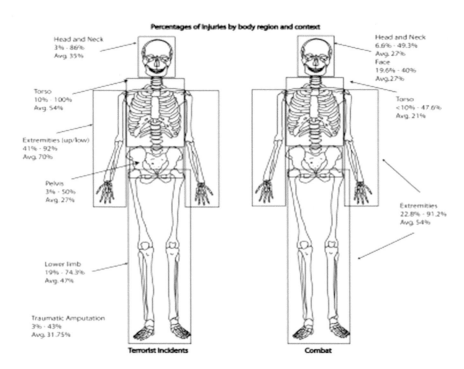

Fig. 2.2 Percentages of injuries by body region and context [22, 23]

Table 2.1 Structural consideration in the pediatric population [39]

Skin	Scalp	The younger a child is, the thinner and the poorer its ability to cushion against external forces
	Epidermis/ Dermis	Fragile and prone to blistering and tearing
	Subcutaneous fat layer	Easily retains water and microvascular breakdown causes a subcutaneous hematoma
	Galea aponeurotica	Blood and exudate can accumulate beneath galea
	Periosteum	Cephalic hematoma can be calcified rarely
Cranium	Cranium	The craniofacial ratio is at its greatest Cranial sutures are loose and highly mobile Calvarium is soft and rich in bone marrow, connected with a periosteum, and strongly attached to the bone cortex. The continuity of the skull tends to be well-maintained. Bone fragments are less likely to occur
Brain and nerve fibers	Nerve fibers	In undeveloped myelin sheaths the water content per unit volume of brain tissue is high. Fibers are pliable and less prone to rupture
	Brain/Cortical veins	Cerebral contusion by a direct external force is high because of its softness. Easily extended with accelerated decelerated motion and can cause subdural hematoma with disruption
Neck and cervical spine	Neck	Undeveloped neck muscle and poor head support
	Vertebrae	The fulcrum of the vertebral body is located in the upper cervical spine

features predispose the pediatric population to sustain multiple injuries, suffer higher ISS, and have a greater risk of death following blasts, as described in Table 2.1.

2.5 Injury-Specific Considerations in Pediatrics

2.5.1 Thermal Burns

Thermal burns are a common injury following blasts, with a prevalence ranging from 56 to 70% in pediatric patients of all ages [10, 40]. Thermal energy released from blasts can result directly from the explosion, through superheated gas products, or by secondary fires igniting surrounding vehicles and buildings [41]. Burn severity has been proposed as a prognostic marker for pediatric blast models [42], and severe burns exceeding 30% of the body surface area are the principal cause of death in children under 15 years old [10, 11, 33]. When a large detonation occurs (hundreds to thousands of pounds of explosive materials), the resulting blast wave is accompanied by a large fireball and surrounding flammable materials. The fireball and other secondary fires consume a significant amount of oxygen from the air, reducing its partial pressure to half the normal atmospheric value of 21% oxygen (10–13%). The fireball that emanates from an explosion can reach temperatures of several thousand degrees and lasts for approximately 500 milliseconds. The probability of significant secondary fires, particularly burning vehicles, can further potentiate incendiary effects; the victims' open wounds can be complicated by burns and heavy smoke exposure. This compounding of factors complicates the debridement, surgical management, and healing process of sustained blast wounds. The burns typically encountered in explosion victims are flash and flame burns.

Flash burns are produced by the explosion's radiant heat and sustained by victims in close proximity to the detonation. Due to the short exposure time, they are more superficial than flame burns and are typically found on exposed body parts such as the face (most common), neck, hands, and calves of female victims, indicating the protective value of clothing in blast situations. Flash burns are more extensive and severe in victims of confined space blasts due to the containment of the fireball for a longer time period. Interesting characteristics observed in this type of injury are the charred singeing of scalp hair, eyelashes, and eyebrows. Eyelid burns are the most common injury and account for 96% of all flash burns. Lip burns by blast thermal effects on the mucosa present as singed lips, cyanosed, smoked black, covered by a dry crust of blood, and dry when the oral mucosa's minor salivary glands are affected [9, 16].

Burns are multisystemic insults affecting the dermis as well as the pulmonary, cardiovascular, inflammatory, and metabolic systems [2]. Insulin resistance, increased fracture risk, hepatomegaly, cardiac dysfunction, reduced immune function, and hypermetabolic changes, commonly seen in burn patients, have been demonstrated to persist for up to 3 years following burn exposure in adults [43]. Through systemic alternations such as wound healing impairment, nutritional deficits, and infection risk, burn victims carry an increased risk of hospitalization with higher morbidity and mortality, long after the initial insult [30, 43–45].

Children are predisposed to increased burn severity [46]. Anatomical disproportionality increases the lethality of certain burn patterns: a burn to the face and scalp of an adult comprises only 9% of the total body surface area (TBSA), not requiring IV fluid therapy. Conversely, the same injury in a pediatric patient covers 19% TBSA and requires fluid management [23]. Children under 2 years of age have reduced subcutaneous layers and skin thickness compared to older children and adults. Full-thickness burns, and the resulting rapid fluid, protein, and heat loss, can occur at relatively lower thermal energy levels. Consequently, assessment of clinical severity by burn depth has been shown to be less accurate in young children [29]. Subsequent dehydration, nutritional deficiencies, and hypothermia from full-thickness burns increase morbidity significantly in pediatric victims [46].

Thermal inhalation injuries in pediatric victims are difficult to assess, and symptoms of inhalational injuries such as increased respiratory rate may be incorrectly interpreted in the context of physiological age discrepancies. The pediatric subglottis represents the narrowest section of the upper airway and is quickly affected by burn-induced laryngeal edema, especially in the context of failed intubation attempts [46]. Rapid desaturation occurs following upper airway obstruction due to increased oxygen utilization combined with limited functional residual reserves [31].

Children rarely recover from severe burn injuries without functional sequelae, with limited joint mobility and impaired tactile sensation presenting significant future challenges for rehabilitation [32, 33]. Prolonged rehabilitation and visible aesthetic disfigurement can produce psychosocial morbidity long after the event [34].

Nosocomial infection of the burn eschar, in particular, from *Pseudomonas aeruginosa*, can be prevented by an aggressive debridement and meticulous antimicrobial wound dressings [35]. However, sub-optimal care facilities, delays in wound cleaning, and prolonged transfer times all increase burn infection incidence [36].

In conclusion, pediatric patients should be considered high-risk and require sustained monitoring, optimal treatment, and rehabilitation. Long-term recovery with adequate functional outcomes is achieved by an early return to pre-burn activities and regular multidisciplinary follow-up [43, 45].

2.5.2 Extremity Injuries

Extremity injuries are one of the defining injury patterns observed in adult victims of explosive devices [37]. In the pediatric population, the prevalence of extremity injuries varies greatly from 11 to 85% [12, 38]. The literature establishes a clear age dependence, with only 11% of infants and 20% of children under 7 years old experiencing limb injuries, contrasted with over 50% of older children [38]. Younger children are at increased risk of upper limb injuries, while adolescents predominantly suffer lower limb injuries, in line with data from adult populations [19]. Upper limb traumatic amputations (TA) are commonly associated with the upper torso, neck, and head injuries, and are rarely seen in survivors [40]. Primary, secondary, and tertiary blast injuries result in a variety of extremity wounds, including vascular injuries, long bone fractures, and traumatic amputations.

The long bones of the extremities undergo successive developmental stages which make them more susceptible to trauma when compared to adult bones [41]. The impact tolerance of children's bones is dependent on bone girth and relative proportions of the marrow cavity and bony walls, as well as the relative proportions of organic and inorganic materials that constitute bone tissue (the flexibility or torsional strength of bone is determined by the organic component) [41]. During early bone development, organic components (collagen) outweigh inorganic (minerals) components [41]. The predominance of organic material is maintained through adolescence and is followed by a gradual buildup of inorganic bone materials in early adulthood, with maximal bone strength observed around age 20 years [41]. Children's bones have a lower modulus of elasticity, lower bending strength, and lower bone ash content. They also tend to deflect and absorb more energy, both before and after a fracture starts taking place [42]. That composition may explain the high prevalence of fractures in this demographic following explosive blasts.

Orthopedic trauma resulting from explosive detonations can occur in primary, secondary, tertiary, or quaternary (miscellaneous) blast injuries, in isolation or in combination. Traumatic amputations (TA), or the most severe form of orthopedic trauma, may occur through two mechanisms. The first is diaphyseal stress leading to fracture, flailing of the joint, and transosseous amputation. The second is intra/periarticular stress leading to articular failure, flailing of the joint, and joint amputation [47]. In an explosion, changes in atmospheric pressure caused by the blast wave can fracture bones, followed by limb avulsion at the fracture site by secondary waves (blast winds), resulting in flailing of the extremity [48]. Some studies report that the most common site of amputation was not at the joint, but at different positions along the long bones based on the blast circumstances. The most frequently observed lower limb amputation site was the lower third of the femur and the upper third of the tibia at the level of the tibial tuberosity. In the upper limb, the distal arm was most commonly amputated. This pattern was explained by the shock wave causing a stretch or bend in the mid diaphysis of long bones as it passes through the victim's body and a complete fracture from the following blast wind [48].

Primary blast waves transfer energy at interfaces between tissues with differing acoustic impedance [5] leading to cellular disruption, soft tissue destruction, and bone micro fractures as the stress wave propagates, prior to any displacement [3]. This builds up shearing and axial stress forces that eventually exceed the tensile strength of bone causing fractures. It is suggested that these stress forces, occurring at the site of blast wave-induced bone fracture, are the probable mechanism of traumatic amputation [3]. For example, the most commonly seen proximal tibia fracture occurs when a blast wave penetrates a tibia from a lateral trajectory, and the bending forces exerted interact with the geometry of the tibia, resulting in peak stress applied to the proximal third [3, 5]. Once the bone is fractured by the blast wave, the detonation products exert on the bone additional bending stress [3], clinically manifesting as a traumatic amputation, with the proximal stump containing a short oblique or transverse fracture morphology [3] (Table 2.2).

Secondary blast injury is characterized by penetrating trauma from bomb casing fragments, materials implanted within the explosive (e.g., nails and screws), or from local materials displaced by the energy of the explosion [3, 5]. The projectiles rarely cause direct limb amputations [48], but they can cause fractures, directly or indirectly [5]. Aerodynamic drag on irregularly shaped fragments results in rapid deceleration outward from the point of detonation. Therefore, depending on the distance from the blast, fragments can strike the body with varying velocity, contrary to the streamlining seen in bullets fired through a rifled barrel [48]. In addition to their lack of streamlining, low-velocity fragments from explosive munitions

Table 2.2 Injury mechanisms from the explosion and its interaction with bone [49]

Explosion type	Pathophysiology	Fracture characteristics
Primary	Blast wave-mediated fracture	Traumatic amputation, short oblique/transverse fracture
Secondary	Direct impact of fragment	Highly comminuted multi-fragmentary fractures
Primary and secondary	Direct contact with the seat of the explosion, resulting in blast wave and fragment injury (e.g., antipersonnel landmine explosion)	Traumatic or subtotal amputation with significant soft tissue injury and fragments
Tertiary	Displacement of the causality or objects near the causality	Axial loading, 3-point bending, spinal fracture

Reproduced with the permission of The Royal Society from Ramasamy A et al. (2011) [49]

behave differently than low-velocity bullets. Upon striking tissue, even at low velocity, these fragments may exhibit a tumbling or so-called shimmy effect that can increase the amount of tissue damage [48]. Blast fragments often carry environmental debris into the wound and can inflict more severe tissue injuries than low-velocity bullets [48]. Furthermore, a large, slower projectile can crush a large amount of tissue, and missile fragmentation that may occur within the body can greatly increase temporary cavity effects [48]. A combination of the factors described above most likely accounts for the qualitative differences in tissue damage often seen with explosive fragments, compared to the damage caused by low-velocity gunshot wounds [48]. The direct impacts of high-energy fragments colliding with bone typically result in a highly comminuted fracture with extensive periosteal stripping [5]. Experimental evidence has shown that these injuries result in multiple bone fragments with no periosteal attachment and thus no blood supply [3]. In addition, these direct high-transfer wounds produce significant contamination of the fracture site and the medullary canal, thereby increasing the risk of developing long-term infective complications (osteomyelitis) [3]. As projectiles pass through tissue, they impart radial velocity to the surrounding medium, thereby creating large temporary cavities [3]. After penetrating the bone cortex, a projectile encounters the marrow-filled cancellous bone and propels the marrow radially at high velocity, fracturing the thin trabeculae. After penetrating the second bone cortex, the exit hole is enlarged by cavitation in the cancellous bone [3]. Due to the relatively inelastic nature of bone, the cavity formed in cancellous bone does not collapse and becomes a permanent cavity [3]. With higher velocity impacts (more than 500 m/s^2), the cavitation phenomenon produces widespread destruction of cancellous bone, with increased fragmentation of the cortical bone on the exit hole [3]. Conversely, at slower velocities, full penetration of the bone does not occur and only a single cortex is breached. In these cases, the classical "drill-hole" fracture is produced [3]. Indirect fractures can be caused by high-energy fragments passing in close proximity to bone. Such injuries are caused by the high pressures exerted on the bone surface by the leading edge of a rapidly expanding temporary cavity [3]. These fractures show no bone loss and the fragments retain periosteal attachments and are likely to remain viable [3]. The configuration in these injuries is usually simple (i.e., transverse or oblique) with little comminution, much like primary blast injuries [3, 5] (Table 2.2).

Secondary soft tissue blast effects are due to a propelled fragment colliding with the body that directly damages soft tissue in its path and, if sufficiently energized, generates a high-radial pressure compression wave in the tissues, just as an explosion does in the atmosphere [5]. The wave creates a temporary cavity of subatmospheric pressure as the fragment traverses, which pulls in external debris, increasing the risk of wound contamination [5]. The proportions of temporary and permanent cavities are determined by the kinetic energy of the causative fragment and the nature of the tissue affected. Areas of devitalized tissue can extend several centimeters and the zone of injury is often much greater than the remaining wound track [5]. The irregular morphology of shrapnel in comparison to a uniform bullet, increases the transfer of kinetic energy to surrounding tissues, thereby dealing greater damage

[5]. Consequently, simple surgical debridement of the wound track may not be sufficient to remove all nonviable tissue [5].

Tertiary blast injuries are caused by blast winds that can accelerate bodies as well as objects but do not reach as far as blast projectiles. The injuries sustained are varying in severity and are largely dependent on the distance from the explosion. Often, victims tumble along the ground, sustaining multiple injuries, or may be hurled through the air and struck by objects or impaled by them. Fractures, crush injuries, amputations, severe soft tissue lacerations, and contusions are all possible [48]. Displacement of the victims with force and sudden deceleration against a solid structure can result in significant tertiary orthopedic blast injuries [5] (Table 2.2).

When bone is subjected to external loads, the pressure distributes unevenly due in part to local osseous imperfections. This leads to nucleation, multiplication, and growth of micro-cracks in the weakest areas, and finally to the formation of macroscopic fissures (fracture) as a result of the coalescence of localized micro-cracks in the most densely damaged area [3]. The fracture pattern is a function of the direction and intensity of the load applied, the geometry of the bone involved, and its specific material properties [3]. When pressure is perpendicular to the axis of the bone, the most common fracture reported was a tension wedge, irrespective of the direction of the impact [3]. Tensile wedge fractures originate at a location directly opposite the point of impact, and the wedge segment radiates back through the bone initially forming a 90-degree vertex angle. This suggests failure from direct stress, i.e., axial loading of the bone in tension at the far cortex [3]. The level of comminution at the fracture site was related to higher impact speeds. Spiral fractures only occur when the bones were subjected to additional torsional loads. Severe axial loading of the lower limbs is common with underground explosions, or victims landing on their feet after being thrown by blasts, with comminuted calcaneal (heel) fractures being a prominent injury [3].

Quaternary (miscellaneous) orthopedic blast injuries are much less common than secondary blast injuries and may include burns from the thermal effects of explosions or from secondary fires [5, 48] (Table 2.2).

One of the important determinants of musculoskeletal injuries is the location of the victim relative to the explosion site. For instance, in close proximity to the detonation site, the effects of shock waves and detonation products occur almost instantaneously, leading to mixed primary and secondary blast injuries. This classically occurs with the detonation of anti-personnel mines, which are designed to release explosive energy at point-blank range, with the goal of maiming rather than killing [3]. The mine's blast wave is transmitted directly into the limb causing a brisance (shattering) effect on bone, within 200 milliseconds of the detonation. 1–2 milliseconds post-detonation, the bomb casing, environmental fragments, and other detonation products contact the limbs, causing destruction of traumatized soft tissue and applying maximal stress on bones previously damaged by the blast wave [3]. The end result is a total or sub-total limb amputation, with a zone of soft tissue injury (and significant amounts of foreign debris and fragments) extending more proximally to the damaged bone [3].

As with other types of blast injuries, orthopedic injuries are affected by environmental factors, especially in enclosed vs. open spaces. When a detonation occurs close to but outside of a structure, the resulting blast wave diffracts around and reflects off the obstacle. It also transmits to the interior of the structure with significantly reduced energy and pressure [49], effectively lowering the risk of blast wave-related injuries substantially [49].

In contrast, blast fragments are more likely to result in fractures of victims caught in the open [49]. Studies show that the lower limb is more frequently affected and sustains more tertiary blast injuries from enclosed space detonations [49]. These observations may be attributed to the momentum effects of the explosion that throw victims into the air for long distances before landing on their feet, or secondary to vertical acceleration and local floor pan deformation [49].

2.5.3 Torso Injuries

Chest and abdominal trauma are common following blasts, with an incidence varying between 32 and 50% and a peak in children aged 5–10 years [12, 38]. Primary, secondary, and tertiary blast injuries may impact the abdominal or thoracic structures and viscera. A comparison with unarmored adults [28] suggests that the torso is far more commonly injured in children following landmine and UXO (Unexploded Explosive Ordnance) explosions [28]. This may be due to anatomical susceptibility or unintentional high-risk behavior around explosives. Several structural considerations in pediatric populations lead to distinct patterns of chest injuries [50]. Pediatric thoracic blast injuries usually affect the internal organs due to the lesser protection provided by the developing rib cage [41]. In infants and young children, the thoracic walls are thinner and the ribs are more elastic than their adult counterparts. This greater flexibility is due to incomplete bony ossification, more flexible ligamentous attachments, and less developed supportive musculature, and makes it possible for anterior ribs to be compressed all the way to meet posterior ribs [51]. The anatomical features of the young thorax increase the likelihood of suffering severe parenchymal thoracic injuries such as heart contusion, dislocation, transection, or angulation of the great vessels, tracheal compression, and angulation, esophageal rupture [52], as well as pulmonary contusions with minimal or no signs on superficial examination or admission chest X-rays [41, 50, 51]. Over 80% of children who sustain a thoracic aortic tear will have significant associated injuries to the lung, heart, long bones, abdominal viscera, and central nervous system, although only 50% will present with external evidence of thoracic injury. Rib fractures are much more likely to occur from secondary or tertiary injuries [52]. Primary blast waves powerful enough to fracture flexible ribs usually result in fatal pulmonary trauma [52].

In addition to the structural and size differences, thoracic organs in children exhibit different physiologic characteristics [51]. In early life, the trachea is narrow, short, more compressible, and narrowest at the level of the cricoid cartilage. Therefore, small changes in airway diameter, seemingly inconsequential wounds in the thoracic cage, or small foreign bodies may rapidly lead to respiratory distress [51]. Children also have a lower functional residual capacity coupled with higher oxygen consumption per unit of body mass and are therefore more susceptible to rapid deterioration from hypoxemia [51]. Moreover, they are at particularly high risk for airway obstruction [53] due to several oropharyngeal anatomic features: their tongues are relatively large for their oral cavity, as are the soft palate, oropharyngeal tissues, and the epiglottis, which are relatively longer and stiffer [53]. To complicate matters further, their large heads and occiput relative to body size allow their necks to flex easily when lying supine, exacerbating airway obstruction. These factors make children more susceptible to airway irritation and asphyxiation from the copious amounts of hot dust, sand, particles, debris, smoke, toxic fumes, and gases produced by explosions [7]. Lower respiratory tract and lung burns are rare but can be caused by superheated steam; signs include dyspnea, cough, and crackles from pulmonary edema [7].

Primary blast lung injury (PBLI) is the most common fatal injury following exposure to overpressure waves [2] and presents essentially as pulmonary contusions [52]. The degree of pulmonary pathology is proportional to the velocity of chest wall displacement [52]. A slow steadily applied force to the lungs allows compressed air to vent out through the trachea [52], while the abrupt chest wall compression induced by blast waves does not allow for this equilibration [52]. Pressures within the lung parenchyma and air spaces can match or greatly exceed the blast pressures because lung tissue compresses more slowly than the air in the respiratory tract [52]. Air-tissue interfaces of the pulmonary system are vulnerable to spalling, compression, and shear forces [17]. Barotrauma and volutrauma (overexpansion damage) lead to alveolar hemorrhage, pulmonary contusions, widespread edema, and pneumothoraxes [2, 21]. Depending on the blast load, this varies from scattered petechiae to large confluent hemorrhages involving the entire lung. Pulmonary contusions are more severe on the impact side of blast waves in the open air but tend to be bilateral and diffuse in victims of confined space blasts [52]. Pleural and subpleural petechiae are the mildest pathologies described. Ecchymoses, often in parallel bands corresponding to intercostal spaces, may be seen with larger blast loads [52]. Pneumothoraxes from blast injury are at increased risk of tensioning in infants due to the inherent mobility of the pediatric mediastinum, causing additional mortality [31].

2.5.4 Head and Spinal Injuries

The reported prevalence of pediatric head injuries following blasts varies between 15% and 60% [18, 38]. Patients under 7 years old are almost twice as likely to present with head injuries as older children (28% vs 15%) [18]. Blast-induced traumatic brain injury (bTBI) is more common in victims under 10 years of age compared to adolescents [38]. Head and cervical spine injury is the second most common cause of death in all age groups [18], with one retrospective study conducted on postmortem data reporting skull fractures in 90% of pediatric casualties [54].

Neurosurgical decompression is the most common surgical intervention for blast-related head injuries in children under 3 years old [55].

Child cranial and spinal anatomy undergoes many changes, from the closure of fontanels and cranial sutures to changes in the thickness and pliability of the cranium, anatomy of the vertebra, and the maturity of cervical ligaments and muscles [53]. These structural differences change the fundamental injury mechanism for an infant compared to that of an older child or adult [56]. The child's head and brain are also fundamentally different from adults physiologically and anatomically [53]. Children have larger heads relative to body size, increasing the likelihood of head injuries in pediatric victims [39, 53]. Furthermore, the head is relatively heavy compared to the rest of the body and is supported by a weaker cervical musculature [57], making the head more vulnerable to TBI and resulting in different dynamics of head acceleration in response to external forces [39]. The ratio of head-to-body size gradually declines with age [39].

As children grow and develop, facial development and expansion of the paranasal sinuses progressively provide protection from brain damage [39]: the sinuses play a role as air-filled shock absorbers, partially absorbing energy directed at the skull and brain [39]. At birth the facial portion of the head is smaller than the cranium, with a face-to-cranium ratio of 1:8 (vs. adult ratio of 1:2.5). This pattern is notable in children up to age 8 years [41]. Moreover, the newborn forehead is high and bulged relative to the facial profile, due to the large size of the frontal lobe of the brain [41]. Thus, in newborns and infants, the face is tucked below the larger brain case, and their protruding forehead increases the probability that a force directly impacts the frontal skull and underlying cerebral parenchyma [39]. Furthermore, they lack the protection of fully pneumatized sinus cavities.

The mechanical characteristics of infant and adult skulls are significantly different. Anatomical immaturity in skull composition may increase the risk of bTBI from primary blast waves. Infant and child skulls are considerably more pliable, due to the segmental development and arrangement of skull bones, in addition to the flexibility and thinness of individual bones, possibly leading to greater shear stress and subsequent injury to the underlying brain structures [58]. Reduced calvarium thickness is also likely to provide less protection from penetrating and blunt traumatic injury. Another material property of the calvarium is its elastic modulus: fiber orientations parallel to the long axis have significantly higher elastic moduli than those with fibers perpendicular to the long axis [59]. In adults, cranial bones and sutures have similar properties and adult calvarias deform very little prior to fracture [59]. In contrast, pediatric cranial bones are 35 times stiffer than their cranial sutures and are able to deform 30 times more than older children's cranial bones before failure, and 243 times more than adult bones [59]. The large strains in pediatric bones and sutures result in a skull case that can undergo dramatic shape changes before fracture, potentially causing devastating damage to the brain [59]. In addition, fontanelles are extremely vulnerable to trauma. The skull develops as a loosely joined system of bones formed in the soft tissue matrix surrounding the brain. Interosseous junctions are relatively broad and large, leaving certain areas of the brain covered by a thin fibrous sheath and somewhat exposed to the external environment. They are most obvious in the frontal and posterior skull regions and make the head of the child less resistant to impact trauma [41].

Injury patterns are also determined by the mechanical properties of brain tissue, which is stiffer in children [53]. Infant cerebral white matter contains little myelin, and its distribution is very different compared with adults [39]. The neonatal brain is watery and has a low density, while the fully myelinated adult brain has a much higher density [39]. Different brain regions myelinate at different rates and the resulting density variations can be pronounced at different developmental stages [39]. The degree of myelination results in different absorptions of traumatic forces, with increased susceptibility to TBI in unmyelinated areas [39]. When intracranial volume increases rapidly, as, in blast trauma, the acute increase in ICP can be life threatening. It may be more dangerous in young children than in older children and adults because of the lower normal range of ICP in this age group [53]. Cerebral compliance observed in young children as a result of open fontanelles and unfused sutures can only provide protection to a certain extent [53]. It is also determined by cerebral blood flow (CBF) and volume, and the ratio of cerebrospinal fluid (CSF) volume to brain volume, all of which are age dependent [53]. The CSF-brain ratio reflects the balance between brain tissue and CSF in the ventricles and subarachnoid cisterns of the brain. Although this has not been formally quantified across the age range, radiologists and pediatric specialists are aware of the differences between very young children, older children, and adults with respect to the amount of intracranial CSF that is expected, to reflect the growth of the brain from the neonatal stage through childhood and the gradual atrophy with age [53]. Post-mortem pathoanatomical data provides the majority of evidence for the pathophysiological effects of blast, which include edema, contusions, vasospasm of the internal carotid and anterior cerebral arteries, diffuse axonal injuries, and hematomas [60–64]. Following the blast, cerebral concussion is common, with increasing evidence of association with post-traumatic stress disorder (PTSD) [65–68].

The mechanism of bTBI following primary blast injuries remains incompletely understood [69, 70]; most experimental data originate from laboratory or computer models [66, 69, 71–73]. The overall hypothesis is that brain injuries can occur following overpressure oscillations from the primary blast, pressure on the cranium by the secondary blast winds, and tertiary blast injuries in the form of blunt traumatic or coup-countercoup injuries [74].

Blunt Traumatic brain injury (TBI) in children is caused by one of two mechanisms [56]:

1. Impulsive loading, where the head moves as the result of motion imparted by some other part of the body (e.g., "whiplash").
2. Impact loading, where the head either strikes a stationary object or is struck by a moving object.

These events are mechanically distinct and have very different clinical consequences. Both cannot occur simultaneously, although they may happen sequentially. Impulsive loading of an unsupported head will cause it to rotate around some point in the cervical spine, from the occipital condyles to C7/T1. With such a rotation, the skull will receive the transmitted force faster than the brain, which lags behind because the brain and skull are not rigidly linked [56]. This differential displacement may result in tensile failure of the bridging veins, which can withstand a force up to 30% stronger than their average baseline stretch [56]. It has also been suggested that following brain trauma, pediatric patients are at greater risk of brain injury from enhanced excitotoxicity and impaired cerebral blood flow. Excitotoxic effects may lead to increased neuronal apoptosis [75]. Experimental data using pediatric neurons subjected to non-blast TBI (nbTBI) demonstrated that extrasynaptic N-methyl-D aspartate (NDMA) channels were excited, leading to increased calcium channel influx [76, 77]. Calcium influx is associated with enhancing intracellular cascades and promoting neuroapoptosis [78]. Furthermore, severe nbTBI in children has been associated with impaired cerebral autoregulation and subsequent poor outcomes [79, 80]. In a later study, those under 4 years old were found to be at risk of impaired autoregulation, regardless of nbTBI severity, suggesting an enhanced susceptibility in younger patients. This correlates with animal studies demonstrating prolonged reductions in cerebral blood flow in newborn pigs compared to juvenile pigs following diffuse nbTBI [81].

Significant cognitive, intellectual, and functional sequelae arising from pediatric nbTBI have been described [82–87] and there is a clear need for specific studies on the long-term prognosis of pediatric bTBI. Controversy exists as to whether mild nbTBI is analogous to moderate bTBI in adults [88], and the paucity of pediatric data makes this comparison difficult. Extrapolation of bTBI results from nbTBI data is limited by variable follow-up times, more segmented age groups in pediatric populations, developmental milestones which complicate assessment and differing TBI mechanisms. Early nbTBI data suggest pediatric patients benefit from increased neuroplasticity in the developing brain, allowing recovery of cognitive and intellectual function [82]. However, conflicting studies demonstrated reduced educational performance, increased impulsivity, hyperactivity, and learning disabilities after 2–5 years in children with brain injury [83–86]. A recent study by Shaklai et al. [87] assessed 77 children of ages 2–17 over 10 years following moderate to severe nbTBI and found that 69% were able to fully reintegrate back into regular education following extended rehabilitation. The remaining 31% required additional help (19%) or special education (12%). Previous studies report reintegration of 24–59% of cases [89, 90]. A Higher Glasgow Coma Scale at admission and shorter loss of consciousness correlate with a positive outcome, which is consistent with other reports [91–93].

Pediatric spine injuries affect a modest percentage of children following blast injury (1–3%) [12, 27], with its presentation being almost ubiquitously associated with concurrent head injuries [18]. No data exists for blast-specific pediatric spinal injuries; the literature does, however, describe patterns for non-blast-related spinal trauma: the cervical spine is affected in 60–80% of total pediatric spinal injuries [94], while only in 15–45% of adult spinal injuries [95–97]. This pattern may be explained by progressive changes at the level of the epiphyses which fuse progressively at different times [53]. The biomechanical maturation of the spine only begins to resemble the adult spine after age 8–9 [53]. Prior to the age of 10 years, the relatively large head places the fulcrum of flexion and extension at the upper cervical region, potentially increasing injuries [53]. Cervical spinal fractures are rare while ligamental dislocations are much more common, due to underdeveloped neck musculature, lax interspinous ligaments, and incomplete vertebral ossification. The absence of fractures may partially explain the high rate of spinal cord injury without radiographic abnormalities (SCIWORA) in infants (17%) compared to adolescents (5%) [98]. Other factors also explain the weakness of pediatric cervical spines and their tendency to deform: increased water content of intervertebral disks, unfused epiphyses, shallow facet joints, anteriorly wedged vertebral bodies, and undeveloped uncinate processes [53]. All these contribute to a more malleable spine that puts neural structures at risk, even without bony injury evident on radiographs [53]. Neurological sequelae are largely dependent on the degree of spinal cord injury (SCI) sustained. A high degree of clinical suspicion is thus warranted for pediatric blast victims.

2.5.5   Facial Injuries

Primary blast waves inflict different types of injuries on the maxillofacial region that result from interactions of the blast shockwave with these tissues, resulting in barotrauma [16]. The stress on impacted areas may be concentrated at certain locations called stress points; when tension exceeds their tensile strength, collagen fibers will fracture, and tissues will tear [16]. Primary blast wave impact on the face may result in transverse mandibular fractures, eye rupture, orbital fractures, tympanic membrane rupture, fracture of paranasal sinus walls, facial soft tissue injuries, and scalping injuries. They are usually associated with injuries to the lung, brain, and hollow organs; it is relatively uncommon to find isolated facial injuries in survivors [16]. Exposed wound surfaces are then hit by thermal gases (fireballs) and suffer burns on top of trauma. Blast winds also carry sand and other particles into the damaged soft tissues and exposed fractured bones [16].

When the wave impacts bony processes such as the zygomatic process or mandibular body and symphysis, the energy released can crush soft tissues between the compressed air wave contacting the skin surface, and the internal bone surface, causing skin and subcutaneous contusions. These wounds are characterized by ragged, tattered, and ecchymosed edges [16]. Because facial skin has strong resistance to primary blast waves, most injuries seen on the cheeks, eyelids, and lips are due to the combination of primary and secondary biophysical effects [16]. The suspended hot particles in the blast wave or winds impact a maximally stretched skin at high velocity, resulting in traumatic and deep scratches [16]. These abrasions facilitate the tearing of tightly stretched collagen fibers, resulting in shredding, laceration, or multiple punctures of all layers of skin in the affected area [16]. Scalping blast injuries occur when the blast wave strikes the front of the victim's helmet or scalp and the resultant maximal stretching exceeds the elastic limits of the skin at weak points near the eyelids. This leads to the skin tearing along a line between the eyebrows and eyelashes consisting of the thinnest skin in the region. This can be followed by a degloving of the full thickness of the scalp tissue with separation occurring at another weak attachment at the pericranium and calvarias [16]. The scalping in this case extends posterior to the coronal suture and usually indicates a very powerful blast.

2.5.6 Maxillary Sinus Fracture

Implosion of maxillary sinuses has been proposed as a mechanism of "crushed egg-shell" fractures of the midface, but experimental evidence for primary blasts causing facial fractures directly is lacking. Whether caused by primary blasts or secondary blunt trauma, these types of injuries do occur in victims close to explosions [99]. Rapid external loading of pressure onto the sinus structures compresses the sinus walls and causes them to splinter [6]. Once the high pressure has abated, the air re-expands, effectively creating a miniature explosion within the sinuses [6]. This causes more damage to the delicate structures of the nasal area, and this type of injury occurs when shock waves hit the midface area directly [6]. Alternatively, when a lateral wave impacts the skeletal structures of the cranium, the lateral portion of the maxillary sinuses is less affected due to the thicker zygomatic buttresses deflecting the shock wave more effectively than the thinner maxillary bone with a perpendicular force directly to the front of the face [6].

2.5.7 Mandibular Fracture

The pathophysiology of shock wave impacts at the lateral surface of the body of the mandible is different from non-blast-related trauma and results in a new type of fracture seen only in mandibular blast injuries [100]. Most civilian mandibular fractures are vertical to the longitudinal axis of the mandible, as seen in the body, angle, symphysis, ramus, condyle, and coronoid processes. These fractures are produced by high tensile strain caused by a traumatic impact, which leads to vertically orientated deformation patterns at points of weakness, causing tensile failure [100]. In the case of a transverse impact from a blast, wave-particle displacement is perpendicular to the direction of propagation of the wave, and they oscillate up and down around their individual axis. When the wave encounters the transverse middle part of the body of the mandible, part of it is reflected at the rigid boundaries (upper and lower borders) and the other part is transmitted across a less rigid middle part. A structural difference exists between the different mandibular sections because of solid cortical bone and the alveolar region, which is reinforced by cylindrical sockets and the strength of dental roots [100]. This causes a shearing fragmentation of the mandible at the mylohyoid ridge, a weak area in the mandible and attachment point of the mylohyoid muscle, with separation of muscle and bone [6]. The cancellous and cortical bone at this weaker point split transversely due to the differing shock absorbing properties of the impacted bone structures, provided the blast wave is powerful enough [6]. Because of the factors explained above, blast mandibular fractures are a unique type of transverse split fracture occurring at the angle of the mandible [100]. They can manifest as a single line or multiple, almost parallel shearing lines, in the same region where fragmentation occurs [100].

Teeth are designed to withstand vertical forces; the impact of the blast, however, strikes the lateral surfaces uniformly, and much of the energy is reflected because of the convexity of the buccal surface and the hardness of tooth enamel [100]. The root is protected by the cortical bone of the alveolar socket and by its cylindrical shape which can deflect some of the energy. A powerful enough blast wave can lead to flexural failure and shearing (direct or punching shear) at the cementoenamel junction, resulting in sharp transections at the gingival margins. This type of tooth fracture parallels the displacement of the transverse mandibular fracture segments [100]. The effects of the blast and the tooth's structural response depend mainly on the pressure loading rate, the incoming angle of the blast, and the condition of the bony structures [100].

2.5.8   Acoustic Injury

Hearing loss following blast exposure is the most prevalent primary blast injury [101, 102] persisting well after the initial insult [103]. Blast pressures exceeding 104 kPa, approximately 1/5th the pressure required for a lethal injury, damage the tympanic membrane (TM) at the air–tissue interface with a 50% chance of rupture, in addition to middle ear ossicular damage and subsequent conductive hearing loss [104, 105]. The pars tensa is the TM area most frequently injured. Although much less common, dislocation of the incudomalleal or incudostapedial joints can occur, with or without fractures of the individual ossicles. Orientation of the head relative to the blast wave could possibly alter the severity for smaller blast loads that cause isolated auditory injury. Disruption of the ossicular chain may also protect the inner ear from permanent damage by absorbing the bulk of the pressure wave. In most cases, inner ear injury is reversible or treatable; temporary hearing loss and tinnitus are quite common, the severity of which typically decreases at farther distances from the blast. However, severe cochlear damage may occur: sensorineural hearing loss is usually permanent in these cases and occurs following excessive pressure mechanotransduction to the sensitive cochlear hair cells, or through bTBI damaging the auditory cortex [105].

2.5.9   Eye Injury

Despite representing only 0.3% of the anterior body surface area, eyes are often injured following blasts, with as many as 60% of blast victims undergoing minor clearance operations [27, 54, 106]. Eye injuries, including globe perforation, are commonly caused by secondary projectiles after explosions of all sizes. Interestingly, only one case of ocular primary blast injury (causing hyphemia) has been reported in the literature, likely because of the eye's nearly homogenous density. Damage to the eye can result from overpressure waves reflecting off the bony orbit, causing optic nerve and anterior/posterior segment disruption, from secondary injuries caused by bone fragmentation, tertiary facial trauma, and chemical or thermal burns [107, 108]. Mine blasts are thought to cause a high incidence of eye injuries due to high concentrations of explosive particles, especially affecting children whose eyes are closer to the detonation point [7, 106, 109]. As it was described for the torso and upper limb injuries, the curiosity of children and high-risk behavior in the vicinity of explosives may predispose them to facial and ocular injuries. Vision loss confers significant long-term morbidity in children. In infants, visual processing plasticity and binocular vision develop in the first year of life. Monocular visual impairment can lead to further morbidity through amblyopia and visual defects [110, 111]. Without adequate social support, these victims are likely to suffer from developmental and educational deficiencies. This happens because 75% of early learning occurs through vision, and visual impairment at this age translates into future social and economic challenges to both the individual and the society [110, 112].

References

1. National Consortium for the Study of Terrorism and Responses to Terrorism (START). GTD global terrorism database. Start. 2015;63.
2. Wolf SJ, Bebarta VS, Bonnett CJ, Pons PT, Cantrill SV. Blast injuries. Lancet. 2009;374(9687):405–15.
3. Champion HR, Holcomb JB, Young LA. Injuries from explosions: physics, biophysics, pathology, and required research focus. J Trauma. 2009;66(May):1468–77.
4. Boffard KD, MacFarlane C. Urban bomb blast injuries: patterns of injury and treatment. Surg Annu. 1993;25(Pt 1(part 1)):29–47.
5. Ramasamy, Cooper GA, Sargeant ID, Evriviades D, Porter K, Kendrew JM. (i) An overview of the pathophysiology of blast injury with management guidelines. Orthop Trauma. 2013;27(1):1–8. *ISSN 1877-1327.*
6. Dussault MC, Smith M, Osselton D. Blast injury and the human skeleton: an important emerging aspect of conflict-related trauma. J Forensic Sci. 2014;59(3):606–12.
7. Shuker ST. Facial skin-mucosal biodynamic blast injuries and management. J Oral Maxillofac Surg. 2010;68(8):1818 25.
8. Horrocks CL. Blast injuries: biophysics, pathophysiology and management principles. J R Army Med Corps. 2001;147(1):28–40.
9. Knapp JF, Sharp RJ, Beatty R, Medina F. Blast trauma in a child. Pediatr Emerg Care. 1990;6(2):122–6.
10. DePalma RG, Burris DG, Champion HR, Hodgson MJ. Blast injuries. N Engl J Med. 2005;352(13):1335–42.
11. Zuckerman S. Discussion on the problem of blast injuries. Proc R Soc Med. 1941;34:171–88.
12. Waisman Y, Aharonson-Daniel L, Mor M, Amir L, Peleg K. The impact of terrorism on children: a two-year experience. Prehosp Disaster Med. 2003;18(3):242–8.
13. The impact of blast injury on children Hargrave, Lt J F S Millwood 2018.
14. Physical and pathophysiological effects of blast. J Trauma. 1996;40(3 Suppl):S206–11. https://doi.org/10.1097/00005373-199603001-00045.
15. Mechanisms of injury in wartime. J Trauma. 2008;65(3):604–15. https://doi.org/10.1097/TA.0b013e3181454ab4.

16. Facial skin-mucosal biodynamic blast injuries and management. Acta Biomater. 2011;7(1):83–95. https://doi.org/10.1016/j.actbio.2010.06.035. Epub 2010 Aug 21

17. Edwards D., Clasper J. Blast injury mechanism. In: Blast injury science and engineering: a guide for clinicians and researchers. Springer International Publishing Switzerland; 2016. p. 89–103.

18. Edwards MJ, Lustik M, Eichelberger MR, Elster E, Azarow K, Coppola C. Blast injury in children: an analysis from Afghanistan and Iraq, 2002-2010. J Trauma Acute Care Surg. 2012;73(5):1278–83.

19. Bendinelli C. Effects of land mines and unexploded ordnance on the pediatric population and comparison with adults in rural Cambodia. World J Surg. 2009;33(5):1070–4.

20. Breeze J, Lewis EA, Fryer R, Hepper AE, Mahoney PF, Clasper JC. Defining the essential anatomical coverage provided by military body armour against high energy projectiles. J R Army Med Corps. 2016;162(4):284–90.

21. Yeh DD, Schecter WP. Primary blast injuries—an updated concise review. World J Surg. 2012;36(5):966–72.

22. Shi CX. Pediatric wartime injuries in Afghanistan and Iraq : what have we learned ? 2016;(September).

23. Allison K, Porter K. Consensus on the pre-hospital approach to burns patient management. Injury. 2004:734–8.

24. Currey JD, Butler G. The mechanical properties of bone tissue in children. J Bone Jt Surg. 1975;57–A;810–4.

25. Mabrey JD, Fitch RD. Plastic deformation in pediatric fractures: mechanism and treatment. J Pediatr Orthop. 1989;9(3):310–4.

26. Edwards MJ, Lustik M, Eichelberger MR, Elster E, Azarow K, Coppola C. Blast injury in children: an analysis from Afghanistan and Iraq, 2002–2010. J Trauma Acute Care Surg. 2012;73(5):1278–83. https://doi.org/10.1097/TA.0b013e318270d3ee. Erratum in: J Trauma Acute Care Surg. 2014;77(2):389.

27. Creamer KM, Edwards MJ, Shields CH, Thompson MW, Yu CE, Adelman W. Pediatric wartime admissions to US military combat support hospitals in Afghanistan and Iraq: learning from the first 2,000 admissions. Trauma. 2009;67(4):762–9.

28. Matos RI, Holcomb JB, Callahan C, Spinella PC. Increased mortality rates of young children with traumatic injuries at a US Army combat support hospital in Baghdad, Iraq, 2004. Pediatrics. 2008;122(5):e959–66.

29. Wang XQ, Mill J, Kravchuk O, Kimble RM. Ultrasound assessed thickness of burn scars in association with laser Doppler imaging determined depth of burns in paediatric patients. Burns. 2010;36(8):1254–62.

30. Gore DC, Chinkes D, Heggers J, Herndon DN, Wolf SE, Desai M. Association of hyperglycemia with increased mortality after severe burn injury. J Trauma. 2001;51(3):540–4.

31. Eichelberger MR. Pediatric surgery and medicine for hostile environments. J Pediatr Surg. 2011;46:1683.

32. Sheridan RL, Hinson MI, Liang MH, Nackel AF, Schoenfeld DA, Ryan CM, et al. Long-term outcome of children surviving massive burns. JAMA. 2000;283(1):69–73.

33. Zeitlin REK, Järnberg J, Somppi EJ, Sundell B. Long-term functional sequelae after paediatric burns. Burns. 1998;24(1):3–6.

34. de Sousa A. Psychological aspects of paediatric burns (a clinical review). Ann Burns Fire Disasters. 2010;23:155–9.

35. Peck MD, Weber J, McManus A, Sheridan R, Heimbach D. Surveillance of burn wound infections: a proposal for definitions. J Burn Care Rehabil. 1998;19(5):386–9.

36. Silla RC, Fong J, Wright J, Wood F. Infection in acute burn wounds following the Bali bombings: a comparative prospective audit. Burns. 2006;32(2):139–44.

37. Owens BD, Kragh JF, Wenke JC, Macaitis J, Wade CE, Holcomb JB. Combat wounds in operation Iraqi Freedom and operation enduring freedom. J Trauma. 2008;64(2):295–9.

38. Jaffe DH, Peleg K. Terror Explosive Injuries. Ann Surg. 2010;251(1):138–43.

39. Araki T, Yokota H, Morita A. Pediatric traumatic brain injury: characteristic features, diagnosis, and management. Neurol Med Chir (Tokyo). 2017;57(2):82–93.
40. Patel HDL, Dryden S, Gupta A, Ang SC. Pattern and mechanism of traumatic limb amputations after explosive blast: experience from the 07/07/05 London terrorist bombings. J Trauma Acute Care Surg. 2012;73(1):276–81.
41. Burdi AR, et al. Infants and children in the adult world of automobile safety design: pediatric and anatomical considerations for design of child restraints. J Biomech. 1969;2(3):267–80.
42. Currey JD, Butler G. The mechanical properties of bone tissue in children. J Bone Joint Surg Am. 1975;57(6):810–4.
43. Jeschke MG, Gauglitz GG, Kulp GA, Finnerty CC, Williams FN, Kraft R, et al. Long-term persistence of the pathophysiologic response to severe burn injury. PLoS One. 2011;6:7.
44. García-Avello A, Lorente JA, Cesar-Perez J, García-Frade LJ, Alvarado R, Arévalo JM, et al. Degree of hypercoagulability and hyperfibrinolysis is related to organ failure and prognosis after burn trauma. Thromb Res. 1998;89(2):59–64.
45. Duke JM, Randall SM, Fear MW, Boyd JH, Rea S, Wood FM. Long-term effects of pediatric burns on the circulatory system. Pediatrics. 2015;136(5):e1323–30.
46. Sharma RK, Parashar A. Special considerations in paediatric burn patients. Indian J Plast Surg. 2010;43:S43–50.
47. Singleton JAG. Traumatic amputation. In: Blast injury science and engineering: a guide for clinicians and researchers. 2016. p. 243–8.
48. Covey DC, Born CT. Blast injuries: mechanics and wounding patterns. J Surg Orthop Adv. 2010;19(1):8–12.
49. Ramasamy A, et al. Blast-related fracture patterns: a forensic biomechanical approach. J R Soc Interface. 2011;8(58):689–98.
50. Jakob H, et al. Pediatric Polytrauma Management. Eur J Trauma Emerg Surg. 2010;36(4):325–38.
51. Bliss D, Silen M. Pediatric thoracic trauma. Crit Care Med. 2002;30(11 Suppl):S409-15.
52. Omid R, et al. Gunshot wounds to the upper extremity. J Am Acad Orthop Surg. 2019;27(7):e301–10.
53. Figaji AA. Anatomical and physiological differences between children and adults relevant to traumatic brain injury and the implications for clinical assessment and care. Front Neurol. 2017;8:685.
54. Quintana DA, Jordan FB, Tuggle DW, Mantor PC, Tunell WP. The spectrum of pediatric injuries after a bomb blast. J Pediatr Surg. 1997;32(2):307–11.
55. Edwards MJ, Lustik M, Carlson T, Tabak B, Farmer D, Edwards K, et al. Surgical interventions for pediatric blast injury: an analysis from Afghanistan and Iraq 2002 to 2010. J Trauma Acute Care Surg. 2014;76(3):854–8.
56. Goldsmith W, Plunkett J. A biomechanical analysis of the causes of traumatic brain injury in infants and children. Am J Forensic Med Pathol. 2004;25(2):89–100.
57. Jakob H, Lustenberger T, Schneidmüller D, Sander AL, Walcher F, Marzi I. Pediatric polytrauma management. Eur J Trauma Emerg Surg. 2010;36(4):325–38.
58. Chafi MS, Karami G, Ziejewski M. Biomechanical assessment of brain dynamic responses due to blast pressure waves. Ann Biomed Eng. 2010;38(2):490–504.
59. Coats B, Margulies SS. Material properties of human infant skull and suture at high rates. J Neurotrauma. 2006;23(8):1222–32.
60. Levi L, Borovich B, Guilburd JN, Grushkiewicz I, Lemberger A, Linn S, et al. Wartime neurosurgical experience in Lebanon, 1982-85. II: closed craniocerebral injuries. Isr J Med Sci. 1990;26(10):555–8.
61. Schwartz I, Tuchner M, Tsenter J, Shochina M, Shoshan Y, Katz-Leurer M, et al. Cognitive and functional outcomes of terror victims who suffered from traumatic brain injury. Brain Inj. 2008;22(3):255–63.
62. Svetlov SI, Prima V, Kirk DR, Gutierrez H, Curley KC, Hayes RL, et al. Morphologic and biochemical characterization of brain injury in a model of controlled blast overpressure exposure. J Trauma. 2010;69(4):795–804.

63. Armonda RA, Bell RS, Vo AH, Ling G, DeGraba TJ, Crandall B, et al. Wartime traumatic cerebral vasospasm: recent review of combat casualties. Neurosurgery. 2006;59(6):1215–25.
64. Bell RS, Vo AH, Neal CJ, Tigno J, Roberts R, Mossop C, et al. Military traumatic brain and spinal column injury: a 5-year study of the impact blast and other military grade weaponry on the central nervous system. J Trauma. 2009;66(4 Suppl):S104-11.
65. Okie S. Traumatic brain injury in the war zone. N Engl J Med. 2005;352(20):2043–7.
66. Cernak I, Merkle AC, Koliatsos VE, Bilik JM, Luong QT, Mahota TM, et al. The pathobiology of blast injuries and blast-induced neurotrauma as identified using a new experimental model of injury in mice. Neurobiol Dis. 2011;41(2):538–51.
67. Stein MB, McAllister TW. Exploring the convergence of posttraumatic stress disorder and mild traumatic brain injury. Am J Psychiatry. 2009;166(7):768–76.
68. Taber KH, Warden DL, Hurley RA. Blast-related traumatic brain injury: what is known? J Neuropsychiatry Clin Neurosci. 2006;18(2):141–5.
69. Chen YC, Smith DH, Meaney DF. In-vitro approaches for studying blast-induced. 2009;876(June):861–76.
70. Cernak I. Animal models of head trauma. NeuroRx. 2005;2(3):410–22.
71. Park E, Eisen R, Kinio A, Baker AJ. Electrophysiological white matter dysfunction and association with neurobehavioral deficits following low-level primary blast trauma. Neurobiol Dis. 2013;52:150–9.
72. Park E, Gottlieb JJ, Cheung B, Shek PN, Baker AJ. A model of low-level primary blast brain trauma results in cytoskeletal proteolysis and chronic functional impairment in the absence of lung barotrauma. J Neurotrauma. 2011;28(3):343–57.
73. Pun PBL, Kan EM, Salim A, Li Z, Ng KC, Moochhala SM, et al. Low level primary blast injury in rodent brain. Front Neurol. 2011; *APR*
74. Wightman JM, Gladish SL. Explosions and blast injuries. Ann Emerg Med. 2001;37(6):664–78.
75. Choi DW. Ionic dependence of glutamate neurotoxicity. J Neurosci. 1987;7(2):369–79.
76. Giza CC, Maria NSS, Hovda DA. N -methyl- D -aspartate receptor subunit changes after traumatic injury to the developing brain. J Neurotrauma. 2006;23(6):950–61.
77. McDonald JW, Silverstein FS, Johnston MV. Neurotoxicity of N-methyl-d-aspartate is markedly enhanced in developing rat central nervous system. Brain Res. 1988;459(1):200–3.
78. Rink A, Fung KM, Trojanowski JQ, Lee VM, Neugebauer E, McIntosh TK. Evidence of apoptotic cell death after experimental traumatic brain injury in the rat. Am J Pathol. 1995;147(6):1575–83.
79. Vavilala MS, Muangman S, Tontisirin N, Fisk D, Roscigno C, Mitchell P, et al. Impaired cerebral autoregulation and 6-month outcome in children with severe traumatic brain injury: preliminary findings. Dev Neurosci. 2006;28(4–5):348–53.
80. Vavilala MS, Muangman S, Waitayawinyu P, Roscigno C, Jaffe K, Mitchell P, et al. Neurointensive care; impaired cerebral autoregulation in infants and young children early after inflicted traumatic brain injury: a preliminary report. J Neurotrauma. 2007;24(1):87–96.
81. Armstead WM, Kurth CD. Different cerebral hemodynamic responses following fluid percussion brain injury in the newborn and juvenile pig. J Neurotrauma. 1994;11(5):487–97.
82. Tompkins CA, Holland AL, Ratcliff G, Costello A, Leahy LF, Cowell V. Predicting cognitive recovery from closed head-injury in children and adolescents. Brain Cogn. 1990;13(1):86–97.
83. Wertheimer JC, Hanks RA, Hasenau DL. Comparing functional status and community integration in severe penetrating and motor vehicle-related brain injuries. Arch Phys Med Rehabil. 2008;89(10):1983–90.
84. Perrott SB, Taylor HG, Montes JL. Neuropsychological sequelae, familial stress, and environmental adaptation following pediatric head injury. Dev Neuropsychol. 1991;7(1):69–86.
85. Klonoff H, Low MD, Clark C. Head injuries in children: a prospective five year follow- up. J Neurol Neurosurg Psychiatry. 1977;40(12):1211–9.
86. Chadwick O, Rutter M, Shaffer D, Shrout PE. A prospective study of children with head injuries: IV. Specific cognitive deficits. J Clin Neuropsychol. 1981;3(2):101–20.
87. Shaklai S, Peretz R, Spasser R, Simantov M, Groswasser Z. Long-term functional outcome after moderate-to-severe paediatric traumatic brain injury. Brain Inj. 2014;28(7):915–21.

88. Rosenfeld JV, Ford NL. Bomb blast, mild traumatic brain injury and psychiatric morbidity: a review. Injury. 2010;41:437–43.
89. Koskiniemi M, Kyykkä T, Nybo T, Jarho L. Long-term outcome after severe brain injury in preschoolers is worse than expected. Arch Pediatr Adolesc Med. 1995;149(3):249–54.
90. Brink JD, Imbus C, Woo-Sam J. Physical recovery after severe closed head trauma in children and adolescents. J Pediatr. 1980;97(5):721–7.
91. Catroppa C, Anderson V. Traumatic brain injury in childhood: rehabilitation considerations. Dev Neurorehabil. 2009;12(1):53–61.
92. Avesani R, Salvi L, Rigoli G, Gambini MG. Reintegration after severe brain injury: a retrospective study. Brain Inj. 2005;19(11):933–9.
93. Zuccarello M, Facco E, Zampieri P, Zanardi L, Andrioli GC. Severe head injury in children: early prognosis and outcome. Childs Nerv Syst. 1985;1(3):158–62.
94. Kokoska ER, Keller MS, Rallo MC, Weber TR. Characteristics of pediatric cervical spine injuries. J Pediatr Surg. 2001:100–5.
95. Hasler RM, Exadaktylos AK, Bouamra O, Benneker LM, Clancy M, Sieber R, et al. Epidemiology and predictors of spinal injury in adult major trauma patients: European cohort study. Eur Spine J. 2011;20(12):2174–80.
96. Munera F, Rivas LA, Nunez DB, Quencer RM. Imaging evaluation of adult spinal injuries: emphasis on multidetector CT in cervical spine trauma. Radiology. 2012;263(3):645–60.
97. Stephan K, Huber S, Häberle S, Kanz K-G, Bühren V, van Griensven M, et al. Spinal cord injury—incidence, prognosis, and outcome: an analysis of the TraumaRegister DGU. Spine J. 2015;15(9):1994–2001.
98. Shin JI, Lee NJ, Cho SK. Pediatric cervical spine and spinal cord injury: a national database study. Spine (Phila Pa 1976). 2016;41(4):283–92.
99. Omid R, Stone MA, Zalavras CG, Marecek GS. Gunshot wounds to the upper extremity. J Am Acad Orthop Surg. 2019;27(7):e301–10.
100. Shuker ST. The effect of a blast on the mandible and teeth: transverse fractures and their management. Br J Oral Maxillofac Surg. 2008;46(7):547–51.
101. Fausti SA, Wilmington DJ, Gallun FJ, Myers PJ, Henry JA. Auditory and vestibular dysfunction associated with blast-related traumatic brain injury. J Rehabil Res Dev. 2009;46(6):797–810.
102. August P, Coffey MRA, Force O, Gondusky JS, Reiter MP, Infantry M, et al. Protecting military convoys in Iraq : an examination of Battle injuries sustained by a mechanized battalion during operation Iraqi freedom II. Distribution. 2005;38(6):2001.
103. Catchpole MA, Morgan O. Physical health of members of the public who experienced terrorist bombings in London on 07 july 2005. Prehosp Disaster Med. 2010;25(2):139–44.
104. Garner MJ, Brett SJ. Mechanisms of injury by explosive devices. Anesthesiol Clin. 2007;25:147–60.
105. Il CS, Gao SS, Xia A, Wang R, Salles FT, Raphael PD, et al. Mechanisms of hearing loss after blast injury to the ear. PLoS One. 2013;8:7.
106. Muzaffar W, Khan MD, Akbar MK, Malik AM, Durrani OM. Mine blast injuries: ocular and social aspects. Br J Ophthalmol. 2000;84(6):626–30.
107. Alam M, Iqbal M, Khan A, Khan SA. Ocular injuries in blast victims. J Pak Med Assoc. 2012;62(2):138–42.
108. Ari AB. Eye injuries on the battlefields of Iraq and Afghanistan: public health implications. Optometry. 2006;77(7):329–39.
109. Trimble K, Adams S, Adams M. (iv) Anti-personnel mine injuries. Curr Orthop. 2006;20(5):354–60.
110. Gogate P, Gilbert C, Zin A. Severe visual impairment and blindness in infants: causes and opportunities for control. Middle East Afr J Ophthalmol. 2011;18(2):109–14.
111. Kozma P, Kovács I, Benedek G. Normal and abnormal development of visual functions in children. Acta Biol Szeged Acta Biol Szeged. 2001;45(4):23–4223.
112. Dale N, Salt A. Early support developmental journal for children with visual impairment: the case for a new developmental framework for early intervention. Child Care Health Dev. 2007;33(6):684–90.

Physiologic Considerations in Pediatric Population

3

Ahmad Zaghal and Rebecca Andraos

"Children are not little adults"—PRONCZUK-GABRINO J. Children's Health and Environment: A Global Perspective: A Resource Manual For The Health Sector. World health organization. 2005.

3.1 Introduction

The pediatric population: Who are they?

The pediatric population includes all individuals between birth and 18 years of age, divided into:

1. Neonates: birth–1 month.
2. Infants: 1 month–2 years.
3. Young children (preschool): 2 years–6 years.
4. Older children (school): 6 years–12 years.
5. Adolescents: 12–18 years.
6. Some references include toddlers 1–3 years [1].

This subdivision of the pediatric population helps guide the management approach in these different age group categories, as they vary in terms of body size and composition, physiology, and biochemistry. A thorough understanding of the normal growth and development of children provides solid bases for proper evaluation and assessment of this age group. From birth until 2 years of age, neonates and infants grow fast:

A. Zaghal (✉) · R. Andraos
Department of Surgery, American University of Beirut Medical Center, Beirut, Lebanon
e-mail: az22@aub.edu.lb; ra281@aub.edu.lb

© Springer Nature Switzerland AG 2023
G. S. Abu-Sittah, J. J. Hoballah (eds.), *The War Injured Child*,
https://doi.org/10.1007/978-3-031-28613-1_3

1. Body weight doubles by 6 months, and triples by the first year of life.
2. Body surface area (BSA) doubles during the first year.
3. Proportions of body water, fat, and protein continuously change.
4. Major organ systems mature in size as well as function.
5. Pathophysiology and pharmacology are different than that of adults [1].

Being a diverse group, children vary greatly in anatomy and physiology with age, rendering pediatric medical care a bit more complicated as compared to adults.

3.2 Anatomy and Physiology

3.2.1 Developmental Milestones: Step by Step

Children change in several aspects while growing. Obviously, trauma and war injuries are not the ideal contexts for the assessment of developmental milestones; spending time on such assessment is inefficient and takes away crucial minutes from possible lifesaving interventions. However, being roughly familiar with the motor, cognitive, language, and social changes during the different stages of development of children is of great help in approaching and evaluating injured children. Table 3.1 summarizes the developmental milestones from birth until 3 years of age] [2].

Table 3.1 Developmental milestones

	Motor	Fine Motor	Cognitive	Speech/Language	Social/Emotional
0-2 months	Demonstrates rooting and stepping reflex Lies on back Holds head in line with body Moves extremities in a more refined way	Blinks defensively Follows with eyes Sucks	Pays attention to faces Cries when uncomfortable Shows preference to social stimuli Reacts to noises	Makes noises Turns head to sound	social smiles self calming tries to look at parents
2-4 months	Lifts head and chest Pushes feet against hard surface	Reaches out to grasp Holds rattle Sucks in preparation for food	Turns head to source of noise Establish hand eye coordination Reaches for things	Babbles Mimics sounds	Smiles to familiar voices Fixes eyes on familiar faces Reacts to familiar situations Mimics facial expressions
4-6 months	Raises head Rolls over Develops parachute reflex	Develops palmar grasp Brings objects to mouth	Searches for toys Looks around Passes things back and forth	Respond to soundsby sounds Responds to name Expresses emotions by sounds	Recognizes strangers Looks at self in the mirror Laughs out loud
6-9 months	Develops sideward, forward and backward protective reflex Bears weights on feet Stands with support Pulls to stand Crawls Sits alone	Stretches to grasp Develops finger-thumb grasp Grasp spoon when fed Holds, bits and chews Picks up tiny objects Transfers toys from hand to hand	Develops causal connections	Says "dad-dad", "mum-mum"... Shouts Understands "no" and "bye bye" Reacts to "where is mammy/daddy" Imitate vocal sounds	Develops resistance Plays "peek a bro" Offers food Develops strangers anxiety
	Walks arround furniture	Puts objects in and out of box	Shows interest in pictures Starts to use things correctly		
12-18 months	Walks independently Stands Crawls upstairs Kneels Runs	Matures release of objects Develops pineer grasp Holds pencil Scribbles Develops hand preference	Uses toys functionally Obeys simple instructions Shows body parts Develops self identity Imitates	Says first words/single words Understands simple instructions Communicates wishes by pinpointing or vocalizing	Develops functional play Acts out Develops separation anxiety Hugs parents
18 months-2 years	Runs safely squats Jumps Climbs Walks upstairs and downstairs Sits on a tricycle	Scribbles circles Turns pages Uses preferred hand	Follows 2 step instructions Matches squares	Forms 2 word combinations Speaks 50+ words Refers to self by name	Recognizing self and familiar adults
2-3 years	Jump with 2 feet together Throws and kicks balls	Draws a circle and horizontal lines in imitation Holds pencil in preferred hand Cuts with toy scissors	Understands action words Responds to social information Matches colors	Pronounces "I" and "YOU" speaks 200+ words Imitates phrases Asks questions	Makes verbalm commentary during play Has tantrums Becomes active Conducts meaningful play Conducts make belief play

3.2.2 Body Habitus: Size, Shape, and Surface Area

Children and toddlers are by nature smaller than adults, with different body dimensions and ratios; this potentially affects the response to injury and consequences of trauma. Children have lower physiologic reserves, hence they tend to deteriorate rapidly; therefore timely and effective hemodynamic support is lifesaving [3].

Children have relatively smaller body masses, hence, any mechanical insult will transmit into a greater force per unit of the body area, leading to a higher energy impact on a body with fewer tissues than that of an adult [4]. Organs are also closer to each other; even seemingly trivial mechanisms of injury may result in significant multisystem damage [5]. Thereby, it is sensible to expect more severe injuries in infants compared to adults sustaining the same injury.

Body surface area is proportionately larger in the pediatric age group as compared to adults; the smaller the patient, the larger the ratio of skin surface area to body mass. This correlates with the basal metabolic rate (basal metabolic decreases by 1.5–2 times from infancy to adulthood [6]) and minute volume (also proportionately higher in children due to increased respiratory rate [7]), which should be taken into consideration in assessing the oxygenation and ventilation needs, nutrition support, fluid resuscitation, and burn assessment. Based on the above, and in addition to the fact that children have thinner skin and under-keratinized epidermis, children are more severely affected by skin injuries [7]. Children have limited ability to control their core temperature caused by the rapid heat exchange with the environment, hence the utmost importance of controlling the temperature of the resuscitation bay and keeping it warm enough to avoid hypothermia [4].

Children and infants have disproportionately larger heads as compared to adults; this results in passive flexion of the neck when the patients are placed supine on a spine board, which may result in airway obstruction and difficult tracheal intubation. This can be overcome by placing a layer of padding under the patient's chest and abdomen thus compensating for the large head and bringing the neck to a neutral position [4]. Individuals in the pediatric population are generally shorter than adults, which makes them closer to the ground, and more vulnerable to aerosolized substances that are heavier than air. They also have a higher proportion of growing tissues, which are more sensitive to ionizing radiation and some other toxic agents [7].

Infants have incompletely calcified skeletons, with multiple growth plates in development, rendering them pliable and unable to provide protection to the internal organs [4]. The pediatric bone can deform and bend in a plastic way, due to its capacity to absorb energy, which usually causes "greenstick" fractures [8]. This also applies to the infantile skull that is anatomically immature, thin, and incompletely ossified, conferring greater shear stress to the brain structures, and as a result, greater injury [8]. It is very important to realize that the absence of a bone fracture does not rule out an underlying internal organ injury in the pediatric population; this is due to the high degree of flexibility of the bony structures in this age group.

3.2.3   Hemodynamic Considerations

In general, the physiologic impact of the injury might not vary significantly between children and adults, however, the younger the patient, the more differences are likely to be encountered. Physicians looking after children with trauma should not be falsely reassured by the fact that this population has plenty of physiologic reserves, because in this age group the increased metabolic rate mandates a prompt approach to resuscitation, particularly in the younger patients, as they are prone to fast physiologic decompensation [9]. It is important to be familiar with the normal ranges in different age groups in order to accurately assess patients, recognize instability early on, and avoid failure to recognize injuries (Tables 3.2 and 3.3).

3.2.4   Approach to Pediatric Trauma: What Is Different?!

The general approach to pediatric trauma is similar to that for adults namely the "ABCDE" acronym, primary, secondary, and tertiary surveys. The concepts underpinning trauma evaluation and management are essentially the same; however, the numerical values, cutoffs, and interpretations in the pediatric population are different due to differences in anatomy and physiology.

A (Airway) Individuals that fall under the pediatric population have relatively larger occiputs, small oral cavities with large tongues, narrow nasal passages, higher and more anterior larynx with floppy and long epiglottis (at vertebral level C3-C4), narrow airways, along with soft neck and airway tissues, the compressible floor of the mouth and short trachea and neck [10]. These anatomic characteristics alter the techniques and instruments required in airway management, specifically intubation, which can lead to more rapid obstructive airway problems because of edema and/or swelling, and render the airways easy to occlude with manipulation, swelling, and secretions; hence, leading to more difficult incubation and higher rates of accidental extubations. Failure to appreciate the short trachea in this population may also lead to one lung ventilation due to right main bronchus intubation, as well as accidental dislodgment and barotrauma.

B (Breathing) Patients in the pediatric age group have compliant chest walls and airways. Ribs provide little support to the lungs, leading to poor maintenance of negative intra-thoracic pressure, and increased work of breathing [10]. In children, thoracic injuries (such as pulmonary contusions) may occur without rib fractures, this is caused by the high complaint and elastic chest wall. This anatomic arrangement also results in suboptimal protection of the thoracic abdominal organs putting the latter at higher risk for injury even with minimal trauma. In young children, the intercostal muscles are still underdeveloped; thus, the diaphragm bares the work of breathing in inspiration and maintains minute ventilation. Children tend to breathe

Table 3.2 Estimated blood volume (EBV) per age

Age	Estimated Blood Volume
Premature Neomate	90-100 ml/kg
Term Neonate	80-90 ml/kg
3 months-1 year	75-80 ml/kg
3-6 years	70-75 ml/kg
>6 years	65-70 ml/kg

This table is derived from the contents of "SHARMA A, COCKEREL H. Mary Sheridan's From Birth to 5 Years, Children Developmental Progress. Fourth edition: Routledge Taylor Francis Group, London and New York; 2014."

rapidly taking smaller tidal volumes, which makes the diaphragmatic muscle fibers prone to fatigue earlier [11]. These anatomic facts are the reason behind the diaphragmatic breathing pattern in the pediatric population, which can by itself cause respiratory failure with gastric distention, diaphragmatic injury, or simple physiologic diaphragmatic fatigue. Individuals under 18 years of age have a lower functional residual capacity (FRC) and high oxygen consumption; this puts them at higher risk of rapid desaturation, especially after pre-oxygenation and during laryngoscopy time. The low FRC is below the closing capacity, which can lead to small airway closure, atelectasis, ventilation/perfusion imbalance, and hemoglobin desaturation [10]. Physicians and nurses looking after injured children need to be aware of the normal range and variations of the respiratory rate with age, so that not to miss or overrate injuries [7]. Higher respiratory rates in younger children, lead to proportionately higher minute volumes, making these individuals more susceptible to injury with inhaled toxic substances. Securing the airways with proper oxygenation and ventilation has always been a crucial step in trauma assessment and management; and it is even more critical in pediatric patients, given that failure to protect the Airway (A) and Breathing (B) are the most common causes of pediatric cardiac arrest [4].

C (Circulation) Children have higher blood volume per body weight, smaller total circulatory volume, and higher cardiac index, which can lead to rapid exsanguination in case of massive bleeding. Less stroke volume variation in this population gives more significance to tachycardia in response to hypovolemia, and the increased cardiovascular compensation to hypovolemia might delay hypotension as a manifestation of hypovolemia. Securing intravenous (IV) access may be difficult in young children, toddlers, and infants due to their small caliber peripheral vessels; therefore, the use of ultrasound, if available, can be extremely helpful in ensuring

Table 3.3 Normal pediatric physiologic ranges

Age	Guide weight (kg)	RR at rest Breaths per min 5th-95th centile	HR beats per min 5th-95th centile	BP Systolic 5th centile	BP Systolic 50th centile	BP Systolic 95th centile
Birth	3.5	25-50	120-170	65-75	80-90	105
1 month	4.5					
3 months	6.5	25-45	115-160			
6 months	8	20-40	110-160	70-75	85-95	
12 months	9.5					
18 months	11	20-35	100-155	70-80	85-100	110
2 years	12	20-30	100-150			
3 years	14		90-140			
4 years	16		80-135			
5 years	18			80-90	90-110	110-120
6 years	21		80-130			
7 years	23					
8 years	25	15-25	70-120			
9 years	28					
10 years	31					
11 years	35					
12 years	43	12-24	65-115	90-105	100-120	125-140
14 years	50		60-110			
Adult	70					

From "Pediatric Blast Injury Field Manual. The Pediatrics Blast Injury Partnership. 2019. Section 5, p. 27. [https://www.imperial.ac.uk/blast-injury/research/networks/the-paediatric-blast-injury-partnership/] York; 2014"
This table is derived from the contents of "CHIDANANDA SWAMY MN, MALLIKARJUN D. Applied Aspects of Anatomy and Physiology of Relevance to Pediatric Anesthesia. Indian J Anaesth. 2004; 48(5):333–339. [http://medind.nic.in/iad/t04/i5/iadt04i5p333.pdf]"

reliable venous access in a timely fashion. Alternative routes for fluid and medication administration, such as intraosseous access, should always be entertained in cases of failed attempts at obtaining peripheral venous access. Pulse rate and blood pressure also vary with age; it is important to be familiar with the normal ranges in different age groups to avoid missing injuries in children.

The systemic response to blood loss in pediatric patients follows the below pattern:

- In mild volume blood loss (<30%), children will have increased heart rate, with a weak thready peripheral pulse, but normal systolic blood pressure and pulse pressure. Skin will be cool, mottled with a prolonged capillary refill, and urine output will be low to very low. The child can be anxious, irritable, or even confused.
- In moderate volume blood loss (30–45%), children will have a markedly increased heart rate, with a weak thready central pulse, a low normal systolic blood pressure, and a narrowed pulse pressure. The skin will be cyanotic, with mar redly prolonged capillary refill. Minimal urine output and the child will be lethargic with dulled response to pain.
- In severe blood volume loss (>45%), children will suffer from tachycardia followed by bradycardia, with very weak to absent central pulse, hypotension, and narrowed pulse pressure (diastolic blood pressure can be undetectable at times). The child will be pale and cold, comatose, with no urine output [4].

D (Disability) Pediatric patients have a higher propensity to develop hypoglycemia due to low glycogen stores and high metabolic rates. They also have a more permeable blood–brain barrier; hence, hypotonic/hyponatremic fluids may lead to cerebral edema, and hence should be avoided as resuscitation fluid choices [12].

E (Exposure) Patients in the pediatric age group lose heat faster than adults due to a higher surface body area-to-weight ratio, and are therefore more susceptible to hypothermia [12].

3.3   Assessment

Just like in adults, the initial assessment of trauma patients should be systematic and as efficient as possible. Primary and secondary surveys should be completed in minutes. However, tasks in assessing children are generally more complex than in adults.

In normal situations, there are communication barriers and maturity challenges in dealing with children, let alone in a state of trauma and war. It is usually not straightforward to obtain proper history and perform physical examinations on children.

The psychological status of children in trauma plays a key role in their assessment. Children are often emotionally unstable in events of stress, pain, and threatening environments, which provokes regressive psychological behavior, and decreases the child's ability to interact with strangers [4]. If possible, do not separate children from their caregivers, use distracting techniques, especially with those in pain, engage the child whenever it is appropriate, and rely on non-verbal cues such as facial expressions, and body posture. It is hard to establish rapport in situations of mass casualty but would be of great help if feasible. We need to keep in mind that these children are afraid, angry, and anxious, on top of being injured; if we approach them with that perspective in mind, we might be able to achieve a more accurate assessment [12].

3.4 Treatment

3.4.1 Equipment

The tools required during pediatric resuscitation differ from those used in the adult population, especially in terms of size and sometimes shape, to adapt to the pediatric anatomy.

Below are a few notes on major pediatric equipment needed [4].

Airway and breathing:

- O2 masks: secure premie, newborn, and pediatric sizes.
- Oral airways: secure infant, small and medium sizes.
- Bag-valves: secure infant and pediatric sizes.
- Laryngoscopes: secure size 0 straight for premies less than 3 kg of weight, size 1 straight for newborns with weight more than 3.5 kg till the age of 3 years, size 2 straight or curved for ages 4 till 10 years.
- ET tubes: secure sizes 2.5–3.0 non-cuffed (premie with weight less than 3 kg), 3.0–3.5 non-cuffed (age 0–6 months with weight more than 3.5 kg), 3.5–4.0 cuffed or non-cuffed (6–12 months of age), 4.5–5.0 cuffed or non-cuffed (ages 1–3 years), 5.0–5.5 non-cuffed (ages 4–7 years), 5.5–6.5 cuffed (ages 8–10 years).
- Stylets: secure sizes 6 Fr (newborns till the age of 3), 14 Fr (ages 4–10).
- Suction catheters: secure sizes 6–8 Fr (premies <3 kg), 8 Fr (newborn - 6 months of age), 8–10 Fr (ages 6 -12 months), 10 Fr (1–3 years of age), 14 Fr (ages 4–10).

Circulation:

- BP cuffs: secure premie, newborn, infant, and child sizes.

- IV angio-catheters: secure sizes 22–24 Ga (premie <3 kg), 22 Ga (newborns of weight > 3.5 kg till 12 months of age), 20–22 Ga (ages 1–3 years), 20 Ga (ages 4–7 years), 18–20 Ga (ages 8–10 years).

  Supplemental equipment:

- Oro-gastric/Nasogastric tubes: Size 8 Fr (premies <3 kg), 10 Fr (newborn >3.5 kg—6 months of age), 12 Fr (ages 6 months—7 years), 14 Fr (8–10 years).
- Chest tubes: Size 10–14 Fr (premies <3 kg), 12–18 Fr (newborn >3.5 kg—6 months of age), 14–20 Fr (ages 6–12 months), 14–24 Fr (ages 1–3 years), 20–28 Fr (ages 4–7 years), 28–32 Fr (ages 8–10 years).
- Urinary catheters: 5 Fr feeding tube or foley catheter (premies <3 kg), 6 Fr or 5–8 Fr feeding tube or foley catheter (newborn >3.5 kg–6 months of age), 8 Fr (ages 6–12 months), 10 Fr (ages 1–3 years), 10–12 Fr (ages 4–7 years), 12 Fr (ages 8–10 years).
- Cervical collars: small and medium sizes.

Adult equipment should also be available for children older than 10 years of age, or with adult height and weight.

3.4.2 Pediatric Doses and Side Effects

Commercially available length-based resuscitation tapes (such as Breslow) are helpful adjuncts to quickly estimate the weight of children in trauma settings to determine proper dosages of medications, resuscitative fluid volumes, and sizes of equipment [4].

3.4.3 Interventions

Given the nature of pediatric anatomy and physiology, interventions should be conducted with care and attention to the important differences as compared to adults.

In regards to airway management, nasopharyngeal airway placement is difficult in children under 1 year of age due to the small diameter of the nares [13]; this is also not easy in children under 8 years due to the physiologic hypertrophy of the adenoids and tonsils [3]. Caution must be exercised when inserting these devices to avoid bleeding, because of the high vascularity and fragility of the nasal mucosa [5]. In adults, oropharyngeal airways are placed backward and then rotated 180 degrees while advancing into the oropharynx; this practice is not favored in smaller children as it may lead to injury of the soft tissues of the oropharynx [4].

In the past, cuffed ET tubes were avoided in infants and young children due to the risk of pressure-induced tracheal ischemic injury. An effective functional seal is obtained from the functional narrowing of the airway at the subglottic level. Yet, new studies have shown that a low-pressure high-volume ETT is safe and effective in the pediatric population. Cuffed tubes have higher chances of correct placement from the first attempt, deliver better tidal volumes due to less leak during ventilation, and have no increased rate in short-term post-extubation respiratory complications, or long-term adverse events [14]. The size of the cuff in these tubes can be also adjusted by air inflation/deflation, in cases of air leak, decreasing the rate of tube changes and re-intubations in children suffering from inadequate oxygenation or ventilation due to air leaks [2]. In addition to the above, and based on the latest ATLS guidelines (2018), the newly designed cuffed endotracheal tubes are safe and less likely to cause mucosal necrosis as originally thought [4]. Hence, cuffed tubes are now used for young individuals, requiring meticulous attention to size, cuff pressure (<30 mmHg), and exact placement [3]. For laryngoscopes, straight blades are wildly used in infants [5], and curved can only be used for older children.

Surgical cricothyroidotomy is not advised under the age of 12 years because of the potential risk for laryngeal injury [4]; and, needle cricothyroidotomy is more difficult in the pediatric population due to their short cricothyroid membrane [3].

Regarding interventions to improve ventilation, needle thoracotomy should be applied with caution, especially in infants and small children using 14–18 gauge over-the-needle catheters, as longer might cause a pneumothorax rather than resolve it [4]. Needle thoracotomy, when indicated, is a lifesaving procedure, and is not harmful when done properly.

When it comes to the diagnostic adjuncts, getting a child to the CT scan might be more challenging than in adults, as children will more often require sedation to prevent movement during imaging and get reliable results. The utility of FAST is still uncertain in pediatric trauma; it remains debatable due to its low sensitivity and high false-negative rates, hence it should not be used as independent diagnostic imaging for intra-abdominal injuries in the pediatric population [4].

In a few words, the pediatric population is distinct from the adult population in multiple aspects, and extrapolation from adult physiology is not an accurate practice. We need to have a thorough understanding of children's bodies and functions, and how to interpret their signs and symptoms for proper diagnosis and management.

References

1. Lu H, Rosenbaum S. Developmental pharmacokinetics in pediatric populations. J Pediatr Pharmacol Ther. 2014;19(4):262–76. [https://www.ncbi.nlm.nih.gov/pmc/articles/PMC4341411/]
2. Sharma A, Cockerel H. Mary Sheridan's from birth to five years, children developmental progress. 4th ed. London and New York: Routledge Taylor Francis Group; 2014.
3. Samuels M, Wieteska S. Advanced pediatric life support, a practical approach to emergencies. 6th ed. Australia and New Zealand: Wiley Blackwell; 2016.
4. Advanced Trauma Life Support. Student course manual. 10th ed. Chicago: American college of surgeons; 2018.
5. Skinner DV, Driscoll PA. ABC of major trauma. 4th ed. London: Wiley-Blackwell, a John Wiley & Sons Ltd Publication; 2013.

6. Son'kin V, Tambovtseva R. Energy metabolism in children and adolescents. Bioenergetics. 2012;5, 121:–142. https://doi.org/10.5772/31457. [https://www.researchgate.net/publication/221926731_Energy_Metabolism_in_Children_and_Adolescents]
7. Markenson DS. Pediatric prehospital care. 1st ed. New Jersey: Prentice Hall; 2002.
8. Millwood Hargrave JF. The impact of blast injury on children, a literature review. Centre for Blast Injury Studies; 2017.
9. O'neill JA. Advances in the Management of Pediatric Trauma. Am J Surg. 2000:180.
10. Chidananda Swamy MN, Mallikarjun D. Applied aspects of anatomy and physiology of relevance to pediatric anesthesia. Indian J Anaesth. 2004;48(5):333–9. [http://medind.nic.in/iad/t04/i5/iadt04i5p333.pdf]
11. Saikia D, Mahanta B. Cardiovascular and respiratory physiology in children. Indian J Anaesth. 2019;63(9):690–7. [https://www.ncbi.nlm.nih.gov/pmc/articles/PMC6761775/]
12. Pediatric Blast Injury Field Manual. The pediatrics blast injury partnership. 2019. [https://www.imperial.ac.uk/blast-injury/research/networks/the-paediatric-blast-injury-partnership/].
13. Cameron P, Jelnek G, Everitt I, Browne G, Raftos J. Textbook of paediatric emergency medicine. United Kingdom: Churchill Livingstone; 2006.
14. Nagler J. Emergency endotracheal intubation in children [Up-to-date]. 2019. https://www.uptodate.com/contents/emergency-endotracheal-intubation-in-children

Part II

Acute Management

Resuscitation and Critical Care of the Injured Child

4

Ghadi Abou Daher, Nidale Darjani, and Marianne Majdalani

4.1   Introduction

Resuscitation of war-injured children is challenging. It must be accurate and fast paced. Instant information gathering is crucial for performing rapid diagnostic and therapeutic interventions. The health care providers should immediately differentiate between patients who will and will not need immediate intervention.

The initial evaluation and management of a war-injured child follow well-established international guidelines published such as the Pediatric Advanced Life Support by the American Heart Association or the European Resuscitation Council guidelines [1, 2]. It starts with an initial impression that includes the child's appearance, breathing, and color, that only takes a few seconds. It aims to detect children who need immediate intervention. If the child is unresponsive with no breathing or only gasping, the care provider should activate the emergency response and check for a pulse. For pulseless patients, Cardiopulmonary resuscitation (CPR) must be initiated, and the adopted Pediatric Advanced Life Support algorithm followed [1, 2].

In patients with a pulse and breathing, the initial impression is followed by a primary assessment that quickly estimates the patient's physiologic state. It examines the circulation, airway patency, breathing pattern, disability (to evaluate the neurologic function), and exposure where the child is undressed to perform a focused detailed physical exam of the entire body, looking for signs of bleeding, burns, bruises, and injury to the extremities. This is followed by a secondary head-to-toe assessment to look for other potential injuries.

In this chapter, we will be focusing on the initial resuscitation and cardiovascular system of children presenting after a war injury with special consideration for

G. A. Daher · N. Darjani · M. Majdalani (✉)
Department of Pediatrics and Adolescent Medicine, American University of Beirut Medical Center, Beirut, Lebanon

© Springer Nature Switzerland AG 2023
G. S. Abu-Sittah, J. J. Hoballah (eds.), *The War Injured Child*,
https://doi.org/10.1007/978-3-031-28613-1_4

children who are malnourished. One of the common clinical presentations of children will be in a state of shock.

The primary survey's goal is to recognize and manage rather than define the specific etiology of shock [3]. The aim is the improve oxygen delivery and tissue perfusion and prevent progression to cardiac arrest. Children have a greater physiological reserve; hence, early identification of cardiovascular compromise is more challenging than adults [3]. The health care provider must be alert to warning signs like tachycardia, poor peripheral and weakened central pulses, narrow pulse pressure, and decreased level of consciousness early on. Hypotension is usually a late finding. In fact, up to a 30% decrease in circulating blood volume is needed to cause a diminution in a child's systolic blood pressure.

Victims of war injuries are predisposed to three main types of shock: hypovolemic, obstructive, and neurogenic shocks. Before tackling these three types individually, it is crucial to mention some fundamentals in shock management. Shock is a complex state of circulatory dysfunction that results in failure to deliver or use sufficient amounts of oxygen and other nutrients to meet tissue metabolic demands [3]. Rapid identification and intervention in shock are crucial to improving outcomes. If left untreated, shock may progress rapidly to cardiopulmonary arrest leading to death. In order to optimize the oxygen content of the blood, it is advisable to apply a high concentration of oxygen (non-rebreather mask) immediately even if the child is not exhibiting any signs of respiratory distress. In cases where the child is tachypneic, it will allow decreasing the work of breathing, therefore decreasing the oxygen demand. The caring team can as well decrease oxygen demand by addressing pain, anxiety, fever, and infection (e.g., the patient is hemodynamically stable, allowing him or her to remain sitting in the arms of the caregiver).

4.2   Hypovolemic Shock

4.2.1   Definition and Etiology

Hypovolemic shock in a war-injured child might be a hemorrhagic shock secondary to a definite external or internal blood loss (intrathoracic, gastrointestinal, intra-abdominal, major vessel injury, fractures). It can be as well non-hemorrhagic secondary to plasma leak such as in severe burn cases.

On presentation, patients in hypovolemic shock will be tachycardic and tachypneic. Neither tachycardia nor tachypnea can be used as a criterion for diagnosing cardiovascular compromise, as in children both can be exaggerated secondary to pain or anxiety. They must be combined with other parameters [4] (Table 4.1).

Peripheral pulses are usually weak or absent while the central ones might be normal or weak. In fact, central and peripheral pulses should be palpated as a rapid way to detect hypotension before measuring blood pressure. In hypotension, pulses are progressively lost in the wrist or feet, followed by the groin and then the neck. Thus, palpation for the pulses in all these areas is very essential to estimate the degree of hypotension [3].

Table 4.1 Normal vital functions by age group (Adopted from Advanced Trauma Life Support 10th edition)

Age group	Weight range (in kg)	Heart rate (beats/min)	Blood pressure (mm Hg)	Respiratory rate (breaths/min)	Urinary output (ml/kg/hour)
Infant 0–12 months	0–10	<160	>60	<60	2.0
Toddler 1–2 years	10–14	<150	>70	<40	1.5
Preschool 3–5 years	14–18	<140	>75	<35	1.0
School age 6–12 years	18–36	<120	>80	<30	1.0
Adolescent ≥13 years	36–70	<100	>90	<30	0.5

Initially, the blood pressure might be adequate (compensated shock), with narrow pulse pressure. When taking blood pressure, the appropriate size cuff must be used. It must be taken periodically throughout the resuscitation to ensure hemodynamic stability. As a rule, the lower limit of normal systolic blood pressure in children is 70 mmHg +2 × age in years (e.g., for a 4-year-old child the lower limit for systolic BP would be 78 mm Hg).

Additional findings in patients with hypovolemic shock: delayed capillary refill, cool to cold mottled skin, decreased level of consciousness, and oliguria (low normal for infants is 2 ml/kg/h, 1.5 ml/kg/h in the younger child, 1 ml/kg/h in older children, and 0.5 ml/kg/h in adolescents) (Table 4.1).

4.3 Management

4.3.1 Venous Access

Administration of fluids requires the establishment of intravenous access. Options include peripheral intravenous, intraosseous, or central venous access. The preferred route is the peripheral percutaneous one. If access is unsuccessful after two attempts, the intraosseous (IO) route must be considered [3]. IO access consists of inserting a needle into the marrow cavity of a long bone in an uninjured extremity. It is a rapid procedure that requires minimal training. The preferred site is the anteromedial tibia followed by the distal femur. If no special IO needle is available then an 18-gauge needle is used in infants and a 15-gauge in young children.

When the child is older or when the IO equipment is not available a percutaneous central venous catheter can be placed. The femoral vein is the preferred site for central line insertion in an injured child. It can be placed without interfering with ongoing assessment and management. However, if there is suspicion of intra-abdominal injuries, the femoral route is no longer the site of choice. The external jugular vein access is a good option but experienced staff should perform cannulation preferably. It is recommended to avoid the external jugular vein in case of airway compromise or suspicion of any spinal cord injury. A direct venous cutdown done by an experienced physician is the last resort since this procedure is more time consuming [4].

4.3.2   Fluid Resuscitation

Hemorrhagic hypovolemic shock: Healthy children, with intact compensatory mechanisms, can tolerate acute blood losses of 10–15%. Losing acutely, 25% or more of the circulating blood volume frequently results in hypovolemic hemorrhagic shock that requires immediate, aggressive management [3]. Hemorrhagic shock is classified as mild, moderate, or severe according to the estimated amount of blood loss (Table 4.2).

During the primary survey of a hemorrhagic hypovolemic shock, the caring team has to control external bleeding by direct manual pressure and by applying bandages. Also, they will need to splint the pelvis in case of a suspected bleed.

Fluid resuscitation with rapid infusion of isotonic crystalloid (normal saline or Lactated Ringers—LR) in boluses of 20 ml/kg, reaching up to 60 ml/kg over a few minutes. Each bolus is administered over 5–20 min. The patient should be assessed after each bolus. Note that 60 ml/kg of crystalloid fluids are needed to restore 25% of the lost volume [3, 4].

If the child remains hemodynamically unstable after 2–3 boluses of 20 ml/kg, consider 10 ml/kg PRBC transfusion, O negative type, if crossmatched blood is not available. It is recommended to transfuse PRBC in hemorrhagic shock if

Table 4.2   Systemic response to blood loss in pediatric patients (Adopted from Advanced Trauma Life Support 10th edition)

System	Mild blood volume loss <30%	Moderate blood volume loss 30–45%	Severe blood volume loss >45%
Cardiovascular	• Increased heart rate • Weak, thready peripheral pulses • Normal systolic blood pressure • Normal pulse pressures	• Markedly increased heart rate • Weak, thread central pulses • Absent peripheral pulses • Low normal systolic blood pressure • Narrowed pulse pressure	• Tachycardia followed by bradycardia • Very weak or absent central pulses • Absent peripheral pulses • Hypotension • Narrowed pulse pressure
Central nervous system	• Anxious • Irritable • Confused	• Lethargic • Dulled response to pain	• Comatose
Skin	• Cool, mottled: Prolonged capillary refill	• Cyanotic: Markedly prolonged capillary refill	• Pale and cold
Urine output	• Low to very low	• Minimal	• None

hypotension is refractory to crystalloid or if the amount of blood loss is known to be significant. The involvement of a surgeon at this stage is highly recommended for possible ongoing hemorrhage and the need for surgical intervention.

In case of severe hemorrhage, a massive transfusion protocol should be initiated. The patient would receive PRBC, Fresh Frozen Plasma, and platelets in a 1:1:1 ratio [5] 10 ml/kg each.

Vasoactive agents are not routinely indicated in the management of hypovolemic shock. However, in severe cases, fluid refractory hypotension and shock may benefit from a short-term administration of inotrope-like epinephrine (adrenaline) to improve the cardiac contractility, until appropriate fluid resuscitation is achieved [4].

Signs that indicate good response to fluid resuscitation include:

- Slowing of the heart rate.
- Improved peripheral pulses and warmth of extremities.
- Improving systolic blood pressure and urine output.
- Better level of consciousness.

Inserting a urinary catheter for accurate measurement of urine output is highly recommended as it allows for a better assessment of the child's response to fluid resuscitation.

4.3.3 Non-hemorrhagic Shock

Thermal burns, secondary to blast injuries remain one of the major causes of mortality in war-injured kids. Assessment of burn patients consists of identifying the depth and extent of burnt areas using simplified diagrams as illustrated in Fig. 4.1.

Their management follows that of other thermal injuries. First, stop the burning process, remove the clothing, and wash the burnt area with lukewarm water. Examine the extent and depth of the burn.

Resuscitation is done for infants and children with 10% or greater total body surface area (TBSA) partial or full thickness burns and teenagers with 15% or greater TBSA burns. Guidelines are based on two formulas: The Parkland and the modified Brooke. However, it should always be individualized to every patient, with the aim to restore perfusion without causing fluid overload [4].

The Parkland formula is most commonly used and recommends the total administration of 4 ml/kg/%TBSA burn over the first 24 h post-injury. For the first 8 h, the patient would receive one-half of this volume with the remaining volume delivered during the next 16 hours.

The modified Brooke formula recommends 2 ml/kg/%TBSA burn of balanced salt solution over the first 24 h of injury.

Hence, resuscitation strategies in children should consist of the administration of estimated basal fluid requirements in addition to the replacement of fluid losses secondary to burn injury calculated by the above-mentioned formulas.

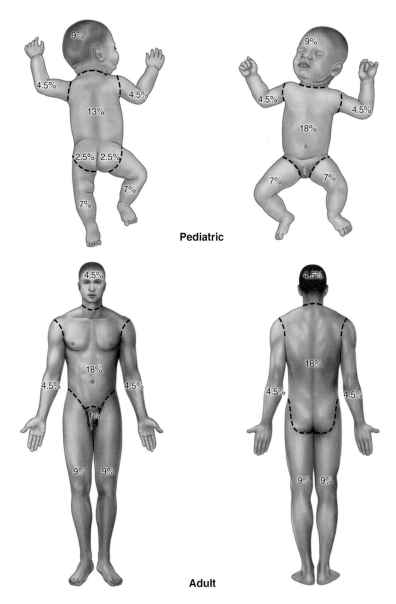

Fig. 4.1 Rule of nines. This practical guide is used to evaluate the severity of burns and determine fluid management. The adult body is generally divided into surface areas of 9% each and/or fractions or multiples of 9% (Adopted from Advanced Trauma Life Support 10th edition)

Very small children (i.e., <30 kg), should receive maintenance fluids of Dextrose 5% Lactated Ringer in addition to the burn resuscitation fluid to avoid hypoglycemia [4].

Colloid use in resuscitation remains controversial. It might be necessary to administer in severe cases due to rapid protein depletion [3].

Fluid infusion must be titrated to avoid under or over-resuscitation. Risks of fluid overload in burn patients include pneumonia, ARDS, bloodstream infection, and compartment syndrome in the extremities and abdomen [3].

Patients with blast injuries are always at risk of sustaining inhalation, blast lung, or chest injury. When these coexist, resuscitation is complicated by conflicting fluid requirements. Thus, fluid infusion in these cases must be tailored to each patient [4].

4.3.4 Additional Considerations

Once the patient is hemodynamically stable, pain control can be achieved with Morphine boluses and continuous infusion if needed, hypoglycemia and hypothermia should be addressed before proceeding to other investigations. Thermoregulation is crucial because hypothermia may affect the central nervous system function, prolong coagulation time and make the child refractory to treatment. Health care providers must always remember to keep the patient covered once the initial survey is done or after any procedure.

If available, laboratory studies can include hemoglobin, blood group, glucose, serum electrolytes, and bleeding profile. X-rays might be needed to rule out fractures and pneumothorax.

If available Point of care ultrasound is a valuable tool to rule out pericardial and pleural effusion as well as abdominal injuries or bleeding.

4.4 Special Population

In war zone areas, malnutrition poses a real threat. For example, a study done in Yemen in 2019 found that 13.3% of all screened children had acute malnutrition [6]. Resuscitation of children with severe acute malnutrition has its own considerations. These patients are at risk of pulmonary edema and cardiogenic shock in case of aggressive fluid resuscitation.

Severe acute malnutrition (SAM) is diagnosed when any of these criteria are met:

• Weight for length/height is less than 3 standard deviation.
• Mid-upper arm circumference is less than 115 millimeters.
• Edema of both feet (Kwashiorkor) or severe wasting (Marasmus).

Oral route rehydration is recommended for patients with SAM not presenting in shock.

For patients with SAM presenting in shock, careful IV resuscitation is done to prevent pulmonary edema and cardiogenic shock. Give fluids 15 ml/kg (LR, or half normal saline plus D5%) over 1 h and re-assess. If hemodynamics of the patient improves and no sign of pulmonary edema, administer a second bolus over 1 h then start oral or nasogastric rehydration with Rehydrating Solution for Malnutrition (oral rehydrating solution with high potassium and low sodium contents) at 10 ml/kg/h up to 10 h. Refeeding can be later started using special formulas if available such as F-100 and F-75 [6]. Close monitoring of temperature and glucose levels should be done, and antibiotics coverage is recommended.

If no improvement after 2 boluses of 15 ml/kg of fluids, start IV maintenance at a rate of 4 ml/kg/h and consider blood transfusion at a rate of 10 ml/kg over 3 h. Then, refeeding with the special formula can be initiated. In case of clinical deterioration, with new signs of cardiogenic shock, stop IV fluids, and consider inotropic support and intubation [7].

4.5   Obstructive Shock

An obstructive shock refers to a condition where blood outflow or return to the heart is physically impaired, despite the normal intravascular volume and cardiac function. The result would be a decrease in cardiac output. The etiologies might be located in the pulmonary or systemic circulation or associated with the heart itself. Examples leading to obstructive shock that are relevant to our topic include pericardial tamponade, tension pneumothorax, or hemothorax.

4.5.1   Cardiac Tamponade

It is an accumulation of fluid, blood, or air in the pericardial space, leading to cardiac compression, reducing ventricular filling, and decreasing the stroke volume and cardiac output. Patients with cardiac tamponade might be in respiratory distress, typically they have muffled or decreased heart sounds and pulsus paradoxus (decrease in systolic blood pressure by more than 10 mmHg during spontaneous inspiration) and distended neck veins. Patients with cardiac tamponade might improve temporarily with fluid resuscitation, to boost the cardiac output. The ultimate treatment is drainage via pericardiocentesis [4].

4.5.2   Tension Pneumothorax or Hemothorax

It is the entry and accumulation of air or blood in the pleural space under pressure. An ongoing leak will create tension. As the pressure increases, it compresses the lung and pushes the mediastinum to the other side of the chest. The high intrathoracic pressure and the compression of vital mediastinal organs obstruct the venous return, ensuing in a rapid decline in cardiac output [4].

It is important to keep tension pneumothorax or hemothorax on the differential. Missing it on the physical exam can lead to unnecessary periods of hypotension and shock that might be life threatening. The physician should look for decreased breath sounds on one side. If highly suspected, inserting a large bore IV cannula with an attached syringe into the second intercostal space in the mid-clavicular line on the side of the pneumothorax will allow for immediate relief and improvement in the child's hemodynamics. This is to be followed by chest tube insertion inserted in the mid-axillary line in the fifth intercostal space.

The diagnosis is clinical in a hemodynamically unstable child and should not be delayed awaiting a chest X-Ray. In a hemodynamically stable (no hypoxia, no respiratory distress, no hypotension) child, however, consider getting an early chest X-Ray as this will prevent the insertion of a potentially unnecessary chest tube and subject the child to a painful procedure.

4.6   Neurogenic Shock: Spinal Cord Injury

Spinal cord injury evaluation in children remains a challenge for any physician; this is due to the differences from adults and the inability of the child to communicate well. The cervical spine is the most vulnerable to injury. Children are at higher risk to sustain spinal cord injury without radiographic abnormalities (SCIWORA). Thus, when there is a high suspicion of a severe cervical spine or spinal cord injury, always immobilize the head and neck, even if X-rays are negative until proper consultation and imaging are done.

Neurogenic shock refers to hypotension usually accompanied by bradycardia secondary to the injury to the autonomic pathways in the spinal cord. The injured areas are usually in the cervical or upper thoracic spinal cord, rarely below T6. This condition leads to loss of vasomotor tone (causing vasodilation and pooling of blood in visceral and lower extremity vessels thus hypotension) and it also causes loss of sympathetic innervation to the heart resulting in bradycardia.

Hypotension secondary to spinal cord injury might not respond to fluid infusion. Vasopressors should be started after moderate volume replacement. Hemodynamically significant bradycardia can be counteracted by atropine or external pacing [3].

4.7   In Summary (Fig. 4.2)

1. If the child is unresponsive or gasping during the initial impression, activate emergency response and check pulse. For pulseless patients start CPR and follow the adopted Pediatric Advanced Life Support Algorithm.
2. If hemodynamically stable, with good urine output and blood pressure, start IV fluids at maintenance rate and admit for further management.
3. If hemodynamically unstable, start IV fluid boluses of isotonic fluid (Normal saline or Lactated Ringers) at 20 ml/kg over 5–20 min. If after three boluses the patient remains hemodynamically unstable, proceed with PRBC transfusion.

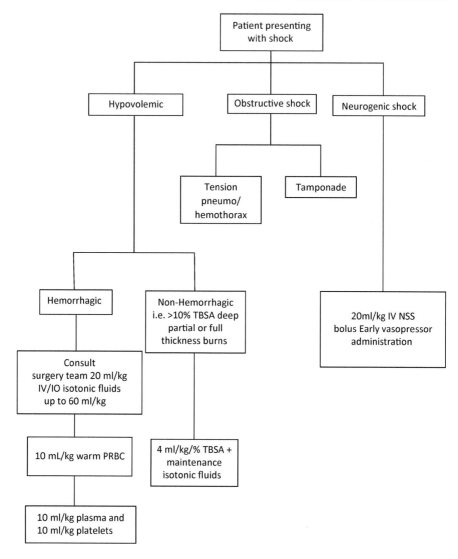

Fig. 4.2 Management algorithm for the pediatric patient presenting in shock in post-war injury

4. If ongoing, blood loss or if hemodynamically unstable, activate massive transfusion protocol and consider early surgery.
5. Titrate to each patient's response (urine output and blood pressure), and avoid under or over-resuscitation.
6. Consider potential inhalation injury with thermal injuries. Consult specialists and consider transfer to specialized centers, if the patient is hemodynamically stable.
7. Immediate needle decompression in case of pneumothorax and pericardiocentesis in case of cardiac tamponade.

References

1. American Heart Association. Pediatric advanced life support. Dallas, TX; 2016.
2. European resuscitation council guidelines for resuscitation 2015Section 6. Paediatric life support. Resuscitation. 2015;95:223–48.
3. Fuhrman BP, Zimmerman JJ (2016) *Pediatric Critical Care Fifth edition.*
4. American College of Surgeons. Advanced trauma life support: student course manual. 10th ed. Chicago, IL; 2018.
5. Spinella PC, Holcomb JB. Resuscitation and transfusion principles for traumatic hemorrhagic shock. Blood Rev. 2009;23(6):231–40. https://doi.org/10.1016/j.blre.2009.07.003.
6. Dureab F, Al-Falahi E, Ismail O, Al-Marhali L, Al Jawaldeh AA, Nuri NN, Safary E, Jahn A. An overview on acute malnutrition and food insecurity among children during the conflict in Yemen. Children. 2019;6:77. https://doi.org/10.3390/children6060077.
7. World Health Organization. Pocket book of hospital care for children: guidelines for the management of common childhood illnesses. Geneva, Switzerland; 2013.

Nursing Management for War Injured Child

5

Nour Nahhas

5.1   Introduction

In times of war, children represent a substantial section of traumatic injuries that come upon in a modern war zone; where many of them are severely injured [1]. In a study done in a conflict zone in Rawanda Chad, where there was the French army, the language was a big barrier between health care workers and native people [1].

Pediatric victims affected by blast injuries constitute an extremely large resource burden on operative workload and the health care system during wars [2]. Refining the consequences of the injured child necessitate individualized approaches since childhood injuries are foreseen as a significant public health issue [3]. Therefore, it is highly important to have a well-prepared health care sector in such environments in order to take care of the vulnerable population [1].

Since the pediatric population are the most commonly encountered casualties in field hospitals during war periods, resuscitating these patients require the presence of pediatric intensivist and nurses with pediatric training [1]. Pediatric nurses often work in a team of pediatric health care professionals [1]. Pediatric nurses are considered very knowledgeable about children's milestones. They know how to interact and care for children with different developmental levels. In addition, they know the importance of engaging parents in the plan of care for the child [2].

N. Nahhas (✉)
Division of Plastic and Reconstructive Surgery, Department of Surgery, American University of Beirut Medical Center, Beirut, Lebanon

© Springer Nature Switzerland AG 2023

G. S. Abu-Sittah, J. J. Hoballah (eds.), *The War Injured Child*,
https://doi.org/10.1007/978-3-031-28613-1_5

5.2   Triage in War Zones

Triage in nursing is very crucial in the management of casualties during wartime or in natural disasters. It is the ethics of doing "the greatest good for the greatest number" [4].

Triage is referred to when the medical care system is burdened. It allows health care workers to have a rational utilization of assets in order to cover a greater number of patients [4]. Many difficulties usually arise when doing triage. In a study done in Rwanda in Chad a conflict zone where the French army was there, it was found that language was a barrier where health care workers were of different nationalities and could not communicate well with patients [4]. As for triage with children, it was even harder, because it is more difficult to communicate with young children, or terrified ones especially if they are without their parents [4].

On battlefields, nurses and physicians usually do triage and the priority of treatment is given to head wounds because craniocerebral injuries are considered the most severe and life-threatening [4]. If children and adults present with similar injuries, children are treated first [5]. Studies show that there is a huge lack of knowledge and responsiveness between nurses and physicians regarding emergency and disaster preparedness plans during war times [6].

Triage in pediatric emergencies is an important means to prioritize critically ill children [5]. It is a method to identify patients who are not in need of urgent care [5]. In a quick assessment of 30–60 seconds, a triage nurse will be able to identify the patient's illness severity, by collecting sufficient information and taking vital signs measures. A triage nurse will also make sure that all pediatric patients are triaged within 10 min of their arrival at the emergency department [5].

The 5-level triage system and nurse-initiated emergency care pathways have been shown to be an approach that facilitates the delivery of care and reduces the risks of mortality in the emergency department [7]. In addition, the Pediatric Emergency Triage, Assessment, and Treatment (ETAT) has been published in 2005 by the World Health Organization (WHO) which includes guidelines and training materials for nurses to do appropriate triage, especially in mass gatherings [6]. Therefore, it is evident that emergency medical services, trauma systems, and disaster response systems should include a pediatric trauma system for it to be successful at local, regional, and national levels [3]. These systems allow for prompt communication, earlier recognition of critical injuries, and continuing education for trauma and emergency care providers [6].

5.3   Emergency Signs in Pediatric Patients

– Obstructed or absent breathing.
– Severe respiratory distress.
– Central cyanosis.
– Signs of shock (defined as cold extremities with capillary refill time > 3 s and weak, fast pulse).

- Coma (or seriously reduced level of consciousness).
- Seizures.
- Signs of severe dehydration in a child with diarrhea with any two of the following signs: lethargy or unconsciousness, sunken eyes, and very slow return of skin after pinching [8].

"Children are not little adults" as per Suzan Hoover in her study about Understanding and managing pediatric trauma [9]. The assessment and management of pediatric victims are different from that of adults because of the anatomical, physiological, and psychological differences between the two [10]. The force of an impact on the child spread widely through the body, resulting in multisystem injuries in almost 50% of children with serious trauma [10]. Therefore, it is important for health care workers especially nurses, to understand the differences in the anatomy and physiology of pediatric patients in order to be able to provide them with optimal care [9].

5.4 Primary and Secondary Assessments

Pediatric nurses in war zones should perform **primary** and **secondary** assessments after the triage.

5.4.1 Primary Assessment

In primary assessment and resuscitation ABCDE should be initiated and followed by nurses and physicians preferably by Pediatric intensivists and pediatric-trained emergency nurses [9].

Primary Assessment: **A** = Airway and cervical spine stabilization; **B** = Breathing; **C** = Circulation; **D** = Disability (Brief Neurological Exam), **E** = Exposure.

- A = Airway and cervical spine stabilization: It is important to maintain a patent airway by intubating and ventilating the patient while ensuring an appropriate alignment of the cervical spine. Nurses should pay attention to tube placement during their post-intubation assessment and should monitor for chest breathing symmetry, and equal bilateral breath sounds. Nurses should directly notify the physician if any tube displacement is suspected [8].
- B=Breathing: In children, it is hard to detect chest wall injuries, so assessing and looking for the breathing pattern of the child is very important. Respiratory rate, chest wall depth evaluation, and auscultation should be performed by nurses upon arrival to the ED. The chest wall of the child should be inspected for symmetry, movement, and expansion. Nurses should pay attention to oxygen saturation if <90% to prepare oxygen supply for immediate use. Oxygen therapy should be given to all war injured children via a facemask or a nasal cannula in order to prevent any rapid deterioration.

- C=Circulation: The heart rate should be assessed by auscultating apical heart rate or Brachial pulses. Tissue perfusion and any signs of bleeding should be assessed for as well. Blood pressure and capillary refill of less than 3 seconds should be checked immediately. Cyanosis or pallor are all signs of hemmorrhage. It is reported that tourniquet use, tranexamic acid administration, and balanced blood transfusion suggest a benefit to the pediatric population [11].
- D = Disability (Brief neurological exam): Level of consciousness should be assessed by doing a brief neurological assessment, in addition to pupillary assessment.
- The pediatric nurse should monitor the neurological status of the patient every 2–4 h. Any alteration in the level of consciousness indicates decreased oxygenation and perfusion, or possible head injury. If a child is suspected to have increased intracranial pressure (ICP) he/she should be intubated and oxygenated at 100%. Signs of increased ICP in the child include severe headache, emesis, irritability, rapidly deteriorating mental status, abnormal posturing, neurological deficits, pupillary abnormalities, and seizures. Infants can also demonstrate bulging fontanels and split sutures.
- E = Exposure: Pediatric nurses are required to do a rapid full inspection and thorough assessment of the body for injuries, such as bruising, bleeding, and abrasions. By following this the nurse will help reduce the chance of lowering the child's temperature. Hypothermia is very common in pediatric patients because of the increased heat loss from their larger body surface area, and trauma can also increase susceptibility to hypothermia. The pediatric patient should be covered as much as possible, exposing only needed body surface areas during any assessment or procedure. To prevent hypothermia, all wet clothing or sheets should be removed, and a warming blanket, and/or a radiant heat source can be used. Active warming may be initiated by using warmed IV fluids and blood to increase the core temperature.

5.4.2 Secondary Assessment

F = Full set of vital signs; **G** = Giving comfort (assessing pain using the age-appropriate pain scale); **H** = Head-to-toe assessment; **I** = Inspection of posterior body.

F = Full set of vital signs: Continuous and frequent readings of vital signs are required until the child is fully stable and the frequency of measuring the vital signs is dependent on the child's condition and the severity of the injury.

G = Giving comfort: Pain assessment is a fundamental aspect of stabilizing a child's condition. Providing comfort by administering adequate painkillers and managing pain speeds up the improvement process of the child's injury. Pain in children is measured using specific pain assessment scales as reporting pain is not as easy as in adults. In Children the most commonly used pain assessment scale is the FLACC scale which is based on observing the behavior of the child, Face, legs, Activity, Cry, and Consolability. This scale is used for children less than 3 years of age. Whereas, the **Wong-baker faces** scale is based on using the drawn faces, where the child chooses the face that describes his pain level, either a smiley face or a sad face. This scale can be used for children more than 3 years of age. As for children more than 9 years of age, the numeric scale is used to determine their level of pain from 0 to 10.

H = Head-to-toe assessment: Nurses should do a head-to-toe assessment in the secondary assessment and obtain a more detailed history after stabilizing the child. They should look for any signs of deterioration, and gather the information that they might have missed during the primary assessment. The head-to-toe assessment of the child includes inspection, auscultation, and palpation.

- Head, face, and neck: The head and face should be inspected for lacerations, depressions, or foreign bodies, and palpated for pain and tenderness. The ears should be checked for bleeding or cerebral spinal fluid leakage. The pupillary reaction should be assessed. The nose should be assessed for any displacement, blood, and cerebral spinal fluid. The neck should be assessed for lacerations, swelling, deformities, and jugular vein distention. The tracheal position should be inspected for any deviations from the midline, and the larynx should be palpated to rule out a fracture. A hoarse voice or cough may be a sign of laryngeal edema and should be taken into consideration if noted.
- Chest: Chest wall movement and expansion should be inspected for symmetry, and assessed for pain during respiration. Retractions or nasal flaring are signs of respiratory distress. The pediatric nurse should inspect the chest for wounds.
- Abdomen: Repeated assessments of the abdomen are highly important since abdominal injuries are usually hard to detect. The nurse should inspect the abdomen for distention, bruising, and lacerations. The abdomen also should be checked for tenderness and pain. In addition to measuring the abdominal girth as a baseline check mark for any abdominal distension.
- Pelvis and Genitourinary: Nurses should inspect the pelvis for any bruising, lacerations, or blood, as well as they should palpate the bony prominences for pain and instability, which may indicate any fracture. A flaccid rectal sphincter may indicate also spinal cord trauma. A urine test should be collected from all trauma children.
- Extremities and Neurological: Nurses should inspect and palpate all extremities for pain, tenderness, deformities, or any signs of soft tissue damage. Pediatric nurses should also evaluate the child's neurological status by examining child's ability to move fingers and toes, the strength of bilateral hand grasps and foot flexion.

The severity of any head injury should be also determined by using the Glasgow Coma Scale which includes an assessment of the motor power, sensory perception, and cranial nerves.

All pediatric patients can compensate and pick up quickly when they are treated properly, yet they can easily deteriorate if they are not well monitored leading to a life-threatening event.

I = Inspection of the posterior body: Inspect for wounds, deformities, discolorations, etc.

5.5   Nursing Assessment and Management

5.5.1   Musculoskeletal Trauma

Nurses should inspect and palpate the extremities for bleeding, deformity, crepitus, circulation, sensory, and motor function. Signs and symptoms of musculoskeletal injury also include swelling, pain, bruising, rigidity, and decreased use of the affected extremity. Nurses should also monitor any indications of a neurovascular compromise. Emergency management of fractures involves assessing damage, avoiding further injury, and providing comfort. Immobilization of the fracture is needed, and realignment may be required. Realignment of the fracture can be either done with closed reduction or open reduction. Splinting, casting, and traction may be performed.

5.5.2   Cardiothoracic Trauma

Identifying a cardiothoracic injury in a child may be difficult since there are no evident visual signs of injury. Thus, 1-to-1 monitoring and assessment by the nurse of the respiratory and cardiac systems of these patients is very crucial. Oxygen saturation assessment, pain management, and restricted fluids are to be followed in blunt traumas. Sometimes, the use of diuretics, intubation, and mechanical ventilation may be essential for severe pulmonary contusions. Treatment of traumatic asphyxia, pneumothorax, and hemothorax may also require oxygen therapy, thoracentesis, chest tubes, mechanical ventilation, restricted fluids, and management of intracranial pressure. Ruptured diaphragm and ventricular or aortic ruptures require surgical repair. Cardiac tamponade is treated with needle aspiration.

5.5.3   Abdominal Trauma

Abdominal traumas in pediatric patients can be fatal and most of the time they are unrecognized. Nurses should look for signs and symptoms of abdominal trauma which include an increase in the abdominal girth, distension/rigidity, pain and tenderness, abnormal bowel sounds, bruising, ecchymosis, abdominal mass, nausea, vomiting, abnormal vital signs, and abdominal pallor/mottling. An X-ray or diagnostic imagining may also show free air in the abdomen or areas of bleeding. The treatment of abdominal trauma is usually dependent on the location and the severity of the injury. Medical management may include insertion of a nasogastric tube, keeping the child NPO, bedridden, fluid management, and total parenteral nutrition. Blood transfusions may also be needed if the child has bleeding or is hemodynamically unstable. Surgical intervention may be required for liver, spleen, pancreatic lacerations, or intestinal perforations.

5.5.4 Traumatic Brain Injury (TBI)

Nurses should look for any clear or pink-tinged CSF leak from the nose and ears of the child as this may indicate a basilar skull fracture. Nurses should also look for any bruising around the ears and the eyes. Nurses also assess the level of consciousness of the child, and they should look for any signs of lethargy, nausea, pallor, diaphoresis, headaches, dizziness, disorientation, and amnesia as all of these indicate TBI [11]. Whereas, loss of consciousness, seizures, bulging fontanels (infants), hypoxia, changes in vital signs (particularly hypertension and bradycardia), vomiting, posturing, changes in pupil size/responsiveness, and apnea are late signs of TBI. Treatment of TBI in children is targeted toward preventing complications, promoting healing, and managing pain. Insertion of drains such as ventricolostomy or VP ventricoperitoneal shunt, medical management of symptoms (including medications for reducing ICP), fluid management, and/or surgical interventions are sometimes required depending on the severity of the TBI [12].

5.5.5 Spinal Cord Trauma

Early detection of spinal cord injury is usually hard to diagnose in children. Signs and symptoms that are associated with spinal cord trauma are abnormal neurological exam, limited mobility of the neck or spine, tenderness, or hypotension. Other signs may include edema, ecchymosis, observable deformity, and muscle spasms. Nurses should be able to identify early signs of spinal cord injury in order to prevent further injuries [13]. Injuries of the spinal cord could be managed by applying skin traction, stabilization and fluid balance. Further medical management of the secondary effects such as neurogenic shock are also potential additional treatments of spinal cord injury. Surgical intervention may be required for decompression, fractures, and dislocations.

5.6 Age-Specific Consideration in Medication Administration

Administering medications to infants and young children requires extra caution. Few studies are conducted on drug safety in children. Pediatric patients are at increased risk for adverse drug events, because of their larger body surface area and immature body systems [14]. Mathematical calculations are often required in preparing pediatric dosages, which also increases the risk of error [11]. In the pediatric population, calculation errors account for 60% of medication errors involving pediatric patients, and almost 70% of medication errors reported involved pediatric patients [12]. Medication errors are three times more common among pediatric patients as compared with adult patients and have 10 times the potential for harm [15].

References

1. Pannell D, Poynter J, Wales P, Tien H, Nathens A, Shellington D. Factors affecting mortality of pediatric trauma patients encountered in Kandahar, Afghanistan. Can J Surg. 2015;58(3):S141–5. https://doi.org/10.1503/cjs.017414.
2. Milwood Hargrave J, Pearce P, Mayhew E, Bull A, Taylor S. Blast injuries in children: a mixed-methods narrative review. BMJ Paediatr Open. 2019;3(1):e000452.
3. Management of Pediatric Trauma. Pediatrics. 2016;138(2):e20161569. https://doi.org/10.1542/peds.2016-1569.
4. Rigal S, Pons F. Triage of mass casualties in war conditions: realities and lessons learned. Int Orthop. 2013;37(8):1433–8. https://doi.org/10.1007/s00264-013-1961-y.
5. van Veen M, Moll H. Reliability and validity of triage systems in paediatric emergency care. Scand J Trauma Resusc Emerg Med. 2009;17(1):38. https://doi.org/10.1186/1757-7241-17-38.
6. Farrag S, ALShmemri M, Rajab O. Pediatric nursing triage in mass gathering: education and training issues. Am J Biomed Sci Res. 2019;5(3):190–6. https://doi.org/10.34297/ajbsr.2019.05.000908.
7. Barata I, Brown K, Fitzmaurice L, Griffin E, Snow S. Best practices for improving flow and care of pediatric patients in the emergency department. Pediatrics. 2014;135(1):e273–83. https://doi.org/10.1542/peds.2014-3425.
8. Paediatric emergency triage, assessment and treatment: care of critically-ill children. 2020. Retrieved 7 May 2020, from https://www.who.int/maternal_child_adolescent/documents/paediatric-emergency-triage-update/en/
9. 2020. Retrieved 7 May 2020, from https://lms.rn.com/getpdf.php/1975.pdf
10. McFadyen J, Ramaiah R, Bhananker S. Initial assessment and management of pediatric trauma patients. Int J Crit Illn Inj Sci. 2012;2(3):121. https://doi.org/10.4103/2229-5151.100888.
11. 2020. Retrieved 7 May 2020, from https://lms.rn.com/getpdf.php/587.pdf
12. Tume LN. The nursing management of children with severe traumatic brain injury and raised ICP. Br J Neurosci Nurs. 2007;3(10):461–7. https://doi.org/10.12968/bjnn.2007.3.10.27273.
13. Oyesanya T, Snedden T. Pediatric nurses' perceived knowledge and beliefs of evidence-based practice in the care of children and adolescents with moderate-to-severe traumatic brain injury. J Spec Pediatr Nurs. 2018;23(2):e12209. https://doi.org/10.1111/jspn.12209.
14. Betancourt T, Meyers-Ohki S, Charrow A, Tol W. Interventions for children affected by war. Harv Rev Psychiatry. 2013;21(2):70–91. https://doi.org/10.1097/hrp.0b013e318283bf8f.
15. Arul G, Reynolds J, DiRusso S, Scott A, Bree S, Templeton P, Midwinter M. Paediatric admissions to the British military hospital at Camp Bastion, Afghanistan. Ann R Coll Surg Engl. 2012;94(1):52–7. https://doi.org/10.1308/003588412x13171221499027.

Airway Management in the War-Injured Child

6

Wissam Maroun and Roland Kaddoum

6.1 Introduction

War injuries in pediatric patients can lead to acute open or closed orofacial trauma, decreased level of consciousness, pneumothorax, hemothorax, airway obstruction, and pulmonary contusions, all of which require prompt airway management. In addition, airway compromise secondary to inadequate airway management is one of the main reasons for early death in pediatric trauma [1, 2], hence the importance of proper airway management.

Compared to airway management in the adult, regular airway management in the pediatric population presents challenges of its own due to different anatomy and physiology. When dealing with the pediatric population with war injuries, additional challenges arise. Considering the airway to be intact, regular trauma precautions and rapid sequence intubation should be considered. In addition, if there is orofacial trauma or airway obstruction, which is quite common in war injury, additional precautions and techniques should be used to secure the airway in these children. Hence, it is pivotal to understand that there are multiple layers of complexity while dealing with airway management in the war-injured pediatric population. The first layer consists of the challenges presented by the regular pediatric anatomy, the second layer consists of the airway considerations for any pediatric emergent case, and the third layer which requires advanced techniques and a lot of expertise consists of dealing with patients that have sustained orofacial or airway trauma. In this chapter, we will explore the various challenges mentioned earlier, in addition to describing basic and advanced techniques to manage the difficult airway of war-injured pediatric patients.

W. Maroun · R. Kaddoum (✉)
Department of Anesthesiology, American University of Beirut Medical Center, Beirut, Lebanon
e-mail: rk16@aub.edu.lb

© Springer Nature Switzerland AG 2023
G. S. Abu-Sittah, J. J. Hoballah (eds.), *The War Injured Child*,
https://doi.org/10.1007/978-3-031-28613-1_6

6.2 Anatomical and Physiological Considerations

6.2.1 Airway Anatomy

The pediatric airway differs significantly from the adult airway impacting airway management. These differences and difficulty in airway management are more pronounced at birth: the most challenging airway is seen in neonates and infants below 1 year of age, as evidenced by suboptimal views during direct laryngoscopy in this age group [3].

The head of pediatric patients is larger relative to body size, along with a more prominent occiput. These anatomical changes become relevant during positioning before intubation, as the neck becomes flexed on a flat surface, leading to airway obstruction in asleep children. Other than neck flexion, multiple other factors lead to airway obstruction and difficult ventilation in children, these include: a large tongue, shorter mandible, frequently prominent adenoids, and tonsils. Therefore, a shoulder roll is required to achieve a neutral position and open up the airway [4]. In addition, calcification of the trachea and larynx does not occur before the teenage years [5]; this flexibility of the tracheal rings can predispose to airway obstruction with negative pressure ventilation or when a partial obstruction already exists [6, 7]. Other than airway obstruction, the larger occiput combined with the shorter neck makes direct laryngoscopy more difficult by preventing proper alignment of the oral, laryngeal, and tracheal axes [8].

In children, the larynx is relatively higher in the neck; the cricoid ring is located at the level of C4 at birth, C5 at age 6 years, and C6 in adults [6]. In addition, the vocal cords are angled in an anterior-inferior to posterior-superior fashion relative to the trachea and are not found at a right angle relative to the trachea [8]. These anatomical differences do not make direct laryngoscopy views suboptimal, however, they make endotracheal tube insertion more difficult and more traumatic; the endotracheal tube has a higher chance to get stuck on the anterior commissure of the vocal cords [4]. Also, in children the epiglottis is "U" shaped, described as omega-shaped, and may lie across the glottis opening [6], hence the use of a straight blade is preferred over the use of a curved blade during regular direct laryngoscopy. Multiple other anatomical differences not mentioned here also complicate airway management in the pediatric population. The point remains simple, because of the airway anatomical differences compared with the adult patient, the pediatric patient by default is problematic when it comes to airway management.

6.2.2 Physiological Considerations

The pediatric patient has also physiological considerations that predispose him/her to hypoxemia as compared to the adult patient. It has been reported that oxygen consumption in children is higher relatively than in adults [7], in addition to lower functional residual capacity in children, this can lead to rapid desaturation during apnea time even with proper preoxygenation [4]. Also, the rate of CO_2 production is increased in children, hence the higher resting respiratory rate in children to achieve higher minute ventilation to eliminate the excess CO_2 [9]. Therefore, during apnea time children are also more prone to CO_2 retention. In addition, the already small pediatric airway could have drastic consequences on respiratory function. The resistance to flow in the airway is governed by Poiseulle's law which states that the resistance to flow is inversely related to the radius of the airway raised to the fourth power. This being said, any narrowing of the airway (hematoma, or airway edema during trauma) would have drastic consequences on airway resistance to flow [4].

6.3   Considerations in the Emergent Airway Management

Airway management in war-injured children should be treated by default like any emergent airway, in addition to the specific considerations that we will elaborate on later in this chapter. It is needless to say that the basic requirements for any airway management case should be ideally present; this includes appropriate and adequate: sized suction catheter and apparatus, oxygen supply, oxygen delivery device, sized airway equipment (nasopharyngeal airways, oral airways, laryngoscope blades [which have been checked, light working], endotracheal tubes, laryngeal mask airways, and bag-valve-mask), medications (sedatives, reversal agents, resuscitation medications), and standard ASA monitoring (pulse oximeter, blood pressure cuffs, ECG, end-tidal CO_2). We will focus in this section on describing briefly the concerns related to emergent airway management in pediatric patients.

6.3.1   Rapid Sequence Intubation

Regardless of the indications for airway management, the goal of intubation is to place an artificial airway in the most effective manner possible. Rapid sequence intubation (RSI) is defined as the simultaneous administration of a sedative agent (the choice of sedative agent is beyond the scope of this discussion, but usually a sedative agent and a paralytic agent are used) for emergent intubation [10]. For pediatric emergent airway management, RSI has been associated with higher success rates at the first attempt and lower rates of adverse events as compared to intubation without medications or with sedatives without paralyzing agents [10]. Hence, it is necessary to consider RSI implying the use of sedative agents and paralytic agents during emergent intubation in the pediatric population. It is important to note that sedatives and paralytic agents use improves the success rate of intubation.

6.3.2   Preoxygenation

Before intubation attempts are made, all pediatric patients should be preoxygenated by the delivery of high-flow 100% oxygen. Due to the physiological concerns explained previously and the apnea created by the use of paralytic agents used in

RSI, without preoxygenation nearly one-third of the patients will have desaturation episodes to less than 90% [11]. Preoxygenation is usually done with 100% oxygen for about 3 min via either a nasal cannula [12] or bag-valve mask or non-rebreather mask, all of which can decrease the chance of rapid desaturation during RSI [13]. Also, apneic oxygenation in a child has been shown to decrease the incidence of hypoxemia during RSI [14]. As a consequence of what has been stated earlier, pre-oxygenation has been shown to be a crucial step in airway management in RSI for trauma patients and hence war-injured pediatric patients.

6.4   The Difficult Airway

As stated previously, airway management in trauma cases starts with preoxygen-ation, followed by endotracheal intubation to secure the airway. War-injured chil-dren may present with neck and face burns, or orofacial trauma. These conditions may lead to distorted anatomy and hence pose a scenario of difficult intubation and sometimes difficult ventilation [15, 16]. These conditions usually require advanced airway techniques and sometimes surgical interventions [15, 16]. For reasons stated before, children with difficult direct laryngoscopy are an especially vulnerable group; multiple guidelines and algorithms describe the management of the unex-pected and expected difficult pediatric airway [17–20]. The main point that one must keep in mind is that if direct laryngoscopy is unsuccessful, ventilation and oxygenation should be established. There are multiple tools and devices that help establish airway access or ventilation, to the point of surgical airway management [17–20]. In the case of a war-injured child with extensive burn injuries or maxillo-facial trauma, this can pose a scenario of difficult intubation and difficult ventila-tion, hence we will proceed to describe techniques that help the anesthesiologist ventilate the patient.

6.4.1   Mask Ventilation

When dealing with a spontaneously breathing patient, one must consider whether to maintain spontaneous ventilation or induce with the use of muscle relaxants during intubation. In the case of the suspected difficult airway (precisely suspected difficult mask ventilation), as is often the case with war-injured children, it is reasonable to either confirm the ability to mask ventilate prior to giving medication that induces apnea or maintain spontaneous ventilation throughout intubation [20]. For patients with maxillofacial trauma, mask ventilation could be difficult because of the dis-torted anatomy, or the airway could be blocked by bleeding: the face mask could not necessarily be fitted to the face for effective ventilation and if there is airway injury this could prevent efficient air transfer from the mask to the lungs [15]. It is, there-fore, crucial to expect that mask ventilation could be problematic in war-injured children and prepare to either preserve spontaneous ventilation during intubation or use devices and techniques to ventilate the patient when mask ventilation fails.

6.4.2   Supraglottic Airway Devices (SGA)

The use of a supraglottic airway device (such as the laryngeal mask airway [LMA]) is an important step in many airway management algorithms [20–22]. A SGA can be used where difficult ventilation, failed intubation, or both occur. In addition, the failure rate of the SGA in the pediatric population is 0.86% [23] which is lower than the failure rate in adults at 1.1% [24]. Hence, in children with difficult airways, an SGA alone can be used to provide adequate airway support with low failure rates, and should definitely be considered with these patients [25]. The use of SGA has been used in trauma cases with successful results even with minimal experience [26, 27]. However, the SGA does not provide a definitive airway in trauma patients and can be displaced especially in patients with facial trauma who might have minimal oropharyngeal space complicating the use of the SGA [15]. Also, fixed neck flexion which happens in the recovered burned patient can limit the use of the SGA [16]. Regardless of the limitations of the SGA, it is still an easy-to-use rescue device for ventilating patients until a definitive airway is provided and therefore has been used in combat victims [28, 29].

6.4.3   Direct Laryngoscopy

Direct Laryngoscopy (DL) is the gold standard for endotracheal intubation in healthy children. The use of Macintosh and Miller blades had the same rate of optimal view in healthy children less than 2 years old [30]. In pediatric patients with a difficult airway, multiple attempts using the direct laryngoscope were associated with high failure rates and severe complications (cardiac arrest, esophageal intubation, airway trauma, bronchospasm, and hypoxemia) [31]. This limits the use of DL in war-injured patients if a difficult airway is anticipated, however the decision to proceed with DL should be based on the expertise and comfort level of the provider.

6.4.4   Video Laryngoscope

The Video Laryngoscope (VL) has more angled blades that can obtain an indirect glottis view without the need to align the oral, pharyngeal, and tracheal axis. VL has been shown to be efficient in providing successful intubation in the pediatric population with difficult airways [32]. However, the successful use of VL relies on a good view of the inner airway which is not the case in most of the trauma patients whose airway view is restricted by blood and secretions [15, 17]. In case of war injuries leading to maxillofacial trauma and distorted anatomy, the VL has limited use except in anatomical distortions that do not affect viewing the epiglottis [15].

6.4.5   The Flexible Fiberoptic

The Flexible Fiberoptic (FF) is considered the gold standard of difficult airway management in pediatric patients. Intubation can be done using different routes (including the mouth, nose, or an SGA), providing versatility for this device [17] making it ideal for patients with normal airway anatomy but extensive facial and neck contractures [16]. However, the use of the FF is impractical when there is distorted anatomy and becomes of no use when blood and secretions obscure the view of its small camera [15, 17], hence its use could be problematic in war-injured children. In addition, the use of this device is expensive and requires a lot of expertise causing additional limitations to its use in war-injured children. The FF can also be used for awake intubation, however, unlike adults, the lack of cooperativity in children makes it more difficult to perform awake intubation. Some case reports have shown the feasibility of awake intubation in pediatric difficult airways [33, 34]; however, this would be difficult in trauma and war injuries where cooperation is not always present.

6.4.6   Rescue Ventilation Using the Endotracheal Tube

When intubation and ventilation fail, the use of the endotracheal tube (ETT), which is readily available and bypasses the tongue or any airway injury of the pediatric patient, can provide safe and efficient rescue ventilation. Zestos et al. described a novel rescue technique for difficult intubation and difficult ventilation using this technique [35]. An endotracheal tube was inserted nasally (can also be inserted orally) and pushed gently and blindly into the hypopharynx where the tip of the endotracheal tube sits just above the vocal cords at the mid-thyroid level. The mouth and nostrils of the patient are sealed by hand and positive pressure ventilation can be initiated with 100% O_2. Effective ventilation can be achieved resulting in appropriate chest rise and end-tidal CO_2 waveform. Zestos et al. showed that this ETT technique can buy some valuable time by assuring oxygenation and ventilation of the patient with 100% oxygen saturation until another trial of intubation can be attempted or alternative airway equipment or help from colleagues become available.

6.4.7   Surgical Airway

In scenarios of "cannot intubate, cannot oxygenate" a surgical airway becomes the last resort to secure the airway. The use of surgical airways in war injuries (not limited to pediatrics) is relatively quite common [28, 29], this should not come as a surprise considering the difficult airway that might be encountered in war injuries. However, the need for surgical airways in infants is very rare and the literature is scarce in this area and limited to animal models using pigs and rabbits [36–39]. In addition, the cricothyroid membrane is small in infants and difficult to identify. Therefore in crises, the best way to oxygenate the lung would be through needle cricothyroidotomy [17]. This technique does not require a scalpel incision; it consists of advancing 14, 16, or 18 G angio-catheters through the cricothyroid membrane until the syringe aspirates air into a 3-ml saline-filled syringe, indicating entry into the trachea. After the air is aspirated, the needle is removed and the catheter is connected to an oxygen or ventilating source [17]. Even though success rates are high with this technique, animal studies showed that needle placement is associated with perforation of the posterior tracheal wall [37, 38]. The use of surgical airways is still controversial in the pediatric population, yet in scenarios where war injuries lead to distorted facial or airway anatomy preventing both ventilation and intubation, needle cricothyroidotomy could be a useful cheap technique that could secure the airway.

6.5   Conclusion

Airway management in war-injured children presents challenges on many different levels. However, it is important to keep in mind that these cases should be treated like any trauma airway management, starting with regular monitoring, preoxygenation, and rapid sequence intubation. In addition, multiple devices are present in case of suspected difficult airway including the VL and the FF; the problem with these devices during trauma and war injury is that even if available, small airway injuries with blood in the airway can make these devices obsolete. When sophisticated devices fail or are not available, the anesthesiologist has to rely on simple cheap techniques like rescue ventilation using the endotracheal tube, supraglottic devices, and needle cricothyroidotomy.

References

1. Luterman A, Ramenofsky M, Berryman C, Talley MA, Curreri PW. Evaluation of pre-hospital emergency medical service (EMS): defining areas for improvement. J Trauma. 1983;23(8):702–7.
2. Ramenofsky ML, Luterman A, Quindlen E, Riddick L, Curreri PW. Maximum survival in pediatric trauma: the ideal system. J Trauma. 1984;24(9):818–23.
3. Heinrich S, Birkholz T, Ihmsen H, Irouschek A, Ackermann A, Schmidt J. Incidence and predictors of difficult laryngoscopy in 11,219 pediatric anesthesia procedures. Paediatr Anaesth. 2012;22(8):729–36.
4. Harless J, Ramaiah R, Bhananker SM. Pediatric airway management. Int J Crit Illn Inj Sci. 2014;4(1):65–70.
5. Hudgins PA, Siegel J, Jacobs I, Abramowsky CR. The normal pediatric larynx on CT and MR. AJNR Am J Neuroradiol. 1997;18(2):239–45.
6. Adewale L. Anatomy and assessment of the pediatric airway. Paediatr Anaesth. 2009;19(Suppl 1):1–8.
7. Mortensen A, Lenz K, Abildstrom H, Lauritsen TL. Anesthetizing the obese child. Paediatr Anaesth. 2011;21(6):623–9.
8. Carr RJ, Beebe DS, Belani KG. The difficult pediatric airway. Semin Anesth Perioper Med Pain. 2001;20(3):219–27.
9. Brambrink AM, Braun U. Airway management in infants and children. Best Pract Res Clin Anaesthesiol. 2005;19(4):675–97.
10. Sagarin MJ, Chiang V, Sakles JC, Barton ED, Wolfe RE, Vissers RJ, et al. Rapid sequence intubation for pediatric emergency airway management. Pediatr Emerg Care. 2002;18(6):417–23.
11. Sakles JC. Improving the safety of rapid sequence intubation in the emergency department. Ann Emerg Med. 2017;69(1):7–9.

12. Hayes-Bradley C, Lewis A, Burns B, Miller M. Efficacy of nasal cannula oxygen as a preoxygenation adjunct in emergency airway management. Ann Emerg Med. 2016;68(2):174–80.
13. Pourmand A, Robinson C, Dorwart K, O'Connell F. Pre-oxygenation: implications in emergency airway management. Am J Emerg Med. 2017;35(8):1177–83.
14. Sakles JC, Mosier JM, Patanwala AE, Dicken JM. Apneic oxygenation is associated with a reduction in the incidence of hypoxemia during the RSI of patients with intracranial hemorrhage in the emergency department. Intern Emerg Med. 2016;11(7):983–92.
15. Barak M, Bahouth H, Leiser Y, Abu El-Naaj I. Airway management of the patient with maxillofacial trauma: review of the literature and suggested clinical approach. Biomed Res Int. 2015;2015:724032.
16. Caruso TJ, Janik LS, Fuzaylov G. Airway management of recovered pediatric patients with severe head and neck burns: a review. Paediatr Anaesth. 2012;22(5):462–8.
17. Huang AS, Hajduk J, Rim C, Coffield S, Jagannathan N. Focused review on management of the difficult paediatric airway. Indian J Anaesth. 2019;63(6):428–36.
18. Weiss M, Engelhardt T. Proposal for the management of the unexpected difficult pediatric airway. Paediatr Anaesth. 2010;20(5):454–64.
19. Black AE, Flynn PE, Smith HL, Thomas ML, Wilkinson KA. Development of a guideline for the management of the unanticipated difficult airway in pediatric practice. Paediatr Anaesth. 2015;25(4):346–62.
20. Apfelbaum JL, Hagberg CA, Caplan RA, Blitt CD, Connis RT, Nickinovich DG, et al. Practice guidelines for management of the difficult airway: an updated report by the American Society of Anesthesiologists Task Force on Management of the Difficult Airway. Anesthesiology. 2013;118(2):251–70.
21. Law JA, Broemling N, Cooper RM, Drolet P, Duggan LV, Griesdale DE, et al. The difficult airway with recommendations for management--part 2--the anticipated difficult airway. Can J Anaesth = Journal canadien d'anesthesie. 2013;60(11):1119–38.
22. Frerk C, Mitchell VS, McNarry AF, Mendonca C, Bhagrath R, Patel A, et al. Difficult airway society 2015 guidelines for management of unanticipated difficult intubation in adults. Br J Anaesth. 2015;115(6):827–48.
23. Mathis MR, Haydar B, Taylor EL, Morris M, Malviya SV, Christensen RE, et al. Failure of the laryngeal mask airway unique and classic in the pediatric surgical patient: a study of clinical predictors and outcomes. Anesthesiology. 2013;119(6):1284–95.
24. Ramachandran SK, Mathis MR, Tremper KK, Shanks AM, Kheterpal S. Predictors and clinical outcomes from failed laryngeal mask airway unique: a study of 15,795 patients. Anesthesiology. 2012;116(6):1217–26.
25. Jagannathan N, Sequera-Ramos L, Sohn L, Wallis B, Shertzer A, Schaldenbrand K. Elective use of supraglottic airway devices for primary airway management in children with difficult airways. Br J Anaesth. 2014;112(4):742–8.
26. Schalk R, Byhahn C, Fausel F, Egner A, Oberndorfer D, Walcher F, et al. Out-of-hospital airway management by paramedics and emergency physicians using laryngeal tubes. Resuscitation. 2010;81(3):323–6.
27. Goliasch G, Ruetzler A, Fischer H, Frass M, Sessler DI, Ruetzler K. Evaluation of advanced airway management in absolutely inexperienced hands: a randomized manikin trial. Eur J Emerg Med. 2013;20(5):310–4.
28. Adams BD, Cuniowski PA, Muck A, De Lorenzo RA. Registry of emergency airways arriving at combat hospitals. J Trauma. 2008;64(6):1548–54.
29. Mabry RL, Frankfurt A. Advanced airway management in combat casualties by medics at the point of injury: a sub-group analysis of the reach study. J Spec Oper Med: a peer reviewed journal for SOF medical professionals. 2011;11(2):16–9.
30. Passi Y, Sathyamoorthy M, Lerman J, Heard C, Marino M. Comparison of the laryngoscopy views with the size 1 Miller and Macintosh laryngoscope blades lifting the epiglottis or the base of the tongue in infants and children <2 yr of age. Br J Anaesth. 2014;113(5):869–74.
31. Fiadjoe JE, Nishisaki A, Jagannathan N, Hunyady AI, Greenberg RS, Reynolds PI, et al. Airway management complications in children with difficult tracheal intubation from the

pediatric difficult intubation (PeDI) registry: a prospective cohort analysis. Lancet Respir Med. 2016;4(1):37–48.

32. Burjek NE, Nishisaki A, Fiadjoe JE, Adams HD, Peeples KN, Raman VT, et al. Videolaryngoscopy versus fiber-optic intubation through a supraglottic airway in children with a difficult airway: an analysis from the multicenter pediatric difficult intubation registry. Anesthesiology. 2017;127(3):432–40.

33. Fraser-Harris E, Patel Y. Awake GlideScope intubation in a critically ill pediatric patient. Paediatr Anaesth. 2012;22(4):408–9.

34. Wong TE, Lim LH, Tan WJ, Khoo TH. Securing the airway in a child with extensive post-burn contracture of the neck: a novel strategy. Burns. 2010;36(5):e78-81.

35. Zestos MM, Daaboul D, Ahmed Z, Durgham N, Kaddoum R. A novel rescue technique for difficult intubation and difficult ventilation. J Vis Exp. 2011;47:1421.

36. Prunty SL, Aranda-Palacios A, Heard AM, Chapman G, Ramgolam A, Hegarty M, et al. The 'can't intubate can't oxygenate'scenario in pediatric anesthesia: a comparison of the Melker cricothyroidotomy kit with a scalpel bougie technique. Pediatr Anesth. 2015;25(4):400–4.

37. Stacey J, Heard AM, Chapman G, Wallace CJ, Hegarty M, Vijayasekaran S, et al. The 'Can't intubate Can't Oxygenate'scenario in Pediatric Anesthesia: a comparison of different devices for needle cricothyroidotomy. Pediatr Anesth. 2012;22(12):1155–8.

38. Holm-Knudsen RJ, Rasmussen LS, Charabi B, Bøttger M, Kristensen MS. Emergency airway access in children–transtracheal cannulas and tracheotomy assessed in a porcine model. Pediatr Anesth. 2012;22(12):1159–65.

39. Paxian M, Preussler NP, Reinz T, Schlueter A, Gottschall R. Transtracheal ventilation with a novel ejector-based device (Ventrain) in open, partly obstructed, or totally closed upper airways in pigs. Br J Anaesth. 2015;115(2):308–16.

Abdominal Injuries

7

Samir Akel and Arwa El Rifai

7.1   Introduction

Trauma in the pediatric population is a significant cause of morbidity and mortality. It is considered to be the leading cause of death in childhood [1]. This is even more true in conflict zones where civilians including children are often victims summing up to 15.3% of the patient population in certain regions [2]. Traumatic injuries are divided into blunt and penetrating injuries. The most common mechanism of injury in urban settings is blunt trauma accounting for up to 80% of cases [3]. The majority of patients are males and road traffic injuries are responsible for more than half of the injuries [4]. In the context of war, the injury pattern shifts dramatically toward penetrating injuries in the battlefield accounting for almost all injuries. However, in civilian injuries in a zone of conflict, blunt trauma from blasts and bombing remains more prevalent [5]. In a study reflecting on the Syrian civil war injuries that were transferred to Turkey, gunshot injuries accounted for 83% of injuries, explosives, and shrapnel injuries accounted for 15% and blunt injuries were only 0.75% [6]. The most commonly injured sites were the head and neck followed by chest and abdomen then the extremities [3]. In the setting of explosive devices, injury to the extremities were most common [7]. Yet, in another series from Turkey reflecting on the Syrian civil war, blunt trauma accounted for 56% of the cases with head injury being the most commonly injured body part in children.

S. Akel
Department of Pediatric Surgery, American University of Beirut Medical Center, Beirut, Lebanon
e-mail: sa37@aub.edu.lb

A. El Rifai (✉)
Department of General Surgery, American University of Beirut Medical Center, Beirut, Lebanon
e-mail: aye03@mail.aub.edu

© Springer Nature Switzerland AG 2023   89
G. S. Abu-Sittah, J. J. Hoballah (eds.), *The War Injured Child*,
https://doi.org/10.1007/978-3-031-28613-1_7

7.2 Initial Assessment and Triage

7.2.1 CABC Paradigm

Refers to the sequence and priorities when handling a trauma patient and it entails Circulation first, Airway, Breathing, and Circulation with re-evaluation after any intervention.

7.2.2 Catastrophic Bleeding

Any obvious major bleeding should be stopped with compression or tourniquet. Children have a great physiologic reserve and will have to lose more than 30% of their blood volume before exhibiting hypotension. The estimated blood volume in a pediatric patient is around 80 ml/kg [6]..

7.2.3 Airway

Examination of the airway starts with clearing and assessing for obstruction by looking, listening, and feeling. Stabilization of the cervical spine should be done simultaneously with the assumption that all patients will have a suspected injury until proven otherwise. In children, it is important to note that they have a relatively large tongue that can easily obstruct their airway, moreover, the larynx is more anterior and the trachea is short in length [8]..

7.2.4 Breathing

After securing the airway, breathing assessment is done by checking the respiratory rate, chest wall expansion, and use of accessory muscles. Assessment for life-threatening injuries such as tension pneumothorax, massive hemothorax, flail chest, and cardiac tamponade needs to be done [6]..

7.2.5 Circulation

Assessment for internal hemorrhage in the chest, abdomen, and pelvis as well as the lower extremities needs to be done [6]. Signs of hemorrhagic shock include tachycardia, altered mental status, pale skin, hypothermia, and ultimately hypotension. Early detection of signs of shock is imperative to start timely resuscitation [6]..

7.2.6 Disability

Evaluation of the level of consciousness, pupillary size, and reactivity as well as the Glasgow Coma Scale (GCS) should be done [6]..

7.2.7 Exposure and Environment

A full examination should be done to evaluate for other injuries with attention to keeping the patient warmed up and covered after each evaluation [6]. Pediatric patients have a large body surface area-to-weight ratio and therefore are prone to fluid loss as well as hypothermia [6]..

7.2.8 Scoring Systems

Several scoring systems in the setting of a polytrauma are available, such as the Injury Severity Score (ISS) which is applicable in the pediatric age group [6]. Other pediatric-specific scoring systems such as the Pediatric Trauma Score (PTS) are also available.

7.3 Adjuncts to Primary Survey

After completion of the CABC assessment, adjuncts to the primary survey allow early identification of injuries and they include a chest X-ray and Focused Assessment with Sonography for Trauma [6]..

7.3.1 Role of FAST in Children

Focused Assessment with Sonography for Trauma (FAST) is a quick ultrasound tool available at the bedside that evaluates the presence of fluid in four locations. The presence of fluids in the right upper and left upper quadrants, suprapubic area, or the sub-xyphoid (pericardium) area is considered a positive FAST [9]. In adults, a positive FAST indicates the need for further imaging or intervention depending on the clinical scenario. In the pediatric population, there is emerging role for FAST in the setting of blunt abdominal injury. In the hemodynamically stable patient, a negative FAST and lack of findings on physical examination can guide the surgeon toward nonoperative management without fear of missing significant injuries [4]..

7.3.2 Role of DPL

In low resource setting, Diagnostic Peritoneal Lavage or DPL is considered a quick and simple technique to assess abdominal injury in blunt and penetrating trauma. After NG decompression and Foley catheter insertion, open or percutaneous DPL can be done. Using the Seldinger technique with percutaneous access to the peritoneal cavity is most commonly used [10]. An open approach can also be used through which the infra-umbilical region is prepared and infiltrated with anesthetic and then access to the peritoneum is gained by dissection through the skin, soft tissues, and linea alba. The peritoneum is then incised and 20 ml/kg of warm saline is infused and directed toward the pelvis in a sterile fashion. Then the saline bag is placed below the level of the patient to allow the lavage to return and be collected. A sample is then sent to the lab for cell count, Gram stain, amylase [10]. A DPL is considered positive if there is contamination with bacteria, bile, or enteric contents. Presence of $10^5/mm^3$ red blood cells or $500/mm^3$ white blood cells [5]..

7.3.3   Intravenous Access

Simultaneously with the primary assessment, an intravenous access should be established. Intravenous access is of particular challenge in the pediatric age group due to smaller vascular structures. The patient will need a large bore, at least, 18-gauge catheter for rapid fluid and blood administration as needed [11]. Allow for two attempts and IV insertion and if they failed then attempt an interosseous access [9]. Rarely, a cut down is necessary, it is done either at the level of the ankle above the medial malleolus utilizing the long saphenous vein root or a median cephalic cut down at the level of the elbow [6]..

7.3.4   Central Line Access

In case a venous access cannot be secured or further access is needed a central line can be inserted. Acceptable locations include the femoral, internal jugular as well as subclavian veins. The risk of infection seems to be unrelated to the site of access. Comparison between subclavian and jugular access seem to have a similar rate of mechanical complications [12]. However, subclavian access still has the highest rate of other complications including pneumothorax [13]..

7.3.5   Laboratory Tests

After the establishment of an IV access, blood tests are taken for complete blood count, cross-matching, creatinine, electrolytes, liver function tests, and coagulation [6].

7.4   Secondary Survey

This is done after the patient is adequately resuscitated and stabilized. It involves a comprehensive history and examination of the skin, body orifices, chest, abdomen, pelvis, extremities, and an in-depth neurologic evaluation. A nasogastric tube and urinary catheter should be placed if there are no contraindications since urine output is an accurate measure of perfusion [6].

7.5   Damage Control Resuscitation

Hemorrhage and coagulopathy are leading causes of death in trauma patients. A balanced resuscitation approach with blood product administration in a 1:1:1 ratio of packed red blood cells: Fresh frozen plasma: platelets are essential [14]. Therefore, massive transfusion protocols (MTP) are crucial in the resuscitation phase of patients in hemorrhagic shock. In the pediatric population, MTP is defined as transfusion of greater than 100% of the child's total blood volume over a 24-hr period [15].

Whole blood (WB) contains red blood cells, plasma as well as platelets, and coagulation factors. There is an increasing role for WB transfusions in the setting of military trauma and recently in civilian trauma in the adult population [16]. There is emerging evidence to support the safety of WB transfusions in severe pediatric injuries in volumes up to 20 ml/kg [17].

7.6   Damage Control Surgery

Hemorrhage is the principal cause of preventable death in trauma and accounts for around a third of trauma-related mortality [14]. In principle, damage control starts immediately at the trauma scene during the initial assessment. Priorities at the time are given for controlling disastrous bleeding, securing the airway, breathing, and circulation [6]..

Damage control surgery (DCS) is also considered as a "bail out" procedure aimed at doing what is needed to keep the patient alive and defer definitive surgery till the patient is more stable. The objective of DCR is to avoid the lethal triad of acidosis, hypothermia, and coagulopathy that starts at the trauma scene and is perpetuated by prolonged surgery [4]..

The basic tenants of DCS are as follows:

1. Control bleeding.
2. Control contamination.
3. Temporary closure of abdomen if required.

Once indications for laparotomy are satisfied and patient is taken to the operating room it is imperative to have the room warmed up. Preparation should include the chest, abdomen, and thighs [4]. A full laparotomy incision should be made from the sub-xyphoid region up to the pubic symphysis to allow exploration of all four quadrants. Reported pitfalls when performing a DCS in a pediatric patient is the delay in activating the massive transfusion protocol, failure to prevent hypothermia, prolonged operating time, and failure to assess priorities in multi-organ injuries [4]..

Temporary abdominal closure can be established in different ways including skin closure only or a negative pressure dressing. Negative pressure dressing can be improvised by using a sterile saline bag or 3 M-Ioban wrapped towel tucked under the fascia with suction drains placed on top and an occlusive dressing [10]..

7.7   Surgical Approach and Consideration for each Organ

The pediatric skeleton is flexible and therefore soft tissue injuries can occur without fractures [6]. The small abdominal cavity increases the chances for multi-organ injury in the setting of trauma with multi-organ involvement can reach up to 79% of cases [8]..

7.7.1   Stomach

Gastric injuries are very rare; they can occur after blunt trauma leading to transection or near total transection [18]. They can present with massive pneumoperitoneum that may require percutaneous decompression prior to laparotomy. Evaluation for gastric injuries should be done by examining the surface anteriorly as well as the posterior wall by opening the gastrocolic ligament. Depending on the severity of the injury the management is guided. If a gastric hematoma is identified, it can be evacuated and the gastric wall sutured. Deeper injuries are closed primarily in two layers [19]. In cases of more extensive damage with devitalized tissues, debridement, partial gastrectomy, and restoration of continuity with end-to-end anastomosis should be done or a gastrojejunostomy in case of an associated duodenal injury.

7.7.2   Diaphragmatic Injuries

Traumatic injuries to the diaphragm are quite rare, patient often presents with respiratory as well as abdominal complaints, especially if the diaphragm was ruptured. Most commonly the left side is affected. The surgical approach for a major diaphragmatic injury includes a laparotomy with a reduction of herniated viscera, which is the preferred option. Laparoscopy and even thoracoscopic/thoracotomy approaches have been described [20]..

7.7.3   Duodenal Injuries

Prevalence of duodenal injuries accounts for 3–5% of trauma cases and are often associated with other injuries due to its deep retroperitoneal location [21]. Injuries can be due to a crush injury against the spine or due to deceleration injuries. Patients present with non-specific epigastric abdominal pain that gradually worsens as well as vomiting and leukocytosis. The injury is confirmed using a contrast CT scan that would show a contrast leak or extra luminal gas. Management of duodenal injuries depends on the extent of tissue loss. If diagnosis of a hematoma has been done, some can opt for conservative management with NG decompression and close observation. Injuries with less than 50% circumferential tissue loss can be amenable to primary repair. More extensive injuries can be repaired using serosal patches, gastric island flaps, or Roux-en-Y duodenojejunostomy with variable outcomes depending on the timing of diagnosis and intervention [10]..

7.7.4 Small Intestine

In penetrating trauma, the small bowel is most likely injured in up to 62% [5]. Bowel injuries including mesenteric hematomas are rare after blunt trauma. A CT scan can help with the diagnosis and would typically show a hematoma, bowel wall thickening, mesenteric fat stranding, or fluid [22]. However, CT scan is diagnostic in only 60% of cases [17]. In case of hemodynamic stability, close observation and serial abdominal exams should be done and if diagnosis is made then surgery should be entertained. If the injury involves more than 50% of the circumference, then segmental resection is necessary, however, less extensive injuries can be primarily repaired [17]..

7.7.5 Colon and Rectal Injuries

Colon injuries most commonly occur as a result of penetrating trauma, however, it occurs in up to 5% of blunt trauma. As a result of blunt trauma, the colon can be crushed or avulsed from the mesentery. These injuries can be difficult to diagnose, however, once a diagnosis of colonic perforation is made the treatment is surgical [23]. The safest option is to divert the fecal stream, especially in the setting of other concomitant injuries. However, recent literature suggest safety of primary repair even for left-sided colonic injuries [24]..

Rectal trauma often occurs in association with pelvic and urinary tract injuries. The timely diagnosis is often challenging and therefore a suggestive mechanism should prompt further investigation [25]. Triple-phase CT and proctoscopy can be used to detect rectal injuries [26]. Management options include a diverting colostomy with drainage of the perineal area to control sepsis [17]..

7.7.6 Spleen

Vast majority of blunt splenic injuries can be managed non-operatively if the child is hemodynamically stable and without peritoneal signs [27] with failure rate of around 7.4% [28]. The spleen in the pediatric population is thought to have a thicker capsule and higher myoepithelial cell content that can explain the high Non-Operative Management (NOM) success rate. If NOM is to be considered there should be the capability of continuous monitoring, available operating room and trained surgeons at all times [29]. Operative interventions are necessitated in the setting of hemodynamic instability. Surgical options include splenectomy for the shattered spleen and for the critically ill child. Organ preserving techniques can be used such as Splenorrhaphy and partial splenectomy. Non-operative management

(NOM) entails serial hematocrit monitoring as well as physical exam to check for any signs of further bleeding. For penetrating splenic injuries not enough data is available that encourage NOM [29]..

The recommendation after NOM is to restrict activity for a period that is calculated using the following: Injury grade + 2 weeks. The role of follow-up imaging is reserved for symptomatic patients rather than being done routinely [30]. It is important to keep in mind the need for vaccination against encapsulated organisms after 2 weeks of a splenectomy for trauma due to the risk of overwhelming postsplenectomy infection (OPSI). Children are at a higher risk of developing OPSI than adult patients [31]. These patients have at least an eightfold increase in risk of developing severe infectious complications half of which present within the first 2 years after the splenectomy [32]. Moreover, there is a role for antimicrobial prophylaxis in the pediatric population who undergo splenectomy be it for trauma or electively in addition to the vaccinations. Antimicrobial prophylaxis is reported to decrease mortality related to infectious diseases from 88% to 47% [33]. Some guidelines refer to the use of prophylactic antibiotics for a minimum of 2 years after the splenectomy [34]. Others recommend prophylaxis till the age of 5 years and a minimum of 1 year post-splenectomy with extension of the duration of prophylaxis to adulthood if the patient has a history of OPSI [35]..

7.7.7 Liver

Most injuries can be managed non-operatively with a failure rate of 8.3% [14]. Operative management for liver injuries follows the damage control principles of adequate packing to tamponade an uncontrollable bleed and prevent coagulopathy and hypothermia. Definitive surgical interventions are only entertained after stabilizing the patient and reversing coagulopathy, those are often required for major vessel injuries requiring reconstruction as well as bile duct injuries [17]..

7.7.8 Pancreas

Pancreatic injuries are rare with an incidence of around 0.4% most commonly occurring after blunt injuries such as motor vehicle collisions and handlebar injuries. The morbidity of such injuries and mortality are significant reaching up to 26% and 5%, respectively. Management options include operative and non-operative approaches depending on the location of parenchymal disruptions and involvement of the pancreatic duct [36]. Around two-third of injuries are managed non-operatively. Surgery is reserved for extensive injuries and distal pancreatic ductal injuries that are treated with distal pancreatectomy done open or laparoscopically [11].

7.7.9 Adrenal

Adrenal trauma is rare, prevalence is up to 1% of trauma cases and is often occurring on the right side and is combined with other abdominal injuries most commonly the kidney then liver and spleen [37]. Diagnosis is best done with a CT scan. Unilateral injuries are unlikely to cause any clinical symptoms and bilateral trauma may cause adrenal insufficiency [11]..

7.7.10 Kidney

The pediatric patient is at a higher risk of sustaining a renal injury in view of the decrease in the fat surrounding the kidney as well as the weaker abdominal muscles and the more flexible thoracic cage. Blunt trauma involves renal injury in around 10–20% of cases [38]. In hemodynamically stable patients with hematuria or mechanism of injury suspicious of renal trauma a CT is considered the standard for evaluation [39]. Most cases, even high-grade injuries, are managed non-operatively with indications for surgery being hemodynamic instability, grade V injury and expanding hematoma [14]. If a contained non-expanding retroperitoneal hematoma was found during exploration for another reason, its advisable not to enter the retroperitoneum for fear of consequent nephrectomy.

Follow-up imaging with CT scan after a renal injury should be done if the patient develops fever, worsening flank pain, or drop in hemoglobin. If patient is clinically stable no need for follow-up images for grades I–III, however, it is indicated for grade IV with injury to the collecting ducts [14]..

Injury to the ureters is, however, the least common type of genitourinary injury most commonly occurring to the distal third. Management is dependent on the severity and location of the ureteric disruption [14]. Preoperative diagnosis can be made with CT scan with delayed images or using retrograde urography which is more sensitive. In case of laparotomy, inspection of the ureters should be done to rule out any injury. If injury is detected, then a minimally invasive approach for management is undertaken namely nephrostomy drainage and ureteric stent insertion. For partial lacerations, primary repair and stent insertion are advocated, while for severe injuries treatment depends on location and length of gap in the ureter [14].

7.7.11 Bladder

Bladder injuries can be intra- or extra-peritoneal in 30% and 60% of cases, respectively. They are often associated with pelvic fractures. The pediatric patient is more susceptible to bladder injuries since it is less protected by the pelvis. Diagnosis is made via cystography or CT cystography. Management of uncomplicated extra-peritoneal injuries consists of bladder drainage and follow-up cystography in 2–3 weeks. For complicated extra-peritoneal injuries, early surgical repair is warranted to prevent fistula complications and to promote healing. For intra-peritoneal injuries, surgical repair is indicated and a suprapubic catheter placement is warranted. Follow-up cystography is recommended after conservative management of extra-peritoneal injuries and after surgically managed complicated extra-peritoneal injuries [14]..

Injury to the urethra often occurs in association with several other injuries. Management entails a urethral catheter if the patient is still able to void, otherwise, suprapubic drainage is indicated. The definitive treatment can be immediate or delayed depending on the clinical scenario [14]..

Scrotal injury due to blunt trauma can cause testicular rupture which manifests as discoloration and swelling. Evaluation is done using ultrasound, if there is suspicion of testicular rupture then exploration is warranted [14]..

7.8   Conclusion

Pediatric trauma remains significant morbidity and mortality, it is important to have a thorough understanding of the different presentations of the various injuries in the context of war. This overview highlights the major peculiarities that pertain to the pediatric age group and emphasizes the management approach.

References

1. Søreide K, Krüger AJ, Ellingsen CL, Tjosevik KE. Pediatric trauma deaths are predominated by severe head injuries during spring and summer. Scand J Trauma Resusc Emerg Med. 2009;17:3.
2. Haverkamp FJ, Gennip LV, Muhrbeck M, Veen H, Wladis A, Tan EC. Global surgery for paediatric casualties in armed conflict. World J Emerg Surg. 2019;14:55. https://doi.org/10.1186/s13017-019-0275-9.
3. Nielsen JW, Shi J, Wheeler K, Xiang H, Kenney BD. Resource use in pediatric blunt and penetrating trauma. J Surg Res. 2016;202(2):436–42. https://doi.org/10.1016/j.jss.2015.06.018. Epub 2015 Jun 18
4. Kundal VK, Debnath PR, Sen A. Epidemiology of pediatric trauma and its pattern in urban India: a tertiary care hospital-based experience. J Indian Assoc Pediatr Surg. 2017;22(1):33–7. https://doi.org/10.4103/0971-9261.194618.
5. Er E, Çorbacıoğlu ŞK, Güler S, Aslan Ş, Seviner M, Aksel G, Bekgöz B. Analyses of demographical and injury characteristics of adult and pediatric patients injured in Syrian civil war. Am J Emerg Med. 2017;35:82–6.
6. Şimşek BK, Dokur M, Uysal E, Çalıker N, Gökçe ON, Deniz IK, Uğur M, Geyik M, Kaya M, Dağlı G. Characteristics of the injuries of Syrian refugees sustained during the civil war. Ulus Travma Acil Cerrahi Derg. 2017;23(3):199–206. https://doi.org/10.5505/tjtes.2016.95525.
7. Terziæ J, Mestrovic J, Dogas Z, Furlan D, Biocic M. Children war casualties during the 1991–1995 wars in Croatia and Bosnia and Herzegovina. Croat Med J. 2001;42:156–60.
8. Mevius H, Dijk M, Numanoglu A, As AB. The management of pediatric polytrauma: review. Clin Med Insights Trauma Intens Med. 2014;5:27–37. https://doi.org/10.4137/CMtiM.s12260.
9. Tummers W, Schuppen JV, Langeveld H, Wilde J, Bamderker E, As A. Role of focused assessment with sonography for trauma as a screening tool for blunt abdominal trauma in young children after high energy trauma. S Afr J Surg. 2016;54:2.
10. Whitfield C, Garner JP. The early management of gunshot wounds part II: the abdomen, extremities and special situations. Trauma. 2007;9:47–71.
11. Gilley M, Beno S. Damage control resuscitation in pediatric trauma. Emerg Crit Care Med. 2018;30(3):338–43. https://doi.org/10.1097/MOP.0000000000000617.
12. Pirat A, Camkiran A, Zeyneloglu P, Ozkan M, Akpek E, Arslan G. Comparison of internal jugular and subclavian access for central venous catheterization in pediatric cardiac surgery. Crit Care. 2012;16(Suppl 1):P210. https://doi.org/10.1186/cc10817.

13. Trieschmann U, Kruessel M, Cate UF, Sreerman N. Central venous catheters in children and neonates—what is important? Images Paediatr Cardiol. 2007;9(4):1–8.
14. Tran A, Campbell BT. The art and science of pediatric damage control. Semin Pediatr Surg. 2017;26:21–6.
15. Diab YA, Wong EC, Luban NL. Massive transfusion in children and neonates. Br J Haematol. 2013;161(1):15–26.
16. Spinella PC, Cap AP. Whole blood: back to the future. Curr Opin Hematol. 2016;23:536–42.
17. Leeper C, Yazer MH, Cladis FP, Saladino R, Triulzi DJ, Gaines BA. Use of uncrossmatched cold-stored whole blood in injured children with Hemorrhagic shock. JAMA Pediatr. 2018;172(5):491–2.
18. Begossi G, Danielson PD, Hirsh MP. Transection of the stomach after blunt injury in the pediatric population. J Pediatr Surg. 2007;42:1604–7.
19. Weinberg JA, Corce MA. Penetrating injuries to the stomach, duodenum, and small bowel. Curr Trauma Rep. 2015;1(2):107–11.
20. Marzona F, Parri N, Nocerino A, Giacalone M, Valentini E, Masi S, Bussolin L. Traumatic diaphragmatic rupture in pediatric age: review of the literature. Eur J Trauma Emerg Surg. 2019;45:49–58. https://doi.org/10.1007/s00068-016-0737-7.
21. Dhua AK, Joshi M. An isolated duodenal perforation in pediatric blunt abdominal trauma: a rare but distinct possibility. Burns Trauma. 2015;3:4. https://doi.org/10.1186/s41038-015-0008-6.
22. Park HC, Kim JW, Kim MJ, Lee BH. Outcomes of selective surgery in patients with suspected small bowel injury from blunt trauma. Ann Surg Treat Res. 2018;94(1):44–8.
23. Guzzu H, Middlesworth W. Hollow viscus blunt abdominal trauma in children, https://www.uptodate.com/contents/hollow-viscus-blunt-abdominal-trauma-in-children#H10392495
24. Dokucu AI, Ozturk H, Yagmur Y, Otcu S, Onen A, Azal OF, Gurkan F, Yucesan S. Colon injuries in children. J Pediatr Surg. 2000;35:1799–804.
25. Bonnard A, Zamakhshary M. Outcomes and management of rectal injuries in children. Pediatr Surg Int. 2007;23:1071–6. https://doi.org/10.1007/s00383-007-1996-5.
26. Clemens MS, Peace KM, Yi F. Rectal trauma: evidence-based practices. Clin Colon Rectal Surg. 2018;31:17–23.
27. Jakob H, Lustenberger T, Schneidmuller D, Sander AL, Walcher F, Marxi I. Pediatric polytrauma management. Eur J Trauma Emerg Surg. 2010;36:325–38.
28. Linnaus ME, Langlais CS, Garcia NM, Alder AC, Eubanks JW 3rd, Maxson RT, Letton RW, Ponsky TA, St Peter SD, Leys C, Bhatia A, Ostlie DJ, Tuggle DW, Lawson KA, Raines AR, Notrica DM. Failure of nonoperative management of pediatric blunt liver and spleen injuries: a prospective Arizona-Texas-Oklahoma-Memphis-Arkansas Consortium study. J Trauma Acute Care Surg. 2017;82:672–9.
29. Coccolini F, Montori G, Catena F, Kluger Y, Biffl W, Ansaloni L. Splenic trauma: WSES classification and guidelines for adult and pediatric patients. World J Emerg Surg. 2017;12:40. https://doi.org/10.1186/s13017-017-0151-4.
30. Updated APSA Blunt liver/spleen injury guidelines 2019.
31. Buzelé R, Barbier L, Sauvanet A, Fantin B. Medical complications following splenectomy. J Visc Surg. 2016;153(4):277–86. https://doi.org/10.1016/j.jviscsurg.2016.04.013.
32. Spijkerman R, Teuben M, Hietbrink F, Kramer W, Leenen L. A cohort study to evaluate infection prevention protocol in pediatric trauma patients with blunt splenic injury in a Dutch level 1 trauma center. Patient Prefer Adherence. 2018;12:1607–17.
33. Jugenburg M, Haddock G, Freedman MH, Ford-Jones L, Ein SH. The morbidity and mortality of pediatric splenectomy: does prophylaxis make a difference? J Pediatr Surg. 1999;34(7):1064–7.
34. Lammers AJ, van der Maas N, Peters EJ, Meerveld-Eggink A, Sanders EA, Kroon FP, De Werkgroep voor Infectiepreventie bij Hyposplenia en Asplenia. Voorkomen van ernstige infecties bij patienten met hypo- of asplenie [Prevention of severe infections in patients with hyposplenism or asplenia]. Ned Tijdschr Geneeskd. 2012;156(44):A4857. Dutch

35. Pasternack MS. Prevention of infection in patients with impaired splenic function https://www.uptodate.com/contents/prevention-of-infection-in-patients-with-impaired-splenic-function#H480281089.
36. Englum BR, Gulack BC, Rice HE, Scarborough JE, Adibe OO. Management of blunt pancreatic trauma in children: review of the National Trauma Data Bank. J Pediatr Surg. 2016;51:1526–31.
37. Aydogdu B, Okur MH, Arslan S, Zeytun H, Basuguy E, Icer M, Goya C, Uygun I, Cigdem MK, Onen A, Otsu S. The adrenal gland: an organ neglected in pediatric trauma cases. Urol J. 2016;13(6):2916–9.
38. Richards CR, Clark ME, Sutherland RS, Woo RK. Retrospective review of Pediatric blunt renal trauma: a single Institution's five year experience. Hawai'i J Med Public Health. 2017;76:5.
39. Bryk DJ, Zhao LC. Guideline of guidelines: a review of urological trauma guidelines. BJU Int. 2016;117:226–34.

Management of Pediatric Vascular Injuries in Blasts

8

Jamal J. Hobballah

8.1 Introduction

Children living in conflict zones suffer from a broad variety of injuries that can be categorized into penetrating injuries, blunt trauma, crush injuries, and burns [1]. These injuries, which are most commonly penetrating, can lead to vascular injuries, which in turn are a substantial constituent of mortality and morbidity in children exposed to armed conflict (Image 8.1) [2, 3].

The peril of vascular injuries in children is due to their direct and indirect health consequences. Vascular injuries cause external and internal hemorrhages that result in ischemia to limbs or vital organs, both of which amplify mortality among children [4, 5]. On the other hand, vascular injuries have long-term effects, such as delayed limb growth, amputations, and neurologic sequelae [6–8]. These detrimental hazards, in addition to the soaring incidence of vascular injuries secondary to armed conflict in the last century [9], demand vascular specialist management that is unique to the pediatric population. In this chapter, an overview of pediatric vascular injuries in conflict zones will be presented with a focus on diagnosis, intraoperative management, and post-operative follow-up.

J. J. Hobballah (✉)
Department of Surgery, American University of Beirut Medical Center, Beirut, Lebanon
e-mail: jh34@aub.edu.lb

© Springer Nature Switzerland AG 2023
G. S. Abu-Sittah, J. J. Hoballah (eds.), *The War Injured Child*,
https://doi.org/10.1007/978-3-031-28613-1_8

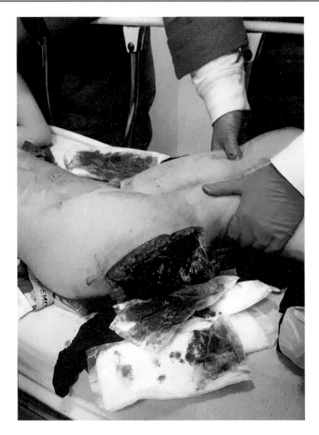

Image 8.1 Exit wound from a high velocity military rifle

8.2   Epidemiology and Anatomical Distribution of Vascular Injuries

In peacetime, the leading cause of death in the pediatric population is trauma [10, 11]. Vascular injuries, as a subcategory of trauma, constitute around 0.3–2% of all traumatic injuries to children [2, 12, 13]. According to the national vascular surgery registry in Sweden, pediatric vascular injuries are relatively uncommon, constituting 1.2% of all traumatic pediatric injuries [14]. These can be due to blunt trauma, penetrating trauma, or iatrogenic injuries, with iatrogenic vascular injuries being the most prevalent in peacetime environments [15–17]. In conflict zones, however, the incidence of vascular injuries climbs to 3–12% [18–20]. The majority are due to penetrating injuries from gunshots and explosions (Images 8.2 and 8.3).

Image 8.2 Severe soft and bony tissue loss in the foot from a blast injury

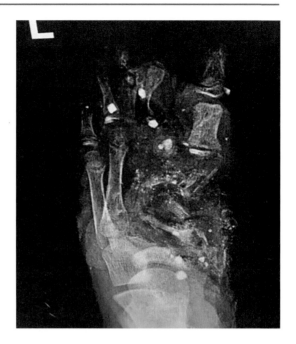

Image 8.3 Multiple shrapnel from a blast injury to the thigh

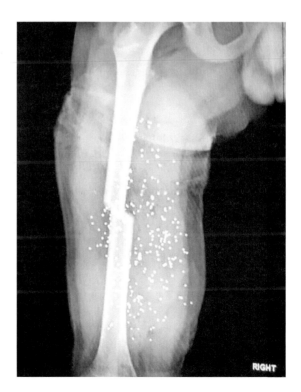

The anatomical distribution of vascular injuries in the pediatric population also differs between war and peacetime environments. In peacetime, more than 60% of vascular injuries are located in the upper extremities, while 29% are in the lower extremities and 7.2% are in the abdomen [21]. In warzones, the anatomical distribution changes to 37.8% in the upper extremities, 28.1% in the lower extremities, 25.4% in the trunk, and 8.6% in the head and neck [21]. Importantly, injuries that are located in the trunk and have damaged the aorta and its branches are the most fatal, constituting 78.1% of children who die from vascular injuries [22–24].

8.3 Types of Vascular Trauma

According to the International Committee of the Red Cross (ICRC) classification, wound ballistics can lead to various types of vascular injuries [25]. These types are:

(i) *Lateral laceration:* occurs when the vascular wall is penetrated, but its continuity remains unaltered [26]. Lateral laceration can lead to a punctate wound with an open laceration, or to a rupture of the vascular wall, which results in a pulsatile hematoma or pseudoaneurysm [25].

(ii) *Avulsion:* is when vascular continuity is interrupted because of direct contact with a projectile. Avulsion injuries are associated with significant damage to nearby tissues [27]. Microscopically, avulsion injuries damage all layers of a vascular wall [25].

(iii) *Isolated Vasospasm:* is a local reflex to penetrating or blunt trauma that carries the risk of causing ischemia to end organs or limbs [28].

(iv) *Contusion:* injures the tunica intima of a vascular wall, which precipitates thrombosis, which leads to ischemia [25].

(v) *Combined arterial and venous injuries*: Post-traumatic arteriovenous fistulae (AVFs) are well-known complications of combined arterial and venous injuries. AVFs lead to local symptoms, like pain and swelling, and systemic manifestations, such as high-output heart failure [29].

8.4 Emergency Care

The need for pre-hospital management is critical and lifesaving, especially that pediatric vascular injury carries significant challenges. These challenges arise from a number of factors, which include:

1. Children have smaller arteries and are at higher risk of vasospasm.
2. Children have less intravascular volume.
3. Children need healthy vessels to follow their growth patterns.
4. Due to their young age, long-term viability, and durability are needed to sustain injured children in their adulthood.

Failure to overcome these challenges increases the incidence of mortality and disability among injured children [30, 31].

It is crucial in the trauma setting to prioritize injuries and to follow a unique protocol. Advanced trauma life support (ATLS) offers guidelines for immediate care in traumatic cases. After securing the airway and breathing, it is crucial to deal with circulatory and vascular injuries. Delayed vascular intervention and timing to get adequate resuscitation are two important obstacles in dealing with war vascular injuries. Controlling external hemorrhage, even in a pre-hospital setting, is crucial and offers survival benefits before reaching the hospital [32]. This can be achieved by applying pressure to the bleeding site or by applying a tourniquet properly proximal to injury in a bleeding extremity. Blood loss and the subsequent shock could increase mortality and morbidity in such cases. Proper Tourniquet application is of high importance and was frequently used in more than half of the pediatric cases reported by Dua et al. [33]. Villamaria et al. reported that all patients whose tourniquets were placed in the field survived but did not prevent amputation in all cases [21]. It is worth noting that the use of pneumatic tourniquets continues to be controversial. Although its usage increases the survival rate and limits resuscitation in pediatric vascular injuries [34]. Pneumatic tourniquets carry the risk of causing local ischemia by cutting off collateral circulation in wounds with self-contained hematoma or isolated ischemic signs [25]. Shock and coagulopathy in cases of pediatric vascular injuries are leading causes of mortality. The triad of acidosis, tachycardia, and hypotension are the presenting signs in children and the targets of adequate resuscitation. Damage control resuscitation is of high importance and permits limb salvage despite injury severity [33]. Dua et al. contributed favorable outcomes in this cohort to total transfused blood components, the ratio of FFP: RBC transfused, and reduced crystalloid amount [33]. After securing intravenous access and initiating adequate resuscitation, a thorough physical examination to rule out internal hemorrhage, retroperitoneal bleeding, intra-thoracic or intra-abdominal bleeding, and deep peripheral vascular injuries should be done [33]. Seat belt sign, Grey Turner sign (flank ecchymosis), and Cullen sign (umbilical ecchymosis) should rise suspicion for internal bleeding. Once stabilized, analgesics, antibiotics, and tetanus prophylaxis should be administered as per protocol [25].

8.5   Diagnosing and Surgical Decision-Making

Diagnosing vascular injuries, particularly arterial, is a strenuous task, especially in a hemodynamically unstable patient. Nevertheless, early diagnosis is vital to facilitate early intervention, preferably within the first 6 h. While doppler ultrasonography and angiography can be used, physical examination is the swiftest and can be sufficient in moments of crisis. Certain findings on physical examination act as cues for surgical exploration. These cues, termed "hard signs," are:

1. Active hemorrhage
2. Pulsatile expanding hematoma

3. Machinery murmur
4. Signs of acute ischemia: 6 P's (pain, pallor, pulselessness, poikilothermia, par-aesthesia, and paralysis)
5. Absence of peripheral pulses despite resuscitation

Conversely, the presence of distal pulses does not exclude proximal vascular injury, due to the possible presence of collaterals that can nourish distal tissues despite major proximal vascular injury. Children, however, are less likely to have developed collateral circulations. In case of a penetrating injury that is close to a major vessel in the absence of "hard signs," observation is warranted. Moreover, para-clinical investigations such as arteriography or doppler ultrasonography (US) can be done in a stable patient to assist and help diagnose and manage suspected pediatric vascular injuries [35].

8.6 Management of Vascular Injuries

8.6.1 Venous Injuries

There is a paucity of recommended management approaches to venous injuries in pediatric trauma [36]. Most of the reported data does not differentiate between the management of penetrating and blunt venous injuries in the pediatric population. Accordingly, the recommendations are directed toward venous injuries in general regardless of etiology.

The management of venous injuries is broadly divided into nonoperative versus operative intervention, with the most vital determiner being hemodynamic instability. Rowland et al. suggest a management algorithm based on evidence-based recommendations. In their algorithm, cases of suspected venous injuries in hemodynamically stable children between 11 and 16 years of age, deserve room for trial of nonoperative management [36]. Virgilio et al. recommend a similar nonoperative approach to thrombotic events too [37].

Operative intervention is recommended for hemodynamic instability, failure of conservative management, and penetrating venous injuries, especially those with concurrent arterial injuries [36, 38]. Early intervention is of high importance in the operative management approach, with the time reported from clinical presentation to intervention as less than 45 minutes as reported by Cox et al. [39].

The operative intervention modalities vary depending on location. These techniques range from open surgical primary repair as the highest used technique, followed in a descending manner by venous ligation, end-to-end anastomosis, saphenous vein interposition grafting, and lateral repair. The lowest reported technique is amputation which is rarely required and is spared for critically injured venous cases with late presentation, which is equivalent to 1% of cases [36].

Operative management depends on the site of injury and the vein injured. The cephalic and tibial veins can be safely ligated whereas ligation is not recommended in cases of major lower extremity veins (femoral/popliteal) and major upper extremity veins (axillary/brachial/basilic) [36]. In these veins, the severity of the injury, timing, and accessibility dictate the adequate surgical technique, where saphenous vein interposition graft, end-to-end anastomosis, and lateral repair are valid surgical options.

Other major venous injuries (subclavian/internal jugular/retro-hepatic inferior vena cava) are technically challenging and data describing the operative approach is limited. Internal jugular venous injuries can be managed by ligation [40]. Subclavian venous injuries can be approached through a median sternotomy and supraclavicular extension [7]. Packing may be required in an attempt for delayed repair in cases of retro-hepatic inferior vena cava injuries [39].

Blunt injuries can cause shear-type venous injuries. These injuries are hard to be controlled surgically and to be repaired primarily as compared to penetrating venous injuries [24]. The end-to-end anastomosis technique of repair requires a maximum discrepancy of 2 cm^3. The anastomosis should be done using absorbable interrupted sutures that do not limit vein growth [41].

Although endovascular techniques of repair are reported in adult venous trauma cases, the data about this approach in children is limited and not described.

In cases of vascular injuries involving arterial and venous systems at the same time, the repair requires venous injuries initially to maintain adequate runoff post-arterial repair and to decrease compartment pressures [38, 39, 41].

8.6.2 Arterial Injuries

Penetrating arterial injuries cross vessel layers with secondary active bleeding or pseudoaneurysm formation [42]. The most frequently injured arteries in the pediatric age group are located in the extremities. Torso vascular injuries are four times more lethal than any other vascular injury pattern [21]. Upper extremity injuries are more common in the younger age group (2–6 years) while lower extremities are more common in the older age group (older than 12 years) [32]. Wahlgren and Kragsterman et al. report that the most injured arteries were the brachial arteries followed by popliteal arteries and then common femoral arteries [32].

Operative techniques vary and include interposition graft, patch, primary repair, bypass, endovascular repair, ligation, thrombectomy, and thromboendarterectomy. These techniques are challenging in children, especially when dealing with small caliber vessels and knowing the need for future vascular growth and long-term patency [30, 43]. Patch angioplasty is the most common repair in younger children, mainly when dealing with the high incidence of upper extremity brachial artery injuries [32]. While in older children, the high incidence of lower extremity injuries whose vessels are of larger caliber, allows for venous interposition and bypass graft [32] (Image 8.4) M. Kirkilas et al. highlight the importance of using interrupted sutures repairs that allow vessel growth rather than running sutures. Kirkalis et al. also discuss the relative contraindication to the use of Polytetrafluoroethylene (PTFE) grafts, other synthetic drafts, and allografts due to the long-term patency rates required in repairing pediatric vascular injuries [44].

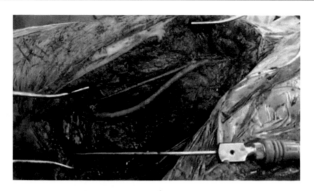

Image 8.4 Vein graft to femoral artery

The small caliber vessels in such cases require precise suturing since imbricating small adventitial flaps at the site of repair could occlude the small vascular lumens [44]. The collateral arterial flow is of high importance and all efforts should be applied in order to preserve them. End-to-side vascular anastomosis is better at sparing collateral circulation when compared to end-to-end anastomosis [6]. Arterial spasm is also a major concern in the small pediatric caliber vessels. This increases the risk of early thrombosis and justifies the helpful use of arterial vasodilators such as papaverine and nitroglycerine.

The use of endovascular modalities in the management of pediatric arterial injuries is significantly increasing and is more frequently used in blunt injuries [45–47]. They can be the treatment modality for head and neck, thoracic, abdominal, and peripheral arterial injuries. They are mostly used, however, in aortic injuries and in older children due to the vascular size that is comparable to adults, allowing adult-sized endovascular devices to be utilized. The two most common modalities used are angioembolization of the internal iliac artery and thoracic endograft [48].

Endovascular repair has many advantages. It permits practitioners to avoid aortic cross-clamping in cases of aortic injuries, open repair associated intracavitary complications, and injury to the nearby nerve structures. Furthermore, it is associated with lower transfusion rates [48].

The contact of a foreign body with the native tissue leading to penetrating arterial injury predisposes the surgical wound to contamination. The most common hospital acute complication in these cases is wound infection despite the use of antibiotics [44]. This highlights the importance of proper debridement, copious irrigation, and excision of necrotic tissue in treating these wounds.

Compartment pressures could increase significantly in case of arterial injuries with secondary tissue edema limiting perfusion pressures despite vascular reperfusion. In such cases, fasciotomy is ideal. The routine fasciotomy performed is four compartment fasciotomy through lateral and medial incisions [2] (Image 8.5).

Many reconstructive modalities including free flaps (Images 8.6 and 8.7), bone grafts (Image 8.8), and skin grafts (Images 8.9 and 8.10) and can be used to cover exposed wounds and traumatic defects. This highlights the importance of multidisciplinary approaches in pediatric war injury vascular cases for immediate vascular interventions and future reconstruction.

Image 8.5 Fasciotomy: 4 compartment fasciotomy through lateral and medial incisions

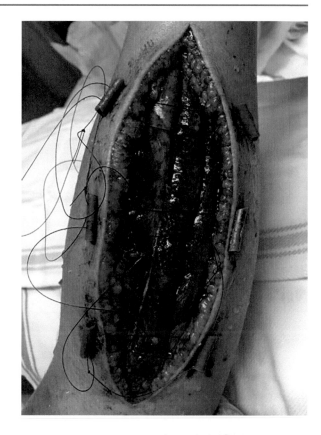

Image 8.6 Reconstructive options: Free Latismus dorsi muscle flap

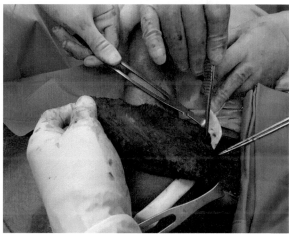

Post-operative care and follow up are also crucial after the acute phase of care. Vascular assessment and clinical signs (pulse, temperature, capillary refill, sensation, and motor powers) are essential in determining the efficiency of vascular repair and the viability of the limb. Adjunctive non-invasive testing such as ankle-brachial

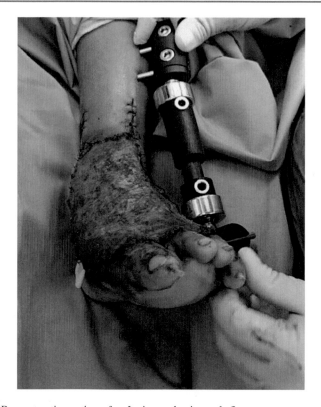

Image 8.7 Reconstructive options: free Latismus dorsi muscle flap

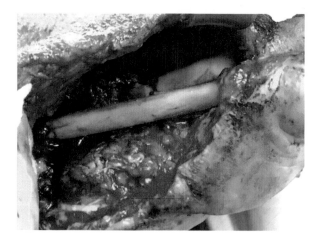

Image 8.8 Reconstructive options: Free fibula osseous flap

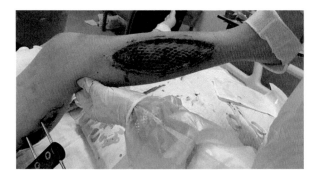

Image 8.9   Reconstructive options: Split Skin Graft – meshed

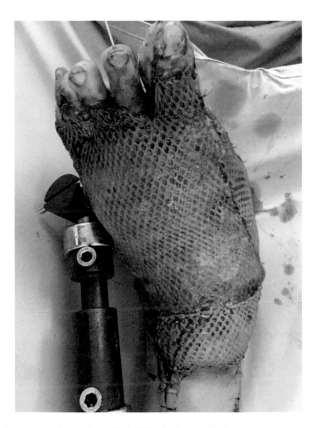

Image 8.10   Reconstructive options: Split Skin Graft – meshed

index and duplex ultrasound appear reliable when assessing the patency of repairs [33].

8.7   Conclusion

Many limitations encounter adequate pediatric vascular injury management. Future studies are required to establish proper clinical guidelines to improve acute surgical care and long-term surveillance.

References

1. Kadir A, Shenoda S, Goldhagen J. Effects of armed conflict on child health and development: a systematic review. PLoS One. 2019;14(1):e0210071.
2. Morão S, Ferreira R, Camacho N, Vital V, Pascoal J, Ferreira M, et al. Vascular trauma in children—review from a major paediatric Center. Ann Vasc Surg. 2018;49:229–33.
3. Sharrock A, Tai N, Perkins Z, White J, Remick K, Rickard R, et al. Management and outcome of 597 wartime penetrating lower extremity arterial injuries from an international military cohort. J Vasc Surg. 2019;70(1):224–32.
4. Elkin D. Vascular injuries of warfare. Ann Surg. 1944;120(3):284–310.
5. Katoch R, Gambhir R. Warfare vascular injuries. Med J Armed Forces India. 2010;66(4):338–41.
6. Whitehouse W. Pediatric vascular trauma. Arch Surg. 1976;111(11):1269.
7. Allison N, Anderson C, Shah S, Lally K, Hayes-Jordan A, Tsao K, et al. Outcomes of truncal vascular injuries in children. J Pediatr Surg. 2009;44(10):1958–64.
8. Friedman R, Jupiter J. Vascular injuries and closed extremity fractures in children. Clin Orthop Relat Res. 1984;188:112–9.
9. Weaver F, Papanicolaou G, Yellin A. Difficult peripheral vascular injuries. Surg Clin N Am. 1996;76(4):843–59.
10. Shah S, Wearden P, Gaines B. Pediatric peripheral vascular injuries: a review of our experience. J Surg Res. 2009;153(1):162–6.
11. Klinkner D, Arca M, Lewis B, Oldham K, Sato T. Pediatric vascular injuries: patterns of injury, morbidity, and mortality. J Pediatr Surg. 2007;42(1):178–83.
12. Coleman D. 3 [Internet]. Mitrauma.org. 2018 [cited 13 May 2020]. https://mitrauma.org/wp-content/uploads/2018/07/PediVasc-Trauma-2018.pdf7
13. Mommsen P, Zeckey C, Hildebrand F, Frink M, Khaladj N, Lange N, et al. Traumatic extremity arterial injury in children: epidemiology, diagnostics, treatment and prognostic value of mangled extremity severity score. J Orthop Surg Res. 2010;5(1):25.
14. Sigvant B, Mani K, Björck M. The Swedish vascular registry Swedvasc 1987–2018. Gefässchirurgie. 2018;24(1):21–6.
15. Besir Y. Surgical approach to vascular iatrogenic injuries in pediatric cases. Turkish J Trauma Emerg Surg. 2016;
16. Rudström H, Bergqvist D, Ögren M, Björck M. Iatrogenic vascular injuries in Sweden. A Nationwide study 1987–2005. J Vasc Surg. 2008;47(2):481.
17. Tonnessen B. Iatrogenic injury from vascular access and endovascular procedures. Perspect Vasc Surg Endovasc Ther. 2011;23(2):128–35.
18. Aharonson-Daniel L, Waisman Y, Dannon Y, Peleg K. Epidemiology of terror-related versus non-terror-related traumatic injury in children. Pediatrics. 2003;112(4):e280.
19. Waisman Y, Aharonson-Daniel L, Mor M, Amir L, Peleg K. The impact of terrorism on children: a two-year experience. Prehosp Disaster Med. 2003;18(3):242–8.

20. Bajec J, Gang R, Lari A. Post gulf war explosive injuries in liberated Kuwait. Injury. 1993;24(8):517–20.
21. Villamaria C, Morrison J, Fitzpatrick C, Cannon J, Rasmussen T. Wartime vascular injuries in the pediatric population of Iraq and Afghanistan: 2002–2011. J Pediatr Surg. 2014;49(3):428–32.
22. Anderson S, Day M, Chen M, Huber T, Lottenberg L, Kays D, et al. Traumatic aortic injuries in the pediatric population. J Pediatr Surg. 2008;43(6):1077–81.
23. Barmparas G, Inaba K, Talving P, David JS, Lam L, Plurad D, Green D, Demetriades D. Pediatric vs adult vascular trauma: a National Trauma Databank review. J Pediatr Surg. 2010;45(7):1404Y1412.
24. Corneille MG, Gallup TM, Villa C, Richa JM, Wolf SE, Myers JG, DentDL SRM. Pediatric vascular injuries: acute management and early outcomes. J Trauma. 2011;70(4):823Y828.
25. Giannou C, Baldan M, Kellenberger J. War surgery. Geneva: International Committee of the Red Cross; 2009.
26. Lateef Wani M, Gani Ahangar A, Ahmad Ganie F, Nabi Wani S, Wani N. Vascular Injuries: Trends in Management. Trauma Mon. 2012;17(2):266–9.
27. Ahmad M, Asghar M, Divecha C, Swain T. A complicated case of innominate artery avulsion and subsequent Aorto-subclavian graft occlusion. Cureus. 2019;
28. Gutstein W. Vasospasm, vascular injury, and atherogenesis: a perspective. Hum Pathol. 1999;30(4):365–71.
29. Nagpal K, Ahmed K, Cuschieri R. Diagnosis and management of acute traumatic arteriovenous fistula. Int J Angiol. 2008;17(04):214–6.
30. Cannon JW, Peck MA. Vascular injuries in the young. Perspect Vasc Surg Endovasc Ther. 2011;23(2):100Y110.
31. Bergqvist D, Karacagil S, Westman B. Paediatric arterial trauma. Eur J Surg. 1998;164(10):723Y731.qrrr.
32. Wahlgren C, Kragsterman B. PS172. Management and outcome of pediatric vascular injuries. J Vasc Surg. 2014;59(6):75S.
33. Dua A, Via K, Kreishman P, Kragh J, Spinella P, Patel B, et al. Early management of pediatric vascular injuries through humanitarian surgical care during U.S. military operations. J Vasc Surg. 2013;58(3):695–700.
34. Fayiga Y, Valentine R, Myers S, Chervu A, Rossi P, Clagett G. Blunt pediatric vascular trauma: analysis of forty-one consecutive patients undergoing operative intervention. J Vasc Surg. 1994;20(3):419–25.
35. Modrall J, Weaver F, Yellin A. Diagnosis and management of penetrating vascular trauma and the injured extremity. Emerg Med Clin North Am. 1998;16(1):129–44.
36. Rowland SP, Dharmarajah B, Moore HM, Dharmarajah K, Davies AH. Venous injuries in pediatric trauma: systematic review of injuries and management. J Trauma Acute Care Surg. 2014;77(2):356–63. https://doi.org/10.1097/ta.0000000000000312.
37. De Virgilio C, Mercado PD, Arnell T, Donayre C, Bongard F, White R. Noniatrogenic pediatric vascular trauma: a ten year experience at a Level I trauma center. Am Surg. 1997;63(9):781Y784.
38. Eren N, Ozgen G, Ener BK, Solak II, Furtun K. Peripheral vascular injuries in children. J Pediatr Surg. 1991;26(10):1164Y1168.
39. Cox CS Jr, Black CT, Duke JH, Cocanour CS, Moore FA, Lally KP, et al. Operative treatment of truncal vascular injuries in children and adolescents. J Pediatr Surg. 1998;33(3):462Y467.
40. Fayiga YJ, Valentine RJ, Myers SI, Chervu A, Rossi PJ, Clagett GP. Blunt pediatric vascular trauma: analysis of forty-one consecutive patients undergoing operative intervention. J Vasc Surg. 1994;20(3):419Y424. discussion 424Y425
41. Goz M, Cakir O, Eren N. Peripheral vascular injuries due to firearms in children. Eur J Vasc Endovasc Surg. 2006;32(6):690Y695.
42. Ravindra VM, Dewan MC, Akbari H, Bollo RJ, Limbrick D, Jea A, Riva-Cambrin JK. Management of penetrating cerebrovascular injuries in pediatric trauma: a retrospective multicenter study. Neurosurgery. 2017;81(3):473–80. https://doi.org/10.1093/neuros/nyx094.

43. St Peter SD, Ostlie DJ. A review of vascular surgery in the pediatric population. Pediatr Surg Int. 2007;23(1):1Y10.
44. Kirkilas M, Notrica DM, Langlais CS, Muenzer JT, Zoldos J, Graziano K. Outcomes of arterial vascular extremity trauma in pediatric patients. J Pediatr Surg. 2016;51(11):1885–90. https://doi.org/10.1016/j.jpedsurg.2016.07.001.
45. Spinella PC, Borgman MA, Azarow KS. Pediatric trauma in an austere combat environment. Crit Care Med. 2008;36(7 Suppl):S293-6.
46. Goz M, Cakir O, Eren N. Peripheral vascular injuries due to firearms in children. Eur J Vasc Endovasc Surg. 2006;32(6):690–5.
47. Moneta G. Blunt intraabdominal arterial injury in pediatric trauma patients: injury distribution and markers of outcome. Yearbook Vasc Surg. 2009;2009:253–4.
48. Branco BC, Naik-Mathuria B, Montero-Baker M, Gilani R, West CA, Mills JL, Chung J. Increasing use of endovascular therapy in pediatric arterial trauma. J Vasc Surg. 2017;66:4. https://doi.org/10.1016/j.jvs.2017.04.072.

Acute Pediatric Burn Management

9

Bachar F. Chaya, Dunia Hatabah, and Amir E. Ibrahim

9.1 Introduction

Thermal injuries remain one of the most common components of armed conflicts [1]. In modern-day conflicts, civilians are becoming major targets. This has led to an increase in pediatric burn injuries. This increase is mainly instigated by global military power advancement and the use of state-of-the-art weaponry such as ballistic rockets, mortar bombs, napalm, and aerial bombing [2, 3]. Although the management of most war-related burn injuries described in the literature is related to military personnel, treatment of pediatric burns in a war environment remains a unique challenge for deployed military and civilian health providers.

9.2 Physiological Differences

Initial management of pediatric burn casualty in the conflict zone requires a strategy of rapid assessment, airway protection, a systematic examination for concomitant injuries, and appropriate imminent resuscitation [1] (Table 9.1).

The key to the treatment of children with burn injuries lies in understanding the physiological differences compared to adults.

B. F. Chaya
Surgery, American University of Beirut Medical Center, Beirut, Lebanon

D. Hatabah
School of Medicine, Emory University, Atlanta, GA, USA
e-mail: dunia.hatabah@emory.edu

A. E. Ibrahim (✉)
Surgery, Division of Plastic & Reconstructive Surgery, American University of Beirut
Medical Center, Beirut, Lebanon
e-mail: ai12@aub.edu.lb

© Springer Nature Switzerland AG 2023
G. S. Abu-Sittah, J. J. Hoballah (eds.), *The War Injured Child*,
https://doi.org/10.1007/978-3-031-28613 1_9

Table 9.1 Initial pediatric burn management [4]

Perform an ABCDE primary survey
A—Airway with cervical spine control
B—Breathing
C—Circulation
D—Neurological status and pain control
E—Environment (heat loss) control
F—Initiate fluid resuscitation

9.2.1 Airway

Anatomically, a shorter trachea with a smaller diameter in pediatric age groups will pose them at a higher risk for airway obstruction. Furthermore, the narrowest portion of the airway is at the cricothyroid membrane with the larynx lying more anteriorly, making intubation more difficult than in adults. This setback can be further intensified by the large tonsils that children might have [5].

9.2.2 Breathing

Until the age of 8 years, an incompletely developed pulmonary reserve will pose pediatric patients with inhalational injuries with a greater impact on their lung function and may prevent further lung development [5]. Add to this, their higher prevalence of asthma and therefore a higher risk of exacerbation when inhaling smoke [6]. On the other hand, children have a higher ability to compensate for hypoxia than adults mainly by increasing their work of breathing and their respiratory rate [7]. In children, an acute respiratory arrest is a major cause of cardiac arrest and once they decompensate it is frequently sudden and complete [7].

9.2.3 Circulation

Similar to the respiratory system, the immature heart of infants and children has limited contractility hence, they can only increase their cardiac output (CO) by mounting a physiological sinus tachycardia. Tachycardia post-burn injuries is a common physiologic inflammatory response secondary to catecholamine release, however, it could be secondary to pain and/or hypovolemia and should not be underestimated [5].

Skin thickness and body surface area (BSA) are two entities of paramount importance to keep in mind. The BSA in children has a different distribution than in adults, with children having a larger head (18% vs 9% of TBSA) and smaller legs (14% vs 18% TBSA) thus, a different method of BSA estimation should be used in children such as the Lund Browder Chart [8]. In addition, the pediatric population has a higher BSA-to-body weight ratio than adults. Therefore, children's intravenous fluid resuscitation requirements per body weight for any area of burn are higher than in adults and they are at a greater risk of developing hypothermia [9].

9.2.4   Neurologic

Different communication strategies are needed with different age groups since their thinking process and behavior change throughout their developmental stages [10]. Neurological status and pain might be difficult to assess in children, especially in infants who still cannot voice out their pain and anxiety. Therefore, the use of age-specific pain scales such as the FLACC and FPS scales is highly recommended. Post-burn injury the child is usually in distress and crying [11]. Consequently, a lethargic child who is minimally responsive warrants instantaneous attention as he might be in shock. Older children should be encouraged to verbalize their pain and thoughts and should be involved in the treatment plan and decisions [10]. In some instances where the parental story does not match the pattern of the burn injury or when there is a delay in seeking treatment, child abuse should be suspected and managed accordingly.

9.2.5   Skin

As previously mentioned, children's skin is much thinner than that of adults. As a result, they are more prone to sustain deeper injuries (increased risk of full-thickness burns) and to develop hypothermia [12]. Preventing hypothermia is critical thus, a warm environment should be maintained, and wet dressings should be avoided. Furthermore, due to the immature immune system that infants and children have, they are more susceptible to infections and sepsis [5].

9.3   Burn Evaluation

9.3.1   Degree of Burns

Clinical classification of burns depends on the depth of injury through the stratum of the skin [4]. Table 9.2 outlines the degree of burn wound with its clinical presentation and associated healing characteristics and management.

Table 9.2 Degree of burns [4]

	Superficial epidermal	Partial thickness superficial	Partial thickness deep	Full thickness
Skin layer involved	Epidermis	Epidermis and papillary dermis	Epidermis and dermis (papillary and reticular)	Entire skin stratum, possibly deeper
Signs	Absence of blisters. Blanches are red and dry	Blanches are pale pink with light blistering	Darkened pink to speckled red. Capillary refill is stagnant to none. In child may be mottling lobster red	Absence of blisters and capillary refill. Thick and leather-like. Charred and waxy white. In child may be mottling lobster red
Sensation	Pain and tenderness upon air exposure	Very painful	Painful or decreased/absent sensation	Absent sensation
Capacity to self-heal	Use of occlusive dressing confers excellent capacity	Proper management confers excellent capacity	Inability to heal alone. Submission to surgery is preferred	Absent healing capacity. Need for surgical management
Duration for skin healing	7 day period	14 day period	Between 14 and 21 days, may be more	Skin does not heal, replaced by scar and contracture
Visible scar	Uncommon	Hypertrophic scarring risk is low to moderate. Color match defects may be present	Hypertrophic scarring risk is moderate to high	Visible scarring present

9.3.2 Extent Evaluation

9.3.2.1 Rule of Nines
The Rule of Nines is a measurement of estimating body surface area by assigning percentages to various body segments. Percentages and subdivisions are outlined in Figs. 9.1 and 9.2 [13].

9.3.2.2 Lund and Browder Chart
The Lund-Browder chart are considered the most accurate method. Its estimations give an accurate assessment of pediatric burn areas as it compensates for discrepancies between body shape and age [14] (Fig. 9.3).

9.3.2.3 Palmar Surface
The Palmar surface technique estimates the patient's palm to be roughly 0.8–1% of TBSA. Large burns >85% TBSA or small burns <15% TBSA can be estimated by the palmar surface. It is inaccurate for medium-sized burns [14].

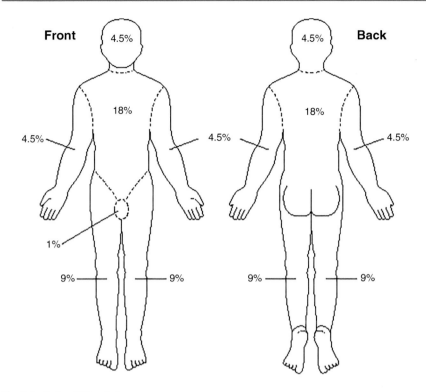

Fig. 9.1 Rule of 9 in adults

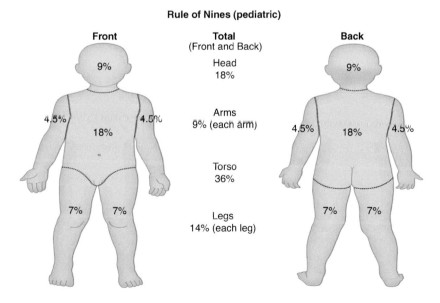

Fig. 9.2 Rule of 9 in pediatrics

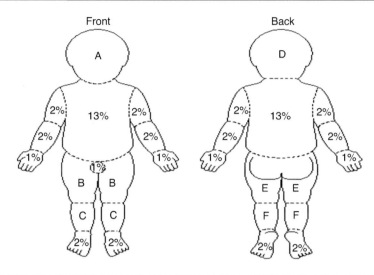

Area	By age in years			
	0	1	5	10
Head (A/D)	10%	9%	7%	6%
Thigh (B/E)	3%	3%	4%	5%
Leg (C/F)	2%	3%	3%	3%

Fig. 9.3 Lund and Browder chart

9.4 Acute Management

9.4.1 Fluid Resuscitation

Fluid resuscitation is a necessity once the burn size exceeds 10–15% of TBSA in order to restore the fluid loss and decrease the risk of a hypovolemic shock [15]. Only the deep partial-thickness burns and the full-thickness burns are included in the calculation of the TBSA [16]. Adult formulas such as the Parkland formula (4 mL × patient's weight (kg) × % TBSA burned) and the modified Brooke formula (2 mL × patient's weight (kg) × %TBSA burned) have been shown to underestimate the fluid needed in the pediatric population compared to the adult population. The most commonly used pediatric burn fluid resuscitation formulas are the Galveston and the Cincinnati [17] (Table 9.3). The preferred and most commonly used crystalloid in all of these formulas is the lactated ringer (LR) [18]. However, children are more prone to develop hypoglycemia due to their limited glycogen reserve, hence LR with 5% dextrose should be used as maintenance fluid [12]. However, these formulas remain a rough estimate of the fluid loss and thus the adequacy of resuscitation should be monitored.

Accurate markers to assess organ and tissue perfusion are the urine output (UO), mean arterial pressure (MAP), and blood lactate (BL) [18]. Common practice uses

Table 9.3 Common pediatric burn fluid resuscitation formula [31]

Formula	Galveston	Cincinnati (young children)	Cincinnati (older children)
Crystalloid	5000 ml/m² burn +2000 ml/m² total BSA of LR	4 ml/kg/%TBSA burn +1500 ml/m² total BSA of LR	4 ml/kg/%TBSA burn +1500 ml/m² total BSA of LR
Colloid	12.5 g of 25% albumin per liter of crystalloid	12.5 g of 25% albumin per 1 liter of crystalloid in the last 8 h of the initial first 24 h post-burn period 5% dextrose as needed	None
Glucose	5% dextrose as needed	5% dextrose as needed	5% dextrose as needed
Administration	1/2 over first 8 h, then 1/2 over next 16 h	To be administered 1/2 over the first 8 h and the second 1/2 over the next 16 h. Fluid composition changes each 8 hours period. (1) first 8 h, add 50 meq/L sodium bicarbonate (2) second 8 h, only LR without additive (3) third 8 h, add albumin	1/2 over first 8 h, then 1/2 over next 16 h

a UO target of 0.5-1 ml/kg/h and a MAP >60 mmHg [19]. In children, a urinary catheter might be necessary in order to have an adequate UO measurement, which will guide our resuscitation. The most accurate guide to resuscitation efficacy is blood lactate levels [20]. Blood lactate levels reflect anaerobic metabolism due to hypoperfusion, and normalizing these levels has been established to improve survival in non-burn shock [20, 21]. In a study performed by Kamolz et al., initial lactate level was found to be an effective parameter in distinguishing survivors from non-survivors [22]. Moreover, in evaluating lactate clearance on day 1, their results demonstrated that when resuscitation produced lactate clearance to normal within 24 hours patients had a better chance of survival [22].

On the other hand, over-resuscitation is also problematic and might worsen the burn injury and lead to the development of compartment syndrome of the extremities or the abdomen in addition to respiratory problems such as acute respiratory distress syndrome [23]. This is known as "Fluid Creep" [24]. The cause of this phenomenon is multifactorial and occurs as a result of:

1. Overestimation of the burn injury size.
2. A large amount of fluid requirements as a result of comorbid conditions such as septic shock or trauma and blood loss.
3. Limited use of colloids.

Fluid resuscitation in children is a dynamic process and hourly titration of fluids based on physical exam (clear lungs, warm extremities, and absence of peripheral mottling), blood pressure, urine output, blood gas analysis (arterial or venous), etc. should be done.

One of the main controversies of fluid resuscitation in burn injuries is whether to use protein-based colloids or not [25]. The most commonly used colloids are Fresh

Frozen Plasma (FFP) (which contains heat-fixed proteins and clotting factors) and albumin (oncotically active plasma protein). These colloids tend to increase the intravascular osmolarity and hence decrease fluid extravasation and third spacing [18]. However, multiple studies have demonstrated that plasma expansion was independent of the type of fluids administered in the first 24 h of resuscitation. Colloids could not increase intravascular oncotic pressure mainly because of the damage to the integrity of the capillaries [17]. Later on, with the emergence of fluid creep as a serious complication of over-resuscitation, it has been hypothesized that colloid use 24 h post-burn may actually increase intravascular osmotic pressure in addition to decreasing capillary leakage and decreasing the total fluid volume required [26]. Faraklas et al. found that administration of colloid protocol (one-third of their fluid requirements was substituted by 5% albumin) in pediatric patients as soon as they started showing signs of fluid overload, increased their intake to urine output ratio (I/O) without any evident complications [27]. They suggest that since the physiological response to resuscitation is tailored to each patient, routine measurement of I/O ratio can be used to institute albumin therapy accordingly and more quickly in patients [28]. Hypertonic saline is another type of fluid that has been used in resuscitation. However, it has fallen out of use once it was linked to a higher rate of acute renal failure [29].

Recently, new devices have been developed to guide the early phase of resuscitation in pediatric burn patients. One such device is PiCCO (pulse contour cardiac output) which is a trans-cardiopulmonary monitoring device that uses thermodilution [30]. It was shown that it decreases the total fluid used and reduces the rate of renal and cardiac failure [30]. However, these devices are still under research and are only present in a few tertiary care centers.

9.4.2 Inhalational Injuries

Due to a more than 15% mortality rate, prompt diagnosis (with a low threshold for suspicion) and management of inhalational injury in pediatric burn patients are crucial [18]. A direct airway insult will lead to severe mucosal swelling and consequently respiratory distress, especially in the pediatric age group where the trachea has a smaller diameter with eventual earlier obstructive airway edema compared to adults [18].

The diagnosis and evaluation of inhalational injury is a multimodal approach relying on accurate history, physical exam (PE), and adjunct diagnostics. A history of burns with secondary smoke occurring in a closed area should alarm for possible inhalation injury. Upon physical examination, singed facial/nasal hair, facial burns, soot around the mouth, hoarseness, and stridor are all suggestive of inhalational injury [32]. While CT Scan findings of atelectasis, ground glass opacities, and interstitial marking are highly specific, fiberoptic bronchoscopy (FOB) is more helpful and is still considered the gold standard for early diagnosis [32, 33]. FOB has a higher sensitivity and allows for severity grading and prognostication of lung injury [32]. Chest X-ray is usually normal in the acute phase and pulse oximetry is

Table 9.4 Inhalation injury stratification [36]

Grade	0	1	2	3	4
Classification of injury	None	Mild	Moderate	Severe	Massive
Description	Absence of carbonaceous deposits, erythema, edema, bronchorrhea, or obstruction	Minor or patchy areas of erythema, carbonaceous deposits in proximal or distal bronchi	Moderate degree of erythema, carbonaceous deposits, bronchorrhea, or bronchial obstruction	Severe inflammation with friability, copious carbonaceous deposits, bronchorrhea, or obstruction	Evidence of mucosal sloughing, necrosis, or endoluminal obliteration

unaffected hence is not helpful in the initial diagnostic phase [31]. Inhalation injury could be secondary to smoke particles reaching the upper or lower airways, incomplete combustion (rare in war injuries, usually affects lower airways), and direct heat injury usually to the upper airways.

Endorf et al. published the Abbreviated Injury Score (AIS) which is now the most widely used severity grading of inhalational injury based on bronchoscopy findings [34]. This score stratifies inhalational injury into five grades outlined in Table 9.4. The higher the grade the poorer the prognosis and the more impaired the gas exchange [33–36].

The acute management of inhalational injury follows the trauma management guidelines ATLS (Advanced Trauma Life Support) [31]. Hence, during the initial assessment, in any burn patient with significant respiratory distress or with extensive burns (>60% TBSA), intubation or a surgical airway should be considered. Once the airway is secured, early management should include oxygen supplementation, aggressive pulmonary toileting (suctioning, chest physiotherapy, and incentive spirometry if feasible), bronchodilators, and racemic epinephrine in order to prevent airway obstruction and bronchospasm [31]. Recent studies have revealed that the use of adjunct therapies such as inhaled heparin and N-acetylcysteine (decrease secretions) will decrease the overall mortality and the reintubation rate of burn patients [37–40]. In pediatric burn patients who remain in distress despite maximal respiratory support, the use of extracorporeal membrane oxygenation (ECMO) has been proven to be safe and efficient [41].

9.4.3   Carbon Monoxide Poisoning

Carbon monoxide (CO) is a special consideration involved in inhalational injury, especially if there is a history that suggests entrapment in a sealed area [31]. In war settings, explosive munitions can lead to burns sustained in closed spaces such as buildings and vehicles, which can lead to inhalation injury. Hypoxia induced by CO toxicity is a rapid and prompt cause of morbidity and mortality in inhalation injury. Smoke from burning wood has high concentrations of CO more so than accelerant, making it a significant component of the smoke inhaled [42].

CO has a much higher affinity for hemoglobin than oxygen [43]. Organ and cellular damage ensues due to reduced perfusion of oxygenated blood to cells and organs [44]. Diagnosis of CO poisoning can be made by measuring the level of carboxyhemoglobin (COHb) in arterial or venous blood by co-oximetry [44]. In acute settings, the most suitable initial management is the immediate administration of 100% fractional inspiration of oxygen (FiO_2) [31]. FiO_2 will decrease the half-life of CO from 4–6 h to 80 min [45]. Hyperbaric oxygen can decreases the half-life of CO to 22 minutes, however, in war settings sealed tanks are often not present, and even in their presence they will impede treatment of often associated burn injuries.

9.4.4 Glycemic Control

One of the metabolic alterations witnessed in post-burn injury is stress-induced hyperglycemia. This is due to both insulin resistance and increased gluconeogenesis and glycogenolysis associated with the exaggerated catecholamine, acute phase protein, cytokine, and hormone release in severe burn injury [46]. Hyperglycemia is associated with an increased risk of fungal and bacterial infection and mortality [47]. This has brought about the need for tight glycemic control which has caused profound changes in standard protocols for ICU care [48]. Maintaining glucose levels between 80 and 110 mg/dl extenuated infections, sepsis, death, and sepsis-associated multiple organ failure [49]. Jeschke et al proposed that an ideal glucose range exists, and avoidance of both hypoglycemia and hyperglycemia would confer better outcomes in pediatric burn patients [47]. Their results show that patients with glucose levels below 130 mg/dl had improved outcomes than patients with glucose above 140 mg/dl [47]. It is also important to consider that pediatric patients are susceptible to hypoglycemia due to their immature liver glycogen storage [50]. For this reason, the administration of fluid in the pediatric burns population often involves 5% dextrose with the lactated ringer [50].

9.4.5 Antibiotics

Systemic antibiotics have not proven to be effective in acute burns, except in the setting of positive wound or blood cultures or burn wound infections that are clinically evident. Topical antimicrobials can play a role in the protection of the dermis decreasing the bacterial burden when there is a loss of the epidermal layer. During the war, topical antimicrobials can be essential when injuries are faced with a transfer delay and should be used in liberation when transfer to burn units takes more than 12 h [3]. One of the most commonly used topical antibiotics is the Silver Sulfadiazine which has a broad-spectrum coverage to most Gram-positive and Gram-negative bacteria along with antifungal coverage; however, it cannot penetrate deep eschars. Other silver-based antimicrobials with a slow release of nano-crystalline silver ions are available as well. Another widely used topical antibiotic is the Mafenide acetate (MA) [51] which has excellent penetration of tissue including eschar but is painful upon application. MA has a broad antibacterial coverage but lacks any antifungal properties hence the addition of topical antifungal such as Nystatin is recommended when prolonged use is needed [52].

9.4.6 Beta-Blockers

A profound catecholamine surge is elicited as part of the hypermetabolic response to extensive burn wounds. Beta-blockers notably propranolol help attenuate this surge [53]. In the pediatric burn population, propranolol is associated with a sustained decrease in cardiac work and an increase in stroke volume over a 12-month period of continued use [54]. Propranolol has multifaceted effects illustrated in Table 9.5 [55]. However, propranolol does not seem to exert any effect on the inflammatory response or respiratory ratio in these patients. In addition, there has been no documented evidence of a difference between propranolol treatment and controls in terms of multi-organ failure, duration of hospital stay, or mortality [53, 56]. Based on findings in burned patients, β-blockade may be the most effective anti-catabolic therapy [57], however, overall patient selection and indications are still to be explored [58].

9.4.7 Testosterone

Loss of lean body mass (LBM) accompanying severe burn injury has a significant impact on patient morbidity and mortality [59]. It has been hypotheised that the predominant hormonal milieu of hypercortisolemia and hypoandrogenemia post-burn injury may be responsible for this loss [60]. In the context of skeletal muscle, the disproportionality in hormonal levels leads to a discrepancy in the anabolic/catabolic ratio trending toward protein breakdown [61]. Testosterone has been shown to increase protein synthesis through the efficient use of intracellular amino acids [62]. Studies have hypothesized that restoration of testosterone to physiologic ranges can help attenuate loss of LBM and increase bone mineral content [63, 64].

A synthetic derivative of 5-alpha dihydrotestosterone, Oxandrolone, is the preferred anabolic agent in pediatric burn patients [65–68]. Reeves et.al report an increase in bone mineral content and a reduction in the loss of lean body mass after

Table 9.5 Propranolol mechanisms of action

Effect	Mechanism
Enhanced deposition of lean body mass	Improves the efficiency of protein synthesis, by inducing an increase in intracellular recycling of free amino acids
Reduced accumulation of central fat	Reduced mesenteric blood flow and peripheral lipolysis
Decreased resting energy expenditure	Reduction of overall hypermetabolic response
Bone loss prevention	Reduction of overall hypermetabolic response

the administration of oxandrolone in their randomized clinical trial [64]. Oxandrolone is a non-aromatizable compound, the structure of which prevents it from being converted to estrogen, as opposed to testosterone. This reduces the risk of premature closure of growth plates in the long bones of pediatric patients, which is estrogen dependent [63, 68]. Virilization and hepatotoxicity are limited with oxandrolone administration as opposed to testosterone [69, 70].

9.4.8 Escharotomy

Full-thickness burns often result in eschar formation in children, characterized by inelastic rigid skin [71]. Circumferential eschar formation around a limb or trunk emulates a tourniquet compromising blood supply and reducing muscle movement. Left untreated and especially after significant edema secondary to acute fluid resuscitation, this can lead to compartment syndrome, distal ischemia, tissue necrosis, respiratory compromise, and death [72].

Compartment syndrome is a disease process where pressure develops in a closed space containing nerves, blood vessels, and muscle, exceeding the vascular perfusion pressure of that compartment resulting in decreased blood flow and ischemia. It can develop in the limb thorax or abdomen [73]. Diagnosis of compartment syndrome is predominantly clinical, characterized by identifying the 6 "P's": pain, pallor, paralysis, paresthesia, pulselessness, and poikothermia [74].

In limb circumferential eschar adjunct use of ultrasonic flowmeter, detecting pulsatile flow in upper limb distal palmar arch vessels and lower limb pedal vessels can aid in the assessment of circulation in the limbs [75]. Pulsatile flow absence is an absolute limb-saving indication for escharotomy [71]. Escharotomy should be performed on all circumferential full-thickness burns whether involving extremities or the trunk and it can be performed without anesthesia through the insensate skin and should be done along the full thickness of the burn to guarantee the sufficient release of vascular compression [75]. The incision cuts through the skin down to the subcutaneous tissue not involving the fascia [73]. Circumferential truncal burns may prompt an escharotomy in the anterior axillary line in the case of respiratory compromise due to impaired diaphragmatic movement or chest expansion. A truncal escharotomy is essentially important in infants below 12 months owing to their predominant abdominal pattern of breathing [72]. When the eschar is not promptly or completely treated limb compartment syndrome can occur. In that case, a fasciotomy should be performed.

A rare but very serious complication of burn injury is abdominal compartment syndrome (ACS). ACS is defined as Intra-abdominal hypertension (Bladder pressure > 10 mmHg) in addition to evidence of end-organ dysfunction [76]. The abdominal cavity has a capacity to accommodate increases in intra-abdominal volume (IAV) sparing increases in IAP. However, in the case of splanchnic edema accompanying massive fluid resuscitation in burn patients, abdominal distention can no longer accommodate the increase in volume and IAP begins to increase. In the presence of an abdominal eschar, abdominal distention is restricted and increased

IAP is achieved with lesser increases in IAV and ACS occurs with less fluid resuscitation volumes. IAP should be closely monitored in patients requiring large amounts of fluids or having abdominal eschars [77]. In these patients, limitation in crystalloid administration is necessary along with escharotomies if circumferential abdominal burns are present.

9.4.9 Early Excision

Early operative intervention through early excision and skin grafting has been shown to decrease infection rates and length of hospital stay and improve burn patients' survival [78]. Once a diagnosis of "deep" injury is established early excision is indicated. Deep injury includes both full-thickness and deep partial-thickness burns. Excision can be performed by two techniques: tangential excision and fascial excision. Tangential excision is the standard operative technique as it preserves body contour through the preservation of underlying viable tissue [79]. Using a Goulian knife or a Watson knife debridement of deep-partial burns proceeds till the appearance of punctate bleeding with a white viable dermis. As for full thickness, debridement proceeds layer by layer until coming upon yellow glistening viable subcutaneous tissue [80]. Following excision, split-thickness autografts are used for wound closure [79]. In the setting of extensive burn injury, there may not be enough viable skin to harvest, several alternatives can be used either to sustain the injury while the donor sites heal or when there is no viable skin left.

Early closure of open wounds is of paramount importance. This is achieved usually with skin autografts, however, sometimes due to the non-availability of skin donor sites in major burns, cadaveric skin allografts are a valuable alternative temporary coverage solution until further donor sites are healed and available again to use. Allografts can either be fresh cadaveric or cryopreserved [81]. Allografts' additional advantage is that they can vascularize when applied, and such can test for wound bed viability and immune rejection [79]. Other temporary skin substitutes can derive from animals, mostly porcine, named xenografts; they are usually used for partial-thickness burns and they do not vascularize [81, 82].

9.4.10 Nutritional Support

The hypermetabolic response in children with major burn injuries increases caloric requirements significantly and sets the patient in a state of negative nitrogen balance. Feeding initiation via a naso-enteral tube is advised within the first 12 h of injury [5]. Recommended caloric intake is shown in Table 9.6. It is important to note that non-protein feeding does not influence lean body mass loss and overfed patients will store the extra calories as fat [5].

Protein requirements in the setting of severe burn injury are markedly increased due to use in gluconeogenesis, wound healing, and increased losses through wound and urine [83]. Optimization of protein synthesis and the offset of the negative

Table 9.6 Recommended caloric intake in the pediatric burn patient

Category	Age (years)	Maintenance (kg)	+ % Burn calories per day
Infants	0–1	98–108	+15 × TBSA
Children	1–3	102	+ 25 × TBSA
	4–6	90	+ 40 × TBSA
	7–10	70	+ 40 × TBSA
Adolescents			
Male	11–14	55	+ 40 × TBSA
	15–18	45	+ 40 × TBSA
Female	11–14	47	+ 40 × TBSA
	15–18	40	+ 40 × TBSA

nitrogen balance is the goal of nutritional support [84]. In the determination of protein requirements, the calculation of nitrogen balance is used [85]. High protein feeding is considered successful in burned patients but increased amino acid availability alone will not reverse protein catabolism [86]. This is due to amino acid transport defects that can be reversed with the use of anabolic agents such as insulin-like growth factor-1 [83].

9.5 Conclusion

Pediatric burn injury in the setting of war has not yet been fully explored. On- and off-site management are still subject to great enhancement and progress to decrease the morbidity and mortality associated with this population. It is important to note that while effective acute management can decrease morbidity and mortality, the years following burn injury are still burdened with metabolic, skeletal, and psychological dysregulation, especially in the setting of war. Management should aim to attenuate both the acute and the chronic sequelae of pediatric burn injury.

References

1. Atiyeh BS, Hayek SN. Management of war-related burn injuries: lessons learned from recent ongoing conflicts providing exceptional care in unusual places. J Craniofac Surg. 2010;21(5):1529–37.
2. Aboutanos MB, Baker SP. Wartime civilian injuries: epidemiology and intervention strategies. J Trauma Acute Care Surg. 1997;43(4):719–26.
3. Atiyeh BS, Gunn S, Hayek S. Military and civilian burn injuries during armed conflicts. Ann Burns Fire Disasters. 2007;20(4):203.
4. Gurtner GC, Neligan PC. Plastic surgery E-book: volume 1 principles. Elsevier Health Sciences; 2017.
5. Palmieri TL. Pediatric burn resuscitation. Crit Care Clin. 2016;32(4):547–59.
6. Dharmage SC, Perret J, Custovic A. Epidemiology of asthma in children and adults. Front Pediatr. 2019;7:246.
7. Atkins DL, Berger S, Duff JP, et al. Part 11: pediatric basic life support and cardiopulmonary resuscitation quality: 2015 American Heart Association guidelines update for cardiopulmonary resuscitation and emergency cardiovascular care. Circulation. 2015;132(18_suppl_2):S519–25.

8. Cc L, Browder NC. The estimation of areas of burns. Surg Gynecol Obstet. 1944;79:352–8.
9. Lund CC. The estimation of areas of burns. Surg Gynecol Obstet. 1944;79:352–8.
10. Playfor S, Jenkins I, Boyles C, et al. Consensus guidelines on sedation and analgesia in critically ill children. Intensive Care Med. 2006;32(8):1125–36.
11. Willis MH, Merkel SI, Voepel-Lewis T, Malviya S. FLACC behavioral pain assessment scale: a comparison with the child's self-report. Pediatr Nurs. 2003;29(3):195.
12. Sharma RK, Parashar A. Special considerations in paediatric burn patients. Indian J Plast Surg. 2010;43(S 01):S43–50.
13. Moore RA, Waheed A, Burns B. Rule of nines. In: *StatPearls [Internet].* StatPearls Publishing; 2019.
14. Hettiaratchy S, Papini R. Initial management of a major burn: II—assessment and resuscitation. BMJ. 2004;329(7457):101–3.
15. Schaefer TJ, Lopez ON. Burn resuscitation and management. In: *StatPearls [Internet].* StatPearls Publishing; 2019.
16. Schulman CI, King DR. Pediatric fluid resuscitation after thermal injury. J Craniofac Surg. 2008;19(4):910–2.
17. Romanowski K, Palmieri T. Paediatric burn resuscitation: past, present, and future. Burns Trauma. 2017;5:26. *This article provides a detailed history of burn resuscitation, relates it to pediatric patients, and then describe some of the issues unique to resuscitation of children*
18. Mehrotra S, Misir A. Special traumatized populations: Burns injuries. Curr Pediatr Rev. 2018;14(1):64–9.
19. Gauglitz GG, Herndon DN, Jeschke MG. Emergency treatment of severely burned pediatric patients: current therapeutic strategies. 2008:761–75.
20. Herndon DN. Total burn care: expert consult-online. Elsevier Health Sciences; 2012.
21. McNelis J, Marini CP, Jurkiewicz A, et al. Prolonged lactate clearance is associated with increased mortality in the surgical intensive care unit. Am J Surg. 2001;182(5):481–5.
22. Kamolz L-P, Andel H, Schramm W, Meissl G, Herndon D, Frey M. Lactate: early predictor of morbidity and mortality in patients with severe burns. Burns. 2005;31(8):986–90.
23. Gibran NS, Wiechman S, Meyer W, et al. American burn association consensus statements. Sam Houston, TX: Army Inst of Surgical Research Fort; 2013.
24. Pruitt Jr BA. Protection from excessive resuscitation: "pushing the pendulum back". In: LWW; 2000.
25. Fodor L, Fodor A, Ramon Y, Shoshani O, Rissin Y, Ullmann Y. Controversies in fluid resuscitation for burn management: literature review and our experience. Injury. 2006;37(5):374–9.
26. James MF. Place of the colloids in fluid resuscitation of the traumatized patient. Curr Opin Anesthesiol. 2012;25(2):248–52.
27. Atiyeh B, Dibo S, Ibrahim A, Zgheib E. Acute burn resuscitation and fluid creep: it is time for colloid rehabilitation. Ann Burns Fire Disasters. 2012;25(2):59.
28. Faraklas I, Lam U, Cochran A, Stoddard G, Saffle J. Colloid normalizes resuscitation ratio in pediatric burns. J Burn Care Res. 2011;32(1):91–7.
29. Huang PP, Stucky FS, Dimick AR, Treat RC, Bessey PQ, Rue LW. Hypertonic sodium resuscitation is associated with renal failure and death. Ann Surg. 1995;221(5).543.
30. Kraft R, Herndon DN, Branski LK, Finnerty CC, Leonard KR, Jeschke MG. Optimized fluid management improves outcomes of pediatric burn patients. J Surg Res. 2013;181(1):121–8.
31. Arbuthnot MK, Garcia AV. Early resuscitation and management of severe pediatric burns. Paper presented at: Seminars in pediatric surgery 2019.
32. Fidkowski CW, Fuzaylov G, Sheridan RL, Coté CJ. Inhalation burn injury in children. Pediatr Anesth. 2009;19:147–54.
33. Walker PF, Buehner MF, Wood LA, et al. Diagnosis and management of inhalation injury: an updated review. Crit Care. 2015;19(1):351.
34. Endorf FW, Gamelli RL. Inhalation injury, pulmonary perturbations, and fluid resuscitation. J Burn Care Res. 2007;28(1):80–3.
35. Jones SW, Williams FN, Cairns BA, Cartotto R. Inhalation injury: pathophysiology, diagnosis, and treatment. Clin Plast Surg. 2017;44(3):505–11.

36. Albright JM, Davis CS, Bird MD, et al. The acute pulmonary inflammatory response to the graded severity of smoke inhalation injury. Crit Care Med. 2012;40(4):1113.

37. Desai M, Mlcak R, Richardson J, Nichols R, Herndon D. Reduction in mortality in pediatric patients with inhalation injury with aerosolized heparin/acetylcystine therapy. J Burn Care Rehabil. 1998;19(3):210–2.

38. Enkhbaatar P, Herndon DN, Traber DL. Use of nebulized heparin in the treatment of smoke inhalation injury. J Burn Care Res. 2009;30(1):159–62.

39. McGinn KA, Weigartz K, Lintner A, Scalese MJ, Kahn SA. Nebulized heparin with N-acetylcysteine and albuterol reduces duration of mechanical ventilation in patients with inhalation injury. J Pharm Pract. 2019;32(2):163–6.

40. Miller AC, Rivero A, Ziad S, Smith DJ, Elamin EM. Influence of nebulized unfractionated heparin and N-acetylcysteine in acute lung injury after smoke inhalation injury. J Burn Care Res. 2009;30(2):249–56.

41. Szentgyorgyi L, Shepherd C, Dunn KW, et al. Extracorporeal membrane oxygenation in severe respiratory failure resulting from burns and smoke inhalation injury. Burns. 2018;44(5):1091–9.

42. Sen S. Pediatric inhalation injury. Burns Trauma. 2017;5:1.

43. Klaassen CD, Amdur MO. Casarett and Doull's toxicology: the basic science of poisons, vol. 1236. New York: McGraw-Hill; 2013.

44. Enkhbaatar P, Sousse LE, Cox RA, Herndon DN. The pathophysiology of inhalation injury. In: Total burn care. Elsevier; 2018:174–183. e174.

45. Juurlink DN, Buckley N, Stanbrook MB, Isbister G, Bennett MH, McGuigan M. Hyperbaric oxygen for carbon monoxide poisoning. Cochrane Database Syst Rev. 2005;1

46. Mecott GA, Al-Mousawi AM, Gauglitz GG, Herndon DN, Jeschke MG. The role of hyperglycemia in burned patients: evidence-based studies. Shock (Augusta, Ga). 2010;33:1.

47. Jeschke MG, Kraft R, Emdad F, Kulp GA, Williams FN, Herndon DN. Glucose control in severely thermally injured pediatric patients: what glucose range should be the target? Ann Surg. 2010;252:3.

48. Van den Berghe G, Wouters P, Weekers F, et al. Intensive insulin therapy in critically ill patients. N Engl J Med. 2001;345(19):1359–67.

49. Van den Berghe G, Wilmer A, Hermans G, et al. Intensive insulin therapy in the medical ICU. N Engl J Med. 2006;354(5):449–61.

50. Jeschke MG, Pinto R, Herndon DN, Finnerty CC, Kraft R. Hypoglycemia is associated with increased post-burn morbidity and mortality in pediatric patients. Crit Care Med. 2014;42(5):1221.

51. Pruitt BA Jr, McManus AT, Kim SH, Goodwin CW. Burn wound infections: current status. World J Surg. 1998;22(2):135–45.

52. Cambiaso-Daniel J, Gallagher JJ, Norbury WB, Finnerty CC, Herndon DN, Culnan DM. Treatment of infection in burn patients. In: Total burn care. Elsevier; 2018:93–113. e114.

53. Herndon DN, Hart DW, Wolf SE, Chinkes DL, Wolfe RR. Reversal of catabolism by beta-blockade after severe burns. N Engl J Med. 2001;345(17):1223–9.

54. Herndon DN, Rodriguez NA, Diaz EC, et al. Long-term propranolol use in severely burned pediatric patients: a randomized controlled study. Ann Surg. 2012;256(3):402.

55. Núñez-Villaveirán T, Sánchez M, Millán P, García-de-Lorenzo A. Systematic review of the effect of propanolol on hypermetabolism in burn injuries. Medicina Intensiva (English Edition). 2015;39(2):101–13.

56. Jeschke MG, Norbury WB, Finnerty CC, Branski LK, Herndon DN. Propranolol does not increase inflammation, sepsis, or infectious episodes in severely burned children. J Trauma Acute Care Surg. 2007;62(3):676–81.

57. Guillory AN, Porter C, Suman OE, Zapata-Sirvent RL, Finnerty CC, Herndon DN. Modulation of the hypermetabolic response after burn injury. In: Total burn care. Elsevier; 2018:301–306. e303.

58. Culnan D, Voigt C, Capek KD, Muthumalaiappan K, Herndon D. Significance of the hormonal, adrenal, and sympathetic responses to burn injury. In: Total burn care. Elsevier; 2018:248–258. e246.

59. Demling R, DeSanti L. Involuntary weight loss and the nonhealing wound: the role of anabolic agents. Adv Wound Care. 1999;12(1 Suppl):1–14. quiz 15-16
60. Ferrando AA, Sheffield-Moore M, Wolf SE, Herndon DN, Wolfe RR. Testosterone administration in severe burns ameliorates muscle catabolism. Crit Care Med. 2001;29(10):1936–42.
61. Lephart ED, Baxter CR, Parker CR Jr. Effect of burn trauma on adrenal and testicular steroid hormone production. J Clin Endocrinol Metabol. 1987;64(4):842–8.
62. Ferrando A, Tipton K, Doyle D, Phillips S, Cortiella J, Wolfe R. Net protein synthesis and amino acid uptake with testosterone injection. FASEB J. 1997;11:3.
63. Murphy KD, Thomas S, Mlcak RP, Chinkes DL, Klein GL, Herndon DN. Effects of long-term oxandrolone administration in severely burned children. Surgery. 2004;136(2):219–24.
64. Reeves PT, Herndon DN, Tanksley JD, et al. Five-year outcomes after long-term oxandrolone administration in severely burned children: a randomized clinical trial. Shock (Augusta, Ga). 2016;45(4):367.
65. Hart DW, Wolf SE, Ramzy PI, et al. Anabolic effects of oxandrolone after severe burn. Ann Surg. 2001;233(4):556.
66. Przkora R, Herndon DN, Suman OE. The effects of oxandrolone and exercise on muscle mass and function in children with severe burns. Pediatrics. 2007;119(1):e109–16.
67. Przkora R, Jeschke MG, Barrow RE, et al. Metabolic and hormonal changes of severely burned children receiving long-term oxandrolone treatment. Ann Surg. 2005;242(3):384.
68. Ulloa-Aguirre A, Blizzard RM, Garcia-Rubi E, et al. Testosterone and oxandrolone, a nonaromatizable androgen, specifically amplify the mass and rate of growth hormone (GH) secreted per burst without altering GH secretory burst duration or frequency or the GH half-life. J Clin Endocrinol Metabol. 1990;71(4):846–54.
69. Ehnholm C, Huttunen JK, Kinnunen PJ, Miettinen TA, Nikkilä EA. Effect of oxandrolone treatment on the activity of lipoprotein lipase, hepatic lipase and phospholipase A1 of human postheparin plasma. N Engl J Med. 1975;292(25):1314–7.
70. Tuvdendorj D, Chinkes DL, Zhang X-J, et al. Long-term oxandrolone treatment increases muscle protein net deposition via improving amino acid utilization in pediatric patients 6 months after burn injury. Surgery. 2011;149(5):645–53.
71. Ramakrishnan KM, Ramachandran B, Ravi R, Mathivanan T, Ravikumar K, Jayaraman V. Decompression escharotomies of burns in children between the ages 0 and 18 years. Indian J Burns. 2018;26(1):99.
72. Zhang L, Hughes PG. Escharotomy. In: StatPearls [Internet]. StatPearls Publishing; 2019.
73. Vincent J-L, Hall JB. Encyclopedia of intensive care medicine. SpringerLink (Online service); 2012.
74. Garner MR, Taylor SA, Gausden E, Lyden JP. Compartment syndrome: diagnosis, management, and unique concerns in the twenty-first century. HSS J. 2014;10(2):143–52.
75. Bowen TE, Bellamy RF. Emergency war surgery. US Department of Defense; 1988.
76. Azzopardi EA, McWilliams B, Iyer S, Whitaker IS. Fluid resuscitation in adults with severe burns at risk of secondary abdominal compartment syndrome—an evidence based systematic review. Burns. 2009;35(7):911–20.
77. Ivy ME, Atweh NA, Palmer J, Possenti PP, Pineau M, D'Aiuto M. Intra-abdominal hypertension and abdominal compartment syndrome in burn patients. J Trauma Acute Care Surg. 2000;49(3):387–91.
78. Aly MEI, Dannoun M, Jimenez CJ, Sheridan RL, Lee JO. Operative wound management. In: Total burn care. Elsevier; 2018:114–130. e112.
79. Mei A, Dannoun M, Jimenez CJ, Sheridan RL, Lee JO. 12 operative wound management. Total Burn Care E-Book; 2017. p. 12114.
80. Klein MB, Hunter S, Heimbach DM, et al. The Versajet™ water dissector: a new tool for tangential excision. J Burn Care Rehabil. 2005;26(6):483–7.
81. Bondoc C, Burke J. Clinical experience with viable frozen human skin and a frozen skin bank. Ann Surg. 1971;174(3):371.
82. Sheridan RL, Tompkins RG. Skin substitutes in burns. Burns. 1999;25(2):97–103.

83. Wise AK, Hromatka KA, Miller KR. Energy expenditure and protein requirements following burn injury. Nutr Clin Pract. 2019;34(5):673–80.
84. Tredget EE, Yu YM. The metabolic effects of thermal injury. World J Surg. 1992;16(1):68–79.
85. Chan MM, Chan GM. Nutritional therapy for burns in children and adults. Nutrition. 2009;25(3):261–9.
86. Meyer N, Muller M, Herndon D. Nutrient support of the healing wound. New Horizons (Baltimore, Md). 1994;2(2):202–14.

Head Trauma in the Pediatric Population

10

Elias Elias and Marwan W. Najjar

10.1 Introduction

Traumatic Brain Injury (TBI) among young patients may lead to detrimental neurological and cognitive deficits, causing an everlasting burden. Mechanisms of TBI alter depending on age category [1], and vary from domestic abuse, and falls, to motor vehicle accidents. TBI Pathology also differs depending on age groups. The younger the child is, the more likely he will endure a subdural hematoma (SDH) and diffuse brain edema compared to contusions and diffuse axonal injury among adolescents [2]. Examining the toddlers and small-aged category is further a difficult task. The clinical presentation is variable depending on the mechanism of trauma, and the pediatric Glasgow Coma Scale is mainly used as an assessment tool [3]. Special care to details should be given to the pediatric population; even scalp bleeders can be a source of significant blood loss and hemorrhagic shock in infants.

Initial emergency management always entails several measures including avoiding hypotension, running primary surveys to rule out another organ injury, head elevation to allow proper jugular venous drainage, and careful manipulation of the cervical spine [4]. In addition, interviewing witnesses and family members is important for understanding the mechanism of injury.

The pediatric skull is different from the adult bone. It has higher plasticity properties, hence leading to better absorptive forces and clinical manifestations [5]. The presence of open sutures in infants can avert an increase in ICP. However, these open suture lines themselves are a risk for growing skull fractures [6]. With respect to skull fractures, linear fractures are more observed over the parietal area, followed by the occipital, frontal, and temporal bones [7]. The presence of extracranial subcutaneous swelling is an indirect diagnosis of such fractures [8].

E. Elias · M. W. Najjar (✉)
Department of Surgery, American University of Beirut, Beirut, Lebanon
e-mail: ee06@aub.edu.lb; mn12@aub.edu.lb

© Springer Nature Switzerland AG 2023
G. S. Abu-Sittah, J. J. Hoballah (eds.), *The War Injured Child*,
https://doi.org/10.1007/978-3-031-28613-1_10

When it comes to the site of brain injury, head-to-body volume or head-to-torso ratio in the pediatric population is higher than in the adult counterpart [9]. This puts the pediatric population at higher risk of head injury [10] due to the bigger forehead protuberance and a higher risk of frontal bone trauma, and frontal lobe contusions.

In the setting of significant head injury, primary objectives in management include maintaining adequate oxygen delivery and proper cerebral perfusion pressure, as well as reduction of intracranial pressure (ICP). In general, ICP in adults ranges normally between 5 and 15 mmHg, however, these values can vary depending on patient age, such as 2–7 mmHg in infants and young children [11].

By and large, the treatment includes two tiers. The first tier approach entails medical management, along with sedation or anesthetics to decrease the metabolic brain demands. This is usually accompanied by ICP monitoring. In case of failure of these strategies, hyperosmolar agents along with controlled ventilation are implemented to decrease the ICP. In the event of medical treatment resistance, escalation to second-tier therapies such as decompressive craniotomies can be used as protective measures to decrease the ICP.

10.2 Mechanisms of Injury

Falls are the most common mechanism in children suffering a head injury, followed by motor vehicle crashes, pedestrian and bicycle accidents, assaults, sports-related trauma, abuse, and projectiles in war conflict areas [12, 13]. These mechanisms cause isolated head trauma in the majority of patients [12]. Infants in general endure more falls and are at increased risk for inflicted injury. Moreover, children who remain in the care of the perpetrator are at significant risk of being injured again.

10.3 Imaging

The aim of neuroimaging is to acquire a quick and sensitive diagnostic assessment of injury extent. A Skull X-ray is not of any value anymore in the presence of other imaging modalities. It only depicts skull fractures but gives no hint regarding the brain parenchyma and extra-axial presence of blood collections. Ultrasound (US) is a bedside modality that is radiation-free and considered a cheap technique. It can accurately diagnose pediatric skull fractures when compared to CT scans, nonetheless, its use is restricted to the neonatal period only [14]. CT scan correlates well with the clinical presentation [15] and is considered the gold standard for TBI diagnosis [16]. MRI is mainly used in the acute stage after head injury in stable patients when CT findings do not explain the neurological symptoms and in the subacute/chronic phases. However, it cannot be utilized in case of foreign bodies penetration, has a longer acquisition time when compared to CT and US, and got a lower sensitivity rate to detect bone fractures and fragments.

10.4   Treatment: Medical

Most cases of mild to moderate TBI may be managed conservatively by simple but important measures. Head elevation is crucial in reducing traumatic congestion of the brain and is imperative in addition to neurologic observation and avoidance of excessive hypotonic fluids. Intracranial pressure (ICP) monitoring is not recommended for most of these cases, but rather in the setting of severe head injury when the Glasgow Coma scale (GCS) is less than 8.

10.5   ICP Monitoring

The intraventricular catheter is the gold standard for ICP measurement. It offers both monitoring and the ability for CSF drainage [17]. The implication of CSF drainage via ventriculostomy or lumbar drain is not well investigated in the literature and is considered level III evidence [18]. Unfortunately, the placement of such catheters is impossible in cases of severe edema and collapsed ventricles.

Intraparenchymal intracranial pressure sensors or intraparenchymal probes can be used as equally sensitive methods for ICP measurement [19]. They were introduced for the first time in the Brain Trauma Foundation Guidelines for TBI in children in 2003 [20, 21]. The main indication was early detection of high ICP among patients with severe TBI, patients with traumatic mass lesions, or in whom the serial neurologic examination is precluded by sedation, neuromuscular blockade, or anesthesia [22]. The presence of an open fontanel and/or sutures or a normal CT scan in an infant with severe TBI does not prevent the development of high ICP or exclude the use of intracranial pressure monitoring. However, ICP monitoring is not regularly suggested in infants/children with mild or moderate head injury [23].

10.6   Cerebral Perfusion Pressure

Although Cerebral Perfusion Pressure (CPP) is currently mentioned in the adult TBI guidelines [24], no large studies have been conducted for the pediatric population. Despite the lack of level I and II evidence regarding the relationship between cerebral perfusion pressure (CPP) and clinical outcome, it is still highly recommended in intensive care unit medical practices to manage both ICP and CPP in pediatric patients with severe TBI [21]. A study conducted by Chambers et al. on a sample of 235 TBI pediatric patients found a correlation between CPP and clinical outcome, after age-stratified critical levels of CPP, among age groups of 2–6, 7–10, and 11–16 years, CPP values of 43, 54, and 58 mmHg, respectively, were associated with good outcomes [25].

10.7 Temperature Control

Hyperthermia should be avoided in order to decrease the brain's metabolic demands, lipid peroxidation, the increase in parenchymal inflammation, and more importantly, to decrease seizure incidence. Hence the importance of a hypothermic state induction, as part of the intracranial hypertension treatment modality, that is considered level II evidence. However, no clear benefit was noted regarding the outcome at 6 months post-severe TBI in the pediatric population [26].

10.8 Hyperosmolar Therapy

Hyperosmolar therapy is the standard treatment to reduce ICP in severe TBI adult patients. Hypertonic saline (HS) and mannitol are the most widely used agents. Common HS solutions are 3%,5%, and 7.5% [27]. There is a difference in the suggested mechanism between mannitol and HS. Mannitol has both a rheological and a vasoconstrictive effect, both of which help in the decrease of ICP [28]. On the other hand, HS acts by creating an osmotic gradient, which is a shift from the intracellular space to the interstitial volume [29]. Despite that, both arms are commonly used in the daily practice among pediatric TBI, where level II and III evidence recommend the use of HS 3% boluses in pediatric patients with high ICP, due to the lack of sufficient data and papers on the use of mannitol [30].

10.9 Anticonvulsants

The pediatric population has lower seizure thresholds when compared to their adult counterparts [31]. What makes the situation worse, is the subtle nature of the seizures, making their detection more difficult to spot [32]. Post-traumatic seizures can be labeled as early seizures when they occur within 7 days of the insult, and late whenever occurrence is after 1 week of the trauma. It is considered a good idea to prevent such seizures, however, the side effects of antiepileptic drugs have an undesirable impact (impaired learning, behavioral changes, skin rash, hematological abnormalities, ataxia, Stevens-Johnson syndrome) and should be avoided [33]. When it comes to early post-traumatic seizures, some data show a benefit in starting antiepileptic drugs (AED) early on especially when GCS is <8. Moreover, level II and III evidence indicates that prophylactic anticonvulsant therapy after 7 days from TBI, did not prevent later post-traumatic seizures [34]. Moreover, no specific guidelines have been approved about the duration of the AED [35, 36]. Further studies should be carried out to assess the outcome in terms of mortality and the effect of the anticonvulsant therapy on different age categories.

10.10 Corticosteroids

The use of steroids in children with traumatic brain injury lacks literature evidence and might inflict harm such as infectious complications, and suppression of endogenous cortisol levels. In addition, its use was not associated with improved outcomes, nor reduction of ICP or mortality rate [37].

10.11 Treatment: Surgical-Decompressive Craniectomy

During trauma, physiologic equilibrium is breached and compensatory mechanisms operate to keep ICP constant [38]. This autoregulation may be disturbed in severe TBI, causing neurological deterioration and brain herniation. A normal ICP in adults is below 15 mmHg. When it reaches a level above 20 mmHg in TBI patients, it is considered pathological and appropriate adjustment is necessary. Once ICP is resistant to medical interventions, second-tier treatment modalities may become necessary.

Surgery is an option whenever ICP is refractory, and brain edema is not resolving. Kocher [39] and Cushing [40] were the first to use Decompressive surgery (DC) as a tool to decrease ICP in TBI cases. It provides a way to physically create more space for the brain allowing it to relax, helps in evacuating the hematomas, and decreases the risk of herniation. Consequently, cerebral blood flow and cerebral perfusion pressure will increase, improving brain tissue oxygenation.

Currently, the evidence describing the benefits of DC in pediatric TBI patients is limited; mostly level II and III evidence [21]. Different techniques have been described for decompressive craniectomies including bifrontal craniectomies, bitemporal, wide unilateral, and bilateral frontotemporoparietal craniectomy [41–43].

For the frontotemporoparietal craniectomy, the patient is placed in a supine position, with the head turned to the contralateral side. A reverse question mark incision is created from the root of the zygoma, around 1 cm in front of the tragus, going around the back of the ear helix reaching approximately 2 cm lateral to the midline (to prevent damage to the superior sagittal sinus) and anterior to the coronal suture. The bone flap should be extended inferiorly toward the floor of the temporal fossa [44]. Insufficient bony decompression will cause mushrooming of the brain parenchyma, and further damage to the brain cortex, and cortical veins engorgement [45]. The bifrontal craniectomy technique is mainly applied in the case of frontal lobe contusions and can be used for generalized cerebral edema. The incision is created from the zygomatic area bilaterally, to around 2 cm from the coronal sutures posteriorly. The craniotomy flap extends to the orbital roofs anteriorly. The superior sagittal sinus will need to be sacrificed anteriorly, by ligating it with stitches and cutting it with scissors. The falx should be also sectioned. This step will allow better brain expansion and prevents the brain from herniating against a tight dural edge. However, surgery comes with a risk of complications such as hydrocephalus, subdural hygroma formation, new hematoma formation or hematoma progression, and wound infection [46].

10.12 Prevention, Future Considerations, and Conclusion

Preventive methods and anticipatory guidance are the most important measures against TBI. Law implementation, such as seat belts, car seats, and helmet use [47]. Education regarding seat use, with correct position, never in the front but in the back seat, and facing the rear of the car, use of head helmets during bicycling, skating, rollerblading, skiing, and practicing martial arts fights is of utmost importance. Future research should be conducted in order to stratify what is normal ICP according to age category. Although randomized controlled trials continue to be the gold standard to provide level I evidence for TBI, we are aware of the lack of sufficient understanding of many basic aspects of TBI which limits the standardization of TBI management [48].

10.13 Case Illustration

A 15-year-old male, previously healthy, endured a motor vehicle accident 24 hours prior to presentation. The patient was on ATV when he was hit by a car. He was not wearing a helmet. As per the family, he lost consciousness and was vomiting before being transferred to another hospital where he was rushed to the operating room for a right-sided decompressive craniectomy.

Upon presentation in the emergency department, he was agitated, moving all four extremities, and the pupils were equal and sluggishly reactive at 3 mm before being fully sedated. After admission to the Pediatric ICU, we recommended head of the bed elevation at 30 degrees, to keep sodium in the range of 145–150 by administering 3% hypertonic saline, PCO_2 in the range of 28–32, and a possibility of an ICP monitor placement based on the CT scan results.

A CT scan showed a left temporal hemorrhagic contusion with a neighboring subdural hematoma, measuring 18 mm in maximum diameter with associated surrounding vasogenic edema and effacement of the adjacent sulci and mass effect on the left hemisphere and left lateral ventricle with a 5-mm shift of the midline structures to the right. This was associated with left uncal herniation, and a hypodensity in the left cerebral peduncle and the genu of the left internal capsule as well as in the medial aspect of the right thalamus that may represent diffuse axonal injury (Fig. 10.1a, b). He was rushed to surgery for a left-sided decompressive craniectomy (Fig. 10.2). After the surgery, a Camino ICP monitor (Integra Life Sciences) was inserted denoting a normal ICP level ranging between 12 and 16 mmHg. One month after the bilateral surgeries, a repeat CT brain showed bilateral subdural hygromas which resolved spontaneously (Fig. 10.3). Two months post-bilateral decompressive surgeries, the patient underwent bilateral cranioplasties and replacement of the bone flaps (Fig. 10.4a, b). Four months post-TBI, the patient is

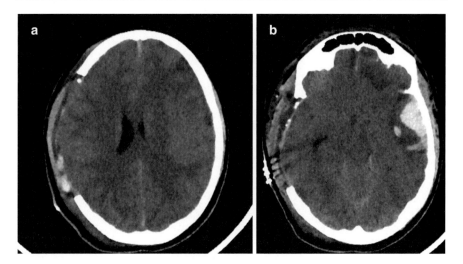

Fig. 10.1 (**a**) CT scan of the upper section of the brain showing right decompressive craniectomy, and left side edema with mass effect on the lateral ventricle. (**b**) lower CT scan cut showing left subdural hematoma and contusions with significant edema and effacement of basal cisterns

Fig. 10.2 CT scan section post-bilateral decompressive craniectomies with some bulging of the brain through the bony defects, but less cerebral edema

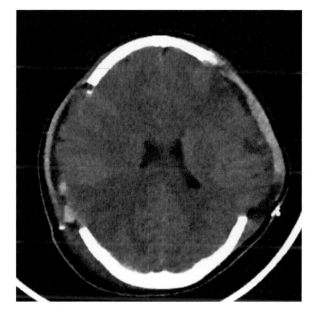

wheelchair bound, still on an NG tube, but able to swallow food, and the tracheostomy was reduced and closed. He wears a diaper, speaks a few words with repetitive anxious behavior, and still suffers from right spastic hemiparesis.

Fig. 10.3 CT scan at
1-month follow-up after
craniectomies showing
widening ventricles and
bilateral subdural
hygromas. The edema is
markedly reduced

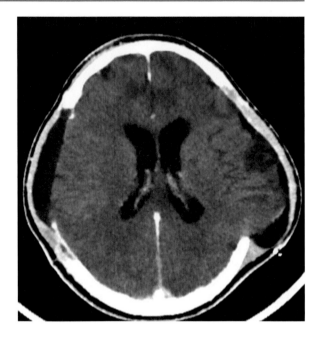

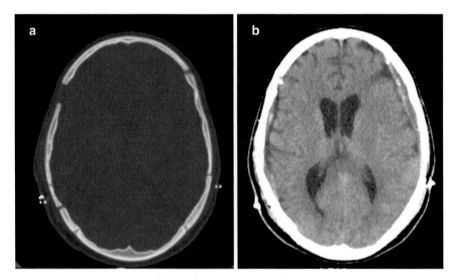

Fig. 10.4 CT scan at 2 months follows up. (**a**) Bone window setting showing replacement of bilateral bone flaps. (**b**) Brain setting showing resolved edema, and minor subdural hygromas

References

1. Araki T, Yokota H, Morita A. Pediatric traumatic brain injury: characteristic features, diagnosis, and management. Neurol Med Chir:82–93.
2. Suh DY, et al. Nonaccidental pediatric head injury: diffusion-weighted imaging findings. Neurosurgery. 2001;49(2):309–18. discussion 318-20
3. Walther AE, et al. Pediatric and adult trauma centers differ in evaluation, treatment, and outcomes for severely injured adolescents. J Pediatr Surg. 2016;51(8):1346–50.
4. Adelson PD, et al. Guidelines for the acute medical management of severe traumatic brain injury in infants, children, and adolescents. Chapter 12. Use of hyperventilation in the acute management of severe pediatric traumatic brain injury. Pediatr Crit Care Med. 2003;4(3 Suppl):S45–8.
5. Ghajar J, Hariri RJ. Management of pediatric head injury. Pediatr Clin N Am. 1992;39(5):1093–125.
6. Sanford RA. Prevention of growing skull fractures: report of 2 cases. J Neurosurg Pediatr. 2010;5(2):213–8.
7. Bonfield CM, et al. Pediatric skull fractures: the need for surgical intervention, characteristics, complications, and outcomes. J Neurosurg Pediatr. 2014;14(2):205–11.
8. Orman G, et al. Pediatric skull fracture diagnosis: should 3D CT reconstructions be added as routine imaging? J Neurosurg Pediatr. 2015;16(4):426–31.
9. Mazzola CA, Adelson PD. Critical care management of head trauma in children. Crit Care Med. 2002;30(11 Suppl):S393–401.
10. Huelke DF. An overview of anatomical considerations of infants and children in the adult world of automobile safety design. Annu Proc Assoc Adv Automot Med. 1998;42:93–113.
11. Dunn LT. Raised intracranial pressure. J Neurol Neurosurg Psychiatry. 2002;73(suppl 1):i23–7.
12. Kuppermann N, et al. Identification of children at very low risk of clinically-important brain injuries after head trauma: a prospective cohort study. Lancet. 2009;374(9696):1160–70.
13. Shravat BP, Huseyin TS, Hynes KA. NICE guideline for the management of head injury: an audit demonstrating its impact on a district general hospital, with a cost analysis for England and Wales. Emerg Med J. 2006;23(2):109–13.
14. Parri N, et al. Ability of emergency ultrasonography to detect pediatric skull fractures: a prospective, observational study. J Emerg Med. 2013;44(1):135–41.
15. Klassen TP, et al. Variation in utilization of computed tomography scanning for the investigation of minor head trauma in children: a Canadian experience. Acad Emerg Med. 2000;7(7):739–44.
16. Blackwell CD, et al. Pediatric head trauma: changes in use of computed tomography in emergency departments in the United States over time. Ann Emerg Med. 2007;49(3):320–4.
17. Guidelines for the management of severe traumatic brain injury. J Neurotrauma. 2007;24(Suppl 1):S1-106
18. Adelson PD, et al. Guidelines for the acute medical management of severe traumatic brain injury in infants, children, and adolescents. Chapter 10. The role of cerebrospinal fluid drainage in the treatment of severe pediatric traumatic brain injury. Pediatr Crit Care Med. 2003;4(3 Suppl):S38–9.
19. Alali AS, et al. Intracranial pressure monitoring among children with severe traumatic brain injury. J Neurosurg Pediatr. 2015;16(5):523–32.
20. Adelson PD, et al. Guidelines for the acute medical management of severe traumatic brain injury in infants, children, and adolescents. Chapter 17. Critical pathway for the treatment of established intracranial hypertension in pediatric traumatic brain injury. Pediatr Crit Care Med. 2003;4(3 Suppl):S65-7.
21. Kochanek PM, et al. Guidelines for the acute medical management of severe traumatic brain injury in infants, children, and adolescents—second edition. Pediatr Crit Care Med. 2012;13(Suppl 1):S1-82.

22. Jagannathan J, et al. Long-term outcomes and prognostic factors in pediatric patients with severe traumatic brain injury and elevated intracranial pressure. J Neurosurg Pediatr. 2008;2(4):240–9.

23. Adelson PD, et al. Guidelines for the acute medical management of severe traumatic brain injury in infants, children, and adolescents. Chapter 5. Indications for intracranial pressure monitoring in pediatric patients with severe traumatic brain injury. Pediatr Crit Care Med. 2003;4(3 Suppl):S19–24.

24. Le Roux P, et al. The International Multidisciplinary Consensus Conference on Multimodality Monitoring in Neurocritical Care: evidentiary tables: a statement for healthcare professionals from the Neurocritical Care Society and the European Society of Intensive Care Medicine. Neurocrit Care. 2014;21(Suppl 2):S297–361.

25. Chambers IR, et al. Age-related differences in intracranial pressure and cerebral perfusion pressure in the first 6 hours of monitoring after children's head injury: association with outcome. Childs Nerv Syst. 2005;21(3):195–9.

26. Hutchison JS, et al. Hypothermia therapy after traumatic brain injury in children. N Engl J Med. 2008;358(23):2447–56.

27. Huh JW, Raghupathi R. New concepts in treatment of pediatric traumatic brain injury. Anesthesiol Clin. 2009;27(2):213–40.

28. Muizelaar JP, Lutz HA 3rd, Becker DP. Effect of mannitol on ICP and CBF and correlation with pressure autoregulation in severely head-injured patients. J Neurosurg. 1984;61(4):700–6.

29. Hinson HE, Stein D, Sheth KN. Hypertonic saline and mannitol therapy in critical care neurology. J Intensive Care Med. 2013;28(1):3–11.

30. Kochanek PM, et al. Guidelines for the management of pediatric severe traumatic brain injury, third edition: update of the brain trauma foundation guidelines, executive summary. Pediatr Crit Care Med. 2019;20(3):280–9.

31. Gross-Tsur V, Shinnar S. Convulsive status epilepticus in children. Epilepsia. 1993;34(Suppl 1):S12-20.

32. Wical BS. Neonatal seizures and electrographic analysis: evaluation and outcomes. Pediatr Neurol. 1994;10(4):271–5.

33. Cramer JA, et al. Adverse effects of antiepileptic drugs: a brief overview of important issues. Expert Rev Neurother. 2010;10(6):885–91.

34. Adelson PD, et al. Guidelines for the acute medical management of severe traumatic brain injury in infants, children, and adolescents. Chapter 19. The role of anti-seizure prophylaxis following severe pediatric traumatic brain injury. Pediatr Crit Care Med. 2003;4(3 Suppl):S72–5.

35. Liesemer K, et al. Early post-traumatic seizures in moderate to severe pediatric traumatic brain injury: rates, risk factors, and clinical features. J Neurotrauma. 2011;28(5):755–62.

36. Tilford JM, et al. Variation in therapy and outcome for pediatric head trauma patients. Crit Care Med. 2001;29(5):1056–61.

37. Adelson PD, et al. Guidelines for the acute medical management of severe traumatic brain injury in infants, children, and adolescents. Chapter 16. The use of corticosteroids in the treatment of severe pediatric traumatic brain injury. Pediatr Crit Care Med. 2003;4(3 Suppl):S60–4.

38. Stocchetti N, Maas AI. Traumatic intracranial hypertension. N Engl J Med. 2014;370(22):2121–30.

39. Hirnerschütterung KT, *hirndruck und chirurgische eingriffe bei hirnkrankheiten*. 1901.

40. Cushing H. The establishment of cerebral hernia as a decompressive measure for inaccessible brain tumors: with the description of intramuscular methods of making the bone defect in temporal and occipital regions. Surg Gynecol Obstet. 1905;1:297–314.

41. Taylor A, et al. A randomized trial of very early decompressive craniectomy in children with traumatic brain injury and sustained intracranial hypertension. Childs Nerv Syst. 2001;17(3):154–62.

42. Jagannathan J, et al. Outcome following decompressive craniectomy in children with severe traumatic brain injury: a 10-year single-center experience with long-term follow up. J Neurosurg. 2007;106(4 Suppl):268–75.

43. Csokay A, et al. The importance of very early decompressive craniectomy as a prevention to avoid the sudden increase of intracranial pressure in children with severe traumatic brain swelling (retrospective case series). Childs Nerv Syst. 2012;28(3):441–4.
44. Aarabi B, et al. Outcome following decompressive craniectomy for malignant swelling due to severe head injury. J Neurosurg. 2006;104(4):469–79.
45. von Holst H, Li X, Kleiven S. Increased strain levels and water content in brain tissue after decompressive craniotomy. Acta Neurochir. 2012;154(9):1583–93.
46. Stiver SI. Complications of decompressive craniectomy for traumatic brain injury. Neurosurg Focus. 2009;26(6):E7.
47. Wesson DE, et al. Trends in pediatric and adult bicycling deaths before and after passage of a bicycle helmet law. Pediatrics. 2008;122(3):605–10.
48. Teng SS, Chong S-L. Pediatric traumatic brain injury—a review of management strategies. J Emerg Crit Care Med. 2018;2:2.

Part III

Reconstruction and Rehabilitation

Management of Soft Tissue Defects in the Limbs

11

Salim Saba and Ahmad Oneisi

11.1 Introduction

Pediatric chronically injured limbs present later than 6 weeks following the initial event and necessitate a specialized approach that goes beyond the "proximal-middle-distal third" paradigm that is often employed for acute traumatic injury. As a tertiary referral center, patients are often referred to the American University of Beirut Medical Center many weeks, and even months, following the initial injury. These patients present a unique challenge in that they did not have access to expert care during the early stages of injury. Thus, many present with chronic wounds or inadequate reconstructions that do not provide adequate coverage or bone stability for ambulation.

A great number of our pediatric patient population arrive with little-to-no previous medical records. Moreover, their parents or guardians only have limited ability to accurately recount the numerous interventions previously undertaken. For this reason, it is vital to illicit clinical details in the proper sequence. A good physical examination can also help piece together a telling history that will help the treating surgeon in formulating a coherent treatment plan moving forward.

S. Saba
Division of Plastic and Reconstructive Surgery, University of Kentucky College of Medicine, Kentucky, Lexington, USA
e-mail: samsaba111@hotmail.com

A. Oneisi (✉)
Plastic and Reconstructive Surgery, American University of Beirut Medical Center, Beirut, Lebanon

© Springer Nature Switzerland AG 2023
G. S. Abu-Sittah, J. J. Hoballah (eds.), *The War Injured Child*,
https://doi.org/10.1007/978-3-031-28613-1_11

When evaluating a chronically injured lower extremity in the child, it is important to glean the patient's functional status. Eliciting the time between injury and presentation allows the surgeon to determine how the patient has compensated in response to their newfound disability. In general, the longer the chronicity of the injury, the more deconditioned the musculature in the affected limb may be, especially if ambulation is severely limited. Not only does this impact surgical planning, but it also implies a protracted recovery post-reconstruction. Proper evaluation, preservation, and reconstruction of the soft tissue of the injured upper or lower extremity are of paramount importance in helping mitigate recovery.

11.2 Epidemiology

Despite advancements in warfare, training, and protective equipment, modern rates of military and civilian extremity injuries are comparable to those seen in major conflicts of the twentieth century. Although these injuries contribute to less overall mortality as compared with injuries to the trunk, abdomen, and head, their effects are often severely debilitating [1–3].

During the conflict, children may be victims of crossfire injuries, military ordnances on their homes, improvised explosive devices (IEDs), or unexploded ordnances or landmines [4, 5]. Between 2009 and 2015, 3746 children died, and 7904 were injured as a result of armed conflict within Afghanistan [6]. IEDs and explosive remnants of war accounted for 29% of child casualties in 2015 [6]. According to the US army databases from Iraq and Afghanistan, pediatric casualties represented 5.8–7.1% of all admissions in battlefield medical treatment facilities (MTFs) [7, 8]. In this patient population, extremity injuries were present in 30–40% of cases and included both penetrating and blunt trauma. Among these, soft tissue injuries, traumatic below-knee amputations, and closed femur fractures were the most common diagnoses [9, 10].

A retrospective analysis of blast injuries collected from the UK Joint Theatre Trauma Registry of emergency pediatric admissions identified 295 cases from June 2006 to March 2013 revealing an overall mortality rate of 18.5% [6]. IEDs (68%) represented the most common blast mechanism and accounted for 80% of fatalities, with the lower extremities representing the most commonly injured region, accounting for 31% of total injuries [6].

11.3 Challenges

The main objective of the initial management of combat-related trauma is to provide life-saving, limb-saving, sight-preserving, and visceral organ-preserving care [11]. An ever-increasing number of both military personnel and civilian casualties are now surviving injuries, that a few decades ago would have proved fatal. Reconstructive surgeons are thus faced with progressively more challenging extremity wounds that warrant reconstruction [11]. Lower extremity reconstruction following modern battlefield trauma poses significant challenges for the reconstructive surgeon compared with lower extremity injuries seen in the civilian population [12, 13]. High-energy blast impact from IEDs leads to an extensive zone of injury, which often results in limited donor site options for reconstruction [14, 15].

11.4   Idiosyncrasies of Modern Combat Trauma

Modern warfare injuries are characterized by high-energy trauma, massive tissue loss, multiple concomitant injuries, and gross bacterial contamination [14, 16, 17]. Therefore, the challenge in treating these wounds compared with those occurring in civilian settings is unquestionable [11]. Inadequate perfusion, heavily contaminated open fractures, exposed bone with stripped periosteum, and devitalized tendons add to the complexity of these cases [11, 18]. These injuries often result in significant and detrimental soft and bony tissue loss, and associated trauma sustained to adjacent tissues means that direct closure or local flaps may not always be feasible [1, 19, 20]. Although amputation is inevitable, and even the preferred treatment in certain cases, successful limb salvage with optimal functional recovery can lead to significant improvement in quality of life for pediatric patients, whose potential for successful adaptation following injury is greater than that for adults [21]. With technological advancements, limb salvage has been reported in as high as 93% of patients from recent conflicts with high-energy ballistic injuries [12, 22].

11.5   Timing

Godina demonstrated that failure and complication rates of free-tissue transfer in civilian patients increase if the operation is performed more than 72 h after injury [23]. However, there are significant differences in combat injuries, which can be contraindications to immediate free-tissue transfer [24]. This is often logistically impossible when taking into account the perilous environment and the difficulties and delays that may be encountered in stabilizing, evacuating, or repatriating patients in combat zones [11]. In recent conflicts, the average time from injury on the battlefield to arrival at a local tertiary medical center was 4–10 days [25]. In addition, the subacute treatment allows time for other more serious injuries to be overcome, which is especially important in the treatment of critically ill patients requiring inotropic support [26]. In contrary to the civilian setting, limb soft tissue reconstruction is usually delayed and addressed in the subacute or delayed phase after addressing more serious life-threatening injuries. Certain schools of thought advocate that a subacute or delayed reconstruction may even be ideal for high-energy wounds as the true zone of trauma may not be immediately apparent and may require time to declare itself and that premature attempts at early reconstruction may compromise flap healing as further debridements may be necessary before definitive surgery [27].

In a systematic review of 11 studies, Theodorakopoulou et al. showed positive short-term outcomes for free-flap reconstruction conducted during the subacute and delayed period [11]. Celikoz et al. identified a cohort of 215 patients with lower limb blast injury, treated 7–21 days post-trauma (subacute period) revealing a 91.8% muscle free-flap success rate and full weight bearing at 4 months (foot trauma) and 8.4 months (leg trauma) [28].

11.6   Polytrauma

War-related injuries are often associated with poly-extremity trauma. Because of heavy casualty loads, it is essential that definitive repairs are performed in a time-efficient and reliable manner, e.g., the use of a single-stage or sequential free-flap repair to address large defects [11]. Multiple free flaps in the same patient for multiple limb salvage have demonstrated a significantly higher failure rate but no significant difference in overall complication rate compared with single limb salvage [29]. In a study by Valerio et al., patients who had sustained simultaneous upper and lower extremity injuries underwent reconstructions of both defects during a single operation with a statistically significant increase in the complication rate but a similar overall flap survival and limb salvage rate compared with the single-flap procedures performed by the group [30].

11.7   Pre-operative Evaluation

Assuming that the patient is ambulatory, the examination actually precedes history by noting how the patient ambulates upon entering the office—the presence of a limp, the need for assistive devices such as a walker or crutches, or assistance from a companion. The patient's ability to ambulate and bear weight on the injured limb portends a good outcome in terms of limb salvage even if the patient is in need of moderate assistance. A good history should elicit the mechanism of injury in addition to other associated injuries. It is also important to note all previous interventions as the challenges faced by previous surgeons lend clues for future interventions.

Examination of the injured limb is first done by looking at both the affected and the non-injured limb concomitantly. I generally begin by taking inventory of all parts, including toes, along with surface anatomy. If the foot is involved, I take stock of the forefoot, the in-step, and the heel as each of these weight-bearing surfaces can be reconstructed differently. I also examine all joints, from the toes to the hip, as limited range of motion in any one of these carries with it various degrees of disability. I note differences in length between feet, legs, and thighs. By combining the latter findings with accompanying scar patterns one might be able to infer diaphyseal, symphyseal, or epiphyseal injury.

I examine the patient's ability to range each joint as that additionally provides information on the functionality of the muscle groups that move them. Disability in movement may stem from muscle, tendon, nerve, or injury to any combination of these. Differences in girth in the legs or thighs are usually due either to missing muscle, atrophied muscle, or both. Of course, a good examination of sensory function may lead to a diagnosis of motor nerve injury by association. While Peroneal nerve injury may be compensated by orthotics to brace the ankle joint, Tibial nerve injury is tolerated to a much lesser degree as plantar sensation is compromised along with the powerful drivers of the posterior compartment muscles of the leg.

11.8 Algorithm

We have devised a straightforward classification to help in the management of these limbs. This algorithm is devised to determine the soft tissue and bony components that need to be reconstructed. We additionally take into account prior surgeries in order to determine the local tissue environment that would dictate the use of local versus distant flap options. We propose a systematic approach to their reconstruction.

Once complete stock of lower extremity function is taken, I then classify the chronic war injury of the extremity into one of the following three categories:

1. Simple: missing skin and/or muscle; surrounding soft tissue is soft and supple; local tissue is available for reconstruction.
2. Intermediate: missing or injured nerves and tendons with or without skin and muscle; surrounding soft tissue is partly or wholly scarred, but local or regional tissue is available for coverage; may be associated with a chronic, draining wound, or sinus.
3. Complex: missing or injured bone with or without any other soft tissue components; significant scarring and/or distortion of surrounding tissue precluding any local or regional options for reconstruction; may be associated with a chronic, draining wound, or sinus.

11.9 Adjunct Therapy

Fleming et al. demonstrated the successful use of dermal substitutes, regenerative matrices, and tissue expansion in single-patient case reports, primarily used as an adjunct to traditional flaps for preserving limb length in war-related amputation stumps [31]. While definitive reconstruction is often delayed, extremity wounds could be managed by aggressive debridements and VAC (Vacuum-assisted closure) dressing changes as merely bridging measures. VAC therapy allows the drainage of exudate, removes metalloproteinases that have been shown to delay wound healing, prevents drying, promotes vascularity, reduces edema, and eliminates the need for bulky dressings that need frequent changing [11].

Intraoperative indo-cyanine green laser angiography (ICGLA) has also been used as a guidance tool for complex debridement in heavily contaminated wounds, soft tissue avulsion injuries, amputation stumps, and flap design and assessment [32]. In a retrospective series, intraoperative plans were modified due to perfusion-related issues in 35 out of 186 (18.8%) patients, as detected by ICGLA [24].

11.10 Flap Selection

Pedicled and free flaps have been precious tools in the armamentarium of reconstructive surgeons when treating pediatric war injuries. Sabino et al. reported
10 years of experiences at Walter Reed National Military Medical Center where 359
flaps were performed for war-related extremity trauma (143 free and 216 pedicled
flaps), including poly-extremity trauma and reconstruction, with outcomes comparable to other military and civilian lower extremity reconstruction [33]. In this
series, 55% of flaps were muscle flaps, and 42% were fasciocutaneous flaps with the
most common free muscle flap being the latissimus dorsi (13%), the most common
free fasciocutaneous flap was the anterolateral thigh (11%), the most common pedicled muscle flap was the gastrocnemius (17%), and the most common pedicled
fasciocutaneous flap was the sural flap (6%) [33].

In a patient who is multiply injured and requires amputations, it is especially
important to bear in mind that the integrity of their girdle, truncal, and core musculature will be necessary for future mobility [33]. Subsequently, Latissimus dorsi and
rectus abdominis flaps may not be ideal for amputees, making anterolateral thigh
flaps more appropriate; however, these flaps may often be in the zone of injury of
lower extremity wounds [11].

Some experts advocate the preferential use of fasciocutaneous and perforator
flaps over abdominal or truncal muscle flaps because of preserved core and girdle
strength for future rehabilitation and mobility and reduced rates of infection in certain centers [30, 34].

Yazar and colleagues reported equal outcomes between muscle and fasciocutaneous flaps in terms of flap survival, postoperative infection, osteomyelitis, primary
and overall bone union, and ambulation without crutches [35]. Thus, donor site
morbidity and its effect on physical rehabilitation can become important considerations in flap selection [33].

Many of the local tissues commonly used as the workhorses of extremity reconstruction are often compromised by the extensive zones of injury and traumatic
amputations associated with a modern blast and war injuries [33].

As reconstructive surgeons continue to develop their skills in harvesting perforators and increasingly smaller pedicles with the advent of super microsurgery, we
will undoubtedly be witnessing a shift in the types of free flaps preferentially used
to reconstruct these defects [11].

11.11 Complex Reconstruction

11.11.1   Vascular Injury

Concomitant vascular injuries are common in ballistic lower extremity wounds. In
a recent report, 24% of patients requiring flap coverage for ballistic lower extremity
wounds had concomitant vascular injuries that required emergent repair [36].

Flap coverage was performed at an average of 31 days following vascular repair with an overall flap failure and complication rate of 8% and 31%, respectively, which was comparable to the complication rate of flaps not requiring vascular repair (10% and 28%, respectively) [36].

Vascular repair does not necessarily precede soft tissue coverage; both issues might be addressed simultaneously using flow-through flaps. Ever since Foucher first described the flow-through variant of the radial forearm-free flap in 1984, [37] other flaps such as the rectus abdominus flap, anterolateral thigh flap, temporoparietal fascial flap, and osteocutaneous fibula flap have all been used as a flow-through flap for simultaneous vascular and wound reconstruction [38]. Flow-through flap reconstruction may have higher patency rates than arterial reconstruction alone due to the increased flow across and through the flap [39, 40].

The additional time needed for the distal anastomosis must be balanced against the patient's condition at the time of operation to achieve a potential benefit [38].

Diagnosis of extremity vascular injuries becomes a critical step in pre-operative planning and choosing the recipient's vessels. An end-to-side arterial anastomosis is indicated in patients with single- or two-vessel limb perfusion, where the distal recipient vasculature must be preserved for adequate blood flow to the foot [41, 42].

11.11.2   Bone Defects

It is hard to discuss the approach to soft tissue reconstruction in the chronically injured lower extremity without taking into account other tissue elements including skeletal support. Bones offer the skeletal support which forms the basis of weight bearing, and ultimately ambulation.

Management of bone defects strongly depends on the length of the existing gap with nonvascularized cancellous bone grafts, best used for nonunions or small bone gaps of less than 5 cm, bone lengthening or distraction osteogenesis for defects of 4–8 cm, and vascularized bone grafts with an average healing time of 6 months ideal for defects greater than 5 cm [43].

11.12 Amputation

Although preservation of a fully intact, functional extremity is an ideal endpoint in such injuries, it is important to consider that amputations still form a significant and necessary management option in these patients [44].

With technological advances in resuscitative trauma care and fracture management, reconstructive options have evolved as well, with more injuries salvaged than ever before [21]. This further adds to the importance of attempting limb salvage at the initial encounter. However, according to the Military Extremity Trauma Amputation/Limb Salvage (METALS) study, those treated with amputation had a better functional outcome than limb salvage at 3 years post-injury, with both groups demonstrating moderate to severe physical and psychosocial disability [45].

The concept of "spare-part" surgery, using uninjured tissue from otherwise unsalvageable extremities, can also be applied as a means of minimizing the creation of new thoracoabdominal donor sites, which further optimizes future rehabilitation and recovery [44, 46]. Where full salvage is not possible, the use of free-tissue transfer can prove an invaluable tool for conferring residual limb length and allowing for the creation of a pain-free, sensate, and resilient stump [31, 44].

Because traditional scoring systems such as the Mangled Extremity Severity Score (MESS) fail to accurately predict the outcome of limb salvage in ballistic wounds, the decision to perform an amputation versus limb salvage is reserved until evacuation and transport to an advanced treatment facility [21]. The UK Joint Theatre Trauma Registry (JTTR) was interrogated to identify all lower extremity traumatic amputations sustained in both Iraq and Afghanistan between January 2003 and the end of UK operations in August 2014 revealing 977 casualties and yielding the largest analysis of combat-related traumatic amputations and confirms that they are associated with significant mortality [47]. More importantly, several specific injury characteristics associated with traumatic amputation have been identified that are associated with an increased mortality rate to include a more proximal amputation level, pelvic fracture, and abdominal injury [47].

References

1. Bhandari PS, Mukherjee MK, Maurya S. Reconstructive challenges in war wounds. Indian J Plast Surg. 2012;45(02):332–9.
2. Coupland RM. The role of reconstructive surgery in the management of war wounds. Ann R Coll Surg Engl. 1991;73(1):21.
3. Dougherty AL, Mohrle CR, Galarneau MR, Woodruff SI, Dye JL, Quinn KH. Battlefield extremity injuries in operation Iraqi freedom. Injury. 2009;40(7):772–7.
4. Gurney I. Paediatric casualties during OP TELIC. BMJ Military Health. 2004;150(4):270–2.
5. Matos RI, Holcomb JB, Callahan C, Spinella PC. Increased mortality rates of young children with traumatic injuries at a US army combat support hospital in Baghdad, Iraq, 2004. Pediatrics. 2008;122(5):e959–e66.
6. Thompson DC, Crooks R, Clasper J, Lupu A, Stapley S, Cloke D. The pattern of paediatric blast injury in Afghanistan. J R Army Med Corps. 2017:jramc-2017-000795.
7. Spinella PC, Borgman MA, Azarow KS. Pediatric trauma in an austere combat environment. Crit Care Med. 2008;36(7):S293–S6.
8. Borgman M, Matos RI, Blackbourne LH, Spinella PC. Ten years of military pediatric care in Afghanistan and Iraq. J Trauma Acute Care Surg. 2012;73(6):S509–S13.
9. Burnett MW, Spinella PC, Azarow KS, Callahan CW. Pediatric care as part of the US Army medical mission in the global war on terrorism in Afghanistan and Iraq, December 2001 to December 2004. Pediatrics. 2008;121(2):261–5.
10. Creamer KM, Edwards MJ, Shields CH, Thompson MW, Clifton EY, Adelman W. Pediatric wartime admissions to US military combat support hospitals in Afghanistan and Iraq: learning from the first 2,000 admissions. J Trauma Acute Care Surg. 2009;67(4):762–8.
11. Theodorakopoulou E, Mason KA, Pafitanis G, Ghanem AM, Myers S, Iwuagwu FC. Free-tissue transfer for the reconstruction of war-related extremity injuries: a systematic review of current practice. Mil Med. 2016;181(1):27–34.
12. Geiger S, McCormick F, Chou R, Wandel AG. War wounds: lessons learned from Operation Iraqi Freedom. Plast Reconstr Surg. 2008;122(1):146–53.

13. Kumar AR. Standard wound coverage techniques for extremity war injury. J Am Acad Orthop Surg. 2006;14(10):S62–S5.
14. Kumar AR, Grewal NS, Chung TL, Bradley JP. Lessons from operation Iraqi freedom: successful subacute reconstruction of complex lower extremity battle injuries. Plast Reconstr Surg. 2009;123(1):218–29.
15. Klem C, Sniezek JC, Moore B, Davis MR, Coppit G, Schmalbach C. Microvascular reconstructive surgery in operations Iraqi and enduring freedom: the US military experience performing free flaps in a combat zone. J Trauma Acute Care Surg. 2013;75(2):S228–S32.
16. Kumar A, Harshbarger R, Martin B. Plastic surgery challenges in war wounded. Adv Wound Care. 2010;1:65–9.
17. Tintle SM, Gwinn DE, Andersen RC, Kumar AR. Soft tissue coverage of combat wounds. J Surg Orthop Adv. 2010;19(1):29–34.
18. Huh J, Stinner DJ, Burns TC, Hsu JR, Team LAS. Infectious complications and soft tissue injury contribute to late amputation after severe lower extremity trauma. J Trauma Acute Care Surg. 2011;71(1):S47–51.
19. Sabino J, Franklin B, Patel K, Bonawitz S, Valerio IL. Revisiting the scapular flap: applications in extremity coverage for our US combat casualties. Plast Reconstr Surg. 2013;132(4):577e–85e.
20. Evriviades D, Jeffery S, Cubison T, Lawton G, Gill M, Mortiboy D. Shaping the military wound: issues surrounding the reconstruction of injured servicemen at the Royal Centre for Defence Medicine. Philos Trans R Soc B: Biol Sci. 2011;366(1562):219–30.
21. Brown KV, Ramasamy A, McLeod J, Stapley S, Clasper JC. Predicting the need for early amputation in ballistic mangled extremity injuries. J Trauma Acute Care Surg. 2009;66(4):S93–S8.
22. Spear M. Outcomes of lower extremity injuries sustained during Operation Iraqi Freedom and Operation Enduring Freedom. Plast Surg Nurs. 2009;29(3):155–7.
23. Godina M. Early microsurgical reconstruction of complex trauma of the extremities. Plast Reconstr Surg. 1986;78(3):285–92.
24. Connolly M, Ibrahim ZR, Johnson ON. Changing paradigms in lower extremity reconstruction in war-related injuries. Mil Med Res. 2016;3(1):9.
25. Chattar-Cora D, Perez-Nieves R, McKinlay A, Kunasz M, Delaney R, Lyons R. Operation Iraqi freedom: a report on a series of soldiers treated with free tissue transfer by a plastic surgery service. Ann Plast Surg. 2007;58(2):200–6.
26. Tajsic NB, Husum H. Reconstructive surgery including free flap transfers can be performed in low-resource settings: experiences from a wartime scenario. J Trauma Acute Care Surg. 2008;65(6):1463–7.
27. Yaremchuk MJ, Brumback RJ, Manson PN, Burgess AR, Poka A, Weiland AJ. Acute and definitive management of traumatic osteocutaneous defects of the lower extremity. Plast Reconstr Surg. 1987;80(1):1–14.
28. Çeliköz B, Şengezer M, Işik S, Türegün M, Deveci M, Duman H, et al. Subacute reconstruction of lower leg and foot defects due to high velocity-high energy injuries caused by gunshots, missiles, and land mines. Microsurgery. 2005;25(1):3–15.
29. Valerio I, Sabino J, Thomas S, Tintle S, Fleming M, Shashikant M, et al. Multiple limbs salvaged using tissue transfers in the same casualty: a cohort comparison study chronicling a decade of war-injured patients. Plast Reconstr Surg. 2014;134(2):333–8.
30. Valerio IL, Sabino J, Bevevino A, Tintle SM, Fleming M, Kumar A. Sequential free tissue transfers for simultaneous upper and lower limb salvage. Microsurgery. 2013;33(6):447–53.
31. Fleming ME, O'Daniel A, Bharmal H, Valerio I. Application of the orthoplastic reconstructive ladder to preserve lower extremity amputation length. Ann Plast Surg. 2014;73(2):183–9.
32. Green JM III, Sabino J, Fleming M, Valerio I. Intraoperative fluorescence angiography: a review of applications and outcomes in war-related trauma. Mil Med. 2015;180(suppl_3):37–43.
33. Sabino J, Polfer E, Tintle S, Jessie E, Fleming M, Martin B, et al. A decade of conflict: flap coverage options and outcomes in traumatic war-related extremity reconstruction. Plast Reconstr Surg. 2015;135(3):895–902.
34. Sabino JM, Shashikant MP, Valerio IL. Muscle versus skin or perforator flaps for extremity salvage: is there a difference? Plast Reconstr Surg. 2012;130(5S-1):59.

35. Yazar S, Lin C-H, Lin Y-T, Ulusal AE, Wei F-C. Outcome comparison between free muscle and free fasciocutaneous flaps for reconstruction of distal third and ankle traumatic open tibial fractures. Plast Reconstr Surg. 2006;117(7):2468–75.
36. Casey K, Sabino J, Jessie E, Martin BD, Valerio I. Flap coverage outcomes following vascular injury and repair: chronicling a decade of severe war-related extremity trauma. Plast Reconstr Surg. 2015;135(1):301–8.
37. Foucher G, Van Genechten F, Merle DM, Michon DJ. A compound radial artery forearm flap in hand surgery: an original modification of the Chinese forearm flap. Br J Plast Surg. 1984;37(2):139–48.
38. Grewal NS, Kumar AR, Onsgard CK, Taylor BJ. Simultaneous revascularization and coverage of a complex volar hand blast injury: case report using a contralateral radial forearm flow-through flap. Mil Med. 2008;173(8):801–4.
39. Karp NS, Kasabian AK, Siebert JW, Eidelman Y, Colen S. Microvascular free-flap salvage of the diabetic foot: a 5-year experience. Plast Reconstr Surg. 1994;94(6):834–40.
40. Banis JJ, Richardson J, Derr JJ, Acland R. Microsurgical adjuncts in salvage of the ischemic and diabetic lower extremity. Clin Plast Surg. 1992;19(4):881–93.
41. Albertengo JB, Rodriguez A, Buncke HJ, Hall EJ. A comparative study of flap survival rates in end-to-end and end-to-side microvascular anastomosis. Plast Reconstr Surg. 1981;67(2):194–9.
42. Godina M. Preferential use of end-to-side arterial anastomoses in free flap transfers. Plast Reconstr Surg. 1979;64(5):673–82.
43. Parrett BM, Pribaz JJ. Lower extremity reconstruction. Rev Med Clin Condes. 2010;21(1):66–75.
44. Ghali S, Harris PA, Khan U, Pearse M, Nanchahal J. Leg length preservation with pedicled fillet of foot flaps after traumatic amputations. Plast Reconstr Surg. 2005;115(2):498–505.
45. Frisch HM, Andersen CRC, Mazurek CMT, Ficke CJR, Keeling CJJ, Pasquina CPF, et al. The military extremity trauma amputation/limb salvage (METALS) study: outcomes of amputation versus limb salvage following major lower-extremity trauma. JBJS. 2013;95(2):138–45.
46. Flurry M, Melissinos EG, Livingston CK. Composite forearm free fillet flaps to preserve stump length following traumatic amputations of the upper extremity. Ann Plast Surg. 2008;60(4):391–4.
47. Webster CE, Clasper J, Stinner DJ, Eliahoo J, Masouros SD. Characterization of lower extremity blast injury. Mil Med. 2018;183(9–10):e448–e53.

The Role of Microsurgery in Pediatric War Injuries

12

Reem A. Karami and Amir E. Ibrahim

12.1   Introduction

War is among the 10 leading causes of death in children around the world. More than 6 million children have been injured or permanently disabled by war over the past decade [1]. Children are particularly a high-risk population for injury due to inherent physical and physiologic vulnerability [2]. It is unfortunate that these injuries are not only civilian injuries but sometimes military injuries. Children are often recruited for military duty due to their helplessness and emotional immaturity [3].

Like adults, children are prone to penetrating vascular injuries, head and neck injuries, and injuries to the thorax and abdomen. Injury to the extremities remains to be a very common form of injury in war [4]. Limb injury has implications for a growing child increasing the need for revision surgery compared to adults. Battlefield trauma and war injuries are significantly different than civilian trauma. These injuries usually cause extensive soft tissue defects, bone fractures, and injury to nerves, tendons, and vessels that pose an overwhelming reconstructive challenge. The surgeon needs to account for wound contamination and large zones of injury with extensive microvascular compromise [5].

Over the past decade, there has been a paradigm shift in trauma care. With better damage control to stabilize critically injured patients, more wounded patients are being evaluated for reconstruction. This improved survival rate, in the setting of increasing severity of injuries, has contributed to an increase in the complexity of the wounds. This translated to an increase in the complexity of treatment modalities in war injured patients [6]. The reconstructive surgeons are often faced with extensive wounds and significant soft tissue and bone loss which drives them to consider procedures that were previously concerning. The aim of treatment no longer focuses

R. A. Karami · A. E. Ibrahim (✉)
Department of Surgery – Division of Plastic and Reconstructive Surgery, American University of Beirut Medical Center, Beirut, Lebanon
e-mail: ai12@aub.edu.lb

© Springer Nature Switzerland AG 2023
G. S. Abu-Sittah, J. J. Hoballah (eds.), *The War Injured Child*,
https://doi.org/10.1007/978-3-031-28613-1_12

solely on life, but a functional reconstruction is becoming a more feasible and realistic endpoint [7].

With advances in microsurgical practice, the role of free tissue transfer in ballistic trauma is rising. This reconstructive option is able to cover large defects with well-vascularized tissue in a single procedure. With microsurgical procedures, open fractures can be covered, enabling a faster recovery and preserving future limb function. A major advantage is that it allows for the transfer of unharmed tissue distant from the zone of injury [8]. The problem is that in a war scenario, it may be difficult to access a surgical service and equipment to perform these procedures. But even in a low-resource setting, a skilled surgeon should be able to perform these procedures; this is where experience becomes extremely relevant [9].

While free tissue transfer is established in the adult age group, its application in the pediatric age group is somehow recent. Anxiety over the feasibility of microsurgery in children remains. There is concern about small vessel size and vasospasm making the anastomosis more difficult and increasing flap failure rates. Limited donor site and donor site morbidity and growth implications should also be considered [10]. Ballistic trauma and subsequent injury to the microvasculature further add to this anxiety. Nevertheless, over the past decade, pediatric microsurgery has proven to have high success rates, making it a reliable reconstructive option [11].

12.2   Location of the Defect

Understanding the injury pattern and characteristics of the ballistic trauma will help guide the clinical decision in the form of reconstruction to be used. It is understood that head and neck trauma is an extremely common war injury in the pediatric age group. This is followed by extremity trauma, and thoracic and abdominal injuries [4].

12.2.1 Upper Extremity

The most common form of injury that might necessitate microsurgical reconstruction is extremity injuries. Compared to adults, children have a higher rate of upper extremity injuries. These vary from simple fractures to more complex traumatic amputations [12]. Mangled upper extremities are particularly challenging. Mutilation of the extremity with high-impact trauma, blast, and crush is associated not only with bony fractures but also with extensive soft tissue loss. Due to the severity of these injuries, microsurgical tissue transfer is often required not only for coverage but also to ensure a good functional outcome. Limb salvage is not the only concern here. Attempts at a functional limb restoration should be fully exhausted [13]. Prior to the era of microsurgery, preservation of mangled upper extremities

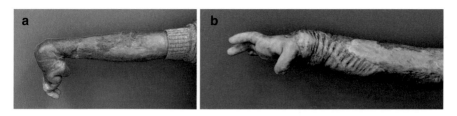

Fig. 12.1 (**a**) A 13-year-old boy with severe wrist contracture. (**b**) After release, wrist fusion, and reconstruction

was not a possibility. With the refinement of surgical technique, a more sophisticated reconstruction is possible (Fig. 12.1). Free flaps can be designed to include multiple types of tissue. Functional muscle transfer has a definite role in the restoration of upper extremity function, especially for recovering finger, wrist, elbow, and shoulder flexion and extension. This can be achieved by the transfer of innervated gracilis of latissimus dorsi flaps [14, 15].

12.2.2 Lower Extremity

Lower extremity injuries are less common than in adults and are mostly seen in landmine strikes [4]. As a general concept, the lower leg has a paucity of soft tissue and so tolerates trauma poorly. Trauma to this area inadvertently leads to soft tissue loss often needing free tissue coverage. The need for free tissue transfer becomes more imminent in cases of Gustilo type IIIB and IIIC open fractures. Conversely, the thigh has a good amount of muscle and soft tissue which allows for local flap coverage as opposed to free tissue transfer [16]. The foot and ankle also need special consideration as they are not amendable to reconstruction with grafts, especially in young children because of the need for weight bearing and free movement of joints and tendons. Local flaps in the foot are small in size rendering them inadequate for coverage of larger defects [17].

Another important issue with the lower extremities is bony growth. Injury to the growth plate is often problematic creating various degrees of growth disturbances. Limb length inequality and angular deformity are sequelae in the future. This issue is further ameliorated in younger children rather than adolescents because of more years of continued growth. Therefore, preservation of the growth plate becomes essential. Microsurgical physeal transfer, even though difficult to achieve, is necessary to allow for longitudinal growth [18].

Complex lower extremity reconstruction requires proper preoperative planning. Even though a single-staged reconstruction is ideal, it may not be practical depending on the situation.

Finally, in the setting of traumatic amputation, free tissue transfers are used to cover the amputation stump. In a growing child, skin grafts and local flaps for stump closure are less optimal choices, as they frequently require revisions. Reliable and durable coverage is the epitome to help improve the quality of life of the patient and decrease ulcerations and complications of the stump [19].

12.2.3 Head and Neck

The vast majority of microsurgical reconstruction of head and neck defects occur after the oncologic resection of neoplasms. There is a limited role of free tissue transfer in traumatic head and neck reconstruction [20].

Most large traumatic head and neck defects in a war setting are actually the result of major burns. Although skin grafts, local flaps, and pedicled flaps are the mainstay of burn reconstruction, they have their limitations in certain anatomic areas [10]. This is readily apparent in anterior neck defects. Anterior neck burns can be covered by skin grafts or by skin substitutes. But often in children, normal skin grows faster than these grafts increasing the risk of contracture and subsequent failure of the reconstruction. Free tissue transfer allows versatile and pliable tissue to be introduced into a heavily burned area. The aim of the reconstruction here is not only to restore esthetic appearance but to also maintain function and range of motion [21].

Even though the majority of free flap reconstruction of burns is used in the delayed setting, for contracture release, its use in the acute setting is also doable. In cases of exposed vital structures such as nerves, vessels, bone, and cartilage, free tissue transfer becomes essential. In addition, early coverage will decrease morbidity, and hospitalization time and will allow for earlier rehabilitation and an eventual better functional recovery [22].

The downside of microsurgical tissue transfer in head and neck reconstruction is the inability to bring in thin tissue with similar thickness to the native facial skin (Fig. 12.2). Prelamination and prefabrication of flaps have been proposed to deal with this issue, but unfortunately, this is not possible in the setting of acute war injuries.

12.2.4 Thorax and Abdomen

The role of microsurgery in the reconstruction of chest and abdominal defects in the acute setting is limited. Due to the abundance of local tissue and muscles, the majority of defects can be closed by pedicled myocutaneous flaps with or without synthetic mesh. Free tissue transfer is infrequent and reserved for situations where no local options are available or in cases of local flap failure [23]. It may also be used in areas where pedicled flaps reach with difficulties, such as the lower thorax and upper epigastric areas. The paucity of local tissue and the ribcage rigidity make local flap mobilization difficult [24]. In general, free tissue transfer is mostly done as a delayed form of reconstruction and is rarely used in the acute war setting.

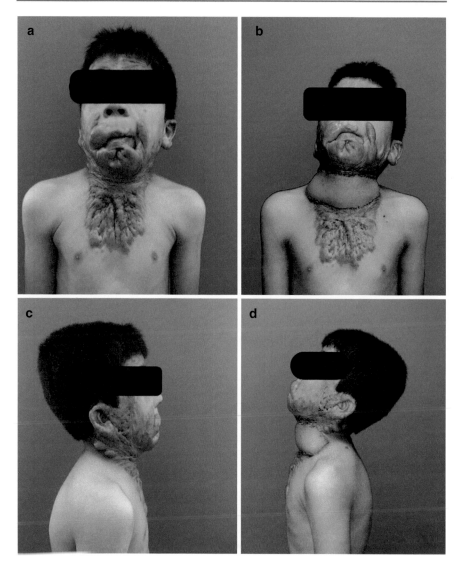

Fig. 12.2 (**a**) A 10-year-old boy with severe neck contracture. The patient had undergone multiple previous release and skin grafting, intralesional steroid injections, and CO_2 laser resurfacing. (**b**) Inhibited full neck extension. American University of Beirut Medical Center, (**c**) After release and reconstruction with a free fasciocutaneous ALT flap. (**d**) Full extension achieved

12.3   Timing of Reconstruction

The timing of reconstruction has long been a controversial topic. The controversy is even more when considering pediatric patients. Godina's landmark paper in 1986 suggested that early flap coverage, within 72 hours, improved outcomes. Coverage in the subacute period, 72 hours to 90 days, had the highest complication and flap failure rates [25]. Three decades after Godinas work, with advances in wound management and microsurgical technique, it seems that reconstructions in the subacute period have an improved success rate. Many studies show that the initial acute period can be extended to 10 days [26]. This is especially important in a war setting since it is not always possible to operate early on. It takes time to transfer patients from the combat zone to a well-equipped trauma center. While the patients await transfer, temporizing interventions such as negative pressure wound therapy can be installed. This influential tool in reconstructive surgery has significantly improved since the time of Godina and has aided in the care of traumatic wounds [27]. If the setting allows, early emergent free flaps can also be an option. This approach will decrease hospital stay, the future need for revision surgeries, and most importantly shortens the period of immobilization [28].

All of these studies were done on adults. The data can be extrapolated to the pediatric age group. The rate of flap loss and flap-related complications in pediatric patients was also lower if the reconstruction was performed within the first 7 days of injury [29]. The basic principle is the same. It is universally accepted that aggressive early debridement, external fixation, early soft tissue coverage with well-vascularized tissue then delayed bone reconstruction are the gold standard. Selecting the proper time for coverage depends on interdependent local and general factors. Surgeon experience and surgical team preparation also play a role.

Delaying reconstruction in the lower extremity is tolerated much better than in the upper extremities. In the upper extremity, prolonged immobilization will probably result in joint stiffness and tendon adhesions. This is why earlier reconstruction is recommended in upper extremity reconstruction [30]. In any case of delay, extensive physical therapy and mobilization should be done to maintain joint motion.

12.4 Choice of Flap

12.4.1 Myocutaneous Flaps

Myocutaneous flaps are ideal when you are reconstructing a large three-dimensional defect. Muscle is able to provide bulk to obliterate dead space. It is also extremely well vascularized and is indicated in heavily contaminated wounds where they provide better antibiotic delivery and better control of bacterial inoculation [31].

The most commonly used free muscle flap in children is the latissimus dorsi (LD) [32]. The LD is a reliable muscle with a reliable blood supply and little anatomic variation. The thoracodorsal artery is of good caliber even in smaller children. The pedicle is also long providing some flexibility in surgery and most importantly allowing the anastomosis to be performed outside the zone of injury without the need for vein grafts [33].

An important thing to be taken into consideration is donor site morbidity. Even though many report no donor site morbidity with the LD, others opt for partial muscle harvesting. Complete removal of the latissimus dorsi muscle may impact chest and shoulder development causing shoulder imbalance. This is why partial preservation of the muscle might be somewhat beneficial [34].

The second most commonly used muscle flap in pediatrics is the rectus abdominus muscle. Again, reasons for its use include consistent and familiar anatomy. The downside is donor site morbidity [35].

The musculocutaneous anterolateral thigh flap, including the vastus lateralis muscle, is also a workhorse flap. The main advantage is easy harvesting and low donor site morbidity. Harvesting can be done in the supine position, limiting the need for repositioning and subsequently operative time. It has a long pedicle with large-sized vessels [36]. Most importantly it can be used as a flow-through flap, which can be useful in cases of ischemic limbs with significant soft tissue loss. The flap can be used to re-establish distal flow and provide coverage at the same time [37].

12.4.2 Fasciocutaneous Flaps

As microsurgical practice is progressing, there has been a shift from concerns about flap survival to concerns about donor site morbidity. When the conditions allow, the use of fasciocutaneous flaps and perforator flaps is advocated. Fasciocutaneous flaps are used for coverage of superficial wounds where no bulk is needed. They are also useful in contour resurfacing. They can be tailored to the defect size. Most importantly they provide an excellent surface for gliding tendons and joints. This is especially important when staged reconstruction is planned; they are easily reelevated to allow tendon transfers and bone grafting [38]. In children, the most commonly used fasciocutaneous flaps were the radial forearm, the groin flap, and the scapular and parascapular flaps [32].

In pediatric patients, fasciocutaneous flaps are associated with a higher rate of debulking surgeries, especially when used to reconstruct foot and ankle defects [17]. Ultimately the reconstructive surgeon must be capable of performing both musculocutaneous and fasciocutaneous flaps depending on the indication.

12.4.3 Perforator Flaps

Microsurgical procedures in children are difficult as is without including the tedious perforator dissection. Many surgeons shy away from perforator flaps in pediatrics. Recent studies show that perforator dissection does not add substantially to the difficulty of the case or duration. Therefore, if one takes into account the decreased donor site morbidity perforator flap becomes a reasonable option [39]. Therefore, the question is no longer whether or not microsurgical procedures can be performed in children, but rather which donor site is the least morbid yet is still able to fulfill the needs of the wound and the patient [40].

Perforator flaps have plenty of advantages including having a sizable source vessel (Fig. 12.3). Proper dissection also provides long pedicle length allowing the

Fig. 12.3 Fasciocutaneous ALT flap based on one perforator

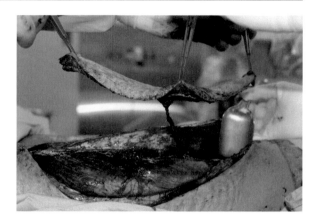

anastomosis to be performed outside of the zone of injury. As in adults, these are very reliable flaps that are often the primary choice in soft tissue reconstruction. The anterolateral thigh flap, the thoracodorsal artery perforator flap, and the deep inferior epigastric artery perforator flap were among the most commonly used flaps [32].

12.4.4 Bone Flaps and Physeal Transfer

In a war zone, the main initial concern is wound coverage rather than bony reconstruction. Management of bone loss in mangled extremities continues to challenge the reconstructive surgeon. Different practices have been described to manage these severe open fractures. Most commonly, early aggressive debridement, skeletal stabilization with an external fixator, and early wound coverage with a flap followed by staged bony reconstruction is performed [8]. Another less popular alternative is a single-staged reconstruction. This has the advantage of a single surgery proving structural stability and promoting a faster bony union. Because the procedure is done early, vessel scaring and inflammation is prevented. With better quality vessels the microanastomosis should become easier [41].

The ideal bone should be vascularized providing osteoinductive, osteoconductive, and osteoprogenitor elements. The vascularized fibula is the most commonly used bone. It can be used to reconstruct long bones and head and neck defects. The resorption rate is relatively low, it provides good strength and should resist infection [42].

Special consideration in pediatric patients is growth. In case of any injury to the growth plate lack of symmetric growth will lead to limb length discrepancy and progressive functional impairment. Vascularized physeal and epiphyseal transfer is possible and allows the potential for future longitudinal growth [43].

The need for flap debulking in general has decreased with the use of thin perforator flaps. Nevertheless, in areas where the native skin is thin such as the hand, foot, anterior leg, and the head and neck area flap debulking becomes essential. The two most common methods for that is direct excision and liposuction, both of which if performed properly and at the correct timing, could be safe procedures [44].

12.5 Radiographic Evaluation

With the extraordinary advances in the field of radiographic imaging, it has become part of the routine practice to obtain preoperative imaging assessment in reconstructive microsurgical cases. Particularly, computed tomography angiography (CTA) has been increasingly employed. Magnetic resonance angiography (MRA) is also another option, with less exposure to both intravenous contrast and radiation [45]. Other sound options are ultrasound and the handheld doppler [46]. In a conflict zone where resources are limited these two options may come in handy.

Generally speaking, preoperative imaging will help map perforators and subsequently shorten operative time and increase the efficacy of flap harvest. Specifically, for high-energy trauma patients, imaging becomes essential to assess not only perforators but recipient's vessels. Screening for arterial injury and aneurysmal pathologies is essential [47].

12.6 Vessel Size and Vasospasm

Surgeons were initially hesitant to perform free flaps on pediatric patients due to the minute vessel diameter and vessel spasticity. Initially, Gilbert suggested that the minimum diameter to perform a safe microanastomosis was 0.7 mm, stating that smaller vessels will create a technical limitation [48]. With skill improvement and the development of ultradelicate microinstruments, supermicrosurgery is being done on vessel sizes between 0.3 and 0.8 mm [49]. This means that surgical technique is not as challenging as it once was. The initial concerns of feasibility fade away. Another important thing is that the relative size of the pedicle vessels compared to the size of the body is larger in children than in adults [39]. This is why body mass index should be considered rather than just chronologic age [35]. Perhaps it is not only the vessel diameter that matters. Pediatric patients inherently have thinner vessel walls making anastomosis more demanding [50].

The true issue with pediatric microvasculature is spasms. Vasospasm is vasoconstriction of the vasculature that can be encountered anytime during the microanastomosis, which is resistant to mechanical dilatation and causes a significant reduction of blood flow [51]. Pediatric vessels are more prone to spasms and so vessel dissection should be kept as minimal as possible to avoid any vessel trauma [52]. Others suggested harvesting a cuff of muscle with the perforator during perforator dissection to minimize vasospasm [17].

It is also reasonable to use local vasodilators such as papaverine and lidocaine. It is really important to control body temperature and pain post-op to help decrease vasospasm [53]. An upside to pediatric vasculature is that since pediatric patients do not suffer from atherosclerosis, peripheral vascular disease, hypertension, diabetes, and smoking, their vessels are pristine and ideal for free tissue transfer [54].

The problem with traumatic war injuries is that often the vasculature is damaged because of the high-energy trauma. This is why it is recommended to perform the anastomosis outside of the zone of injury. There is an inflammatory response in the surrounding soft tissue beyond the margins of the wound that result in perivascular changes in the blood vessels. There is clear-cut margin for the zone of injury at it is difficult to define but it is generally recommended to do an extensive proximal dissection [55]. A tool that might help assess the quality of the vessels is a visual assessment of pulsatile flow [56]. If the pedicle is not long enough, vein grafts may be needed to help stay outside to zone of injury.

12.7   Anesthesia Time

Without question, microsurgical procedures have a long operative time. The time does differ substantially from adults. Because of the heterogeneity of the cases, it is difficult to give an average operative time. Simple fasciocutaneous flaps will take less time than cases that require bony reconstruction [54].

Children can tolerate anesthesia as well as adults. Even though some reports show that increased anesthesia time in pediatrics might have an effect on developmental and behavioral disorders, no conclusion could be drawn about causality [57]. Laryngospasm and airway complications are also something to consider in pediatric patients undergoing prolonged general anesthesia [58].

In the combat zone, where resources are limited, the use of regional anesthesia can be cost-effective. Regional anesthesia is safe and offers the benefit of intra- and postoperative pain control. Specifically, in cases of free tissue transfer, with regional block, there is an increase in circulatory blood flow, maintenance of normal body temperature, and a decrease in the systemic stress response [59]. All these factors improve inflow to the flap and could help decrease vasospasm.

A combination of general and regional anesthesia can be done. When the effect of general anesthesia is over and systemic neurogenous stimuli increase in the early postoperative period, it is wise to have regional anesthesia control to decrease pain and vasospasm [60].

12.8   Flap Outcomes

Reports about flap success rates in children in the literature range between 62 and 100%. The most common cause of flap failure is venous and arterial thrombosis, followed by kinking of the pedicle and vasospasm. Overall flap failure rate averages at 5.01% [61]. This is slightly higher than failure rates in adults which average at 3%. In cases of reexploration, flap salvage occurs on average in two out of three cases explored, which is comparable to the adult population [50].

Without a doubt, microsurgical tissue transfer after blast injury has higher complications than straightforward flaps for all of the above-mentioned reasons. Controlling a number of factors can help improve flap outcomes. The pearls of a successful reconstruction are early aggressive debridement and staying away from the zone of injury. In general, the surgeon must be comfortable with performing flaps in trauma patients. Properly selecting a flap that the surgeons are comfortable with is also crucial.

12.9   Postoperative Anticoagulation

The routine use of anticoagulation postoperatively is controversial. Although over the past 30 years microsurgeons have been using anticoagulation the protocols vary widely. Even though numerous studies have attempted to come up with a protocol, no singular method has been proven to be effective [62]. The use of intraoperative heparin irrigation seems to have a positive effect on the flap with minimal risk to the patient. By consensus, thrombolytics are used in case flow is not immediately reestablished or in case of a difficult anastomosis where revision was needed. Postoperative treatment with aspirin or heparin remains to be controversial [63]. Some authors advocate the use of systemic prophylactic heparin, stating that it might have a role in decreasing postoperative thrombosis [64].

With the current data, an evidence-based decision cannot be made. It remains that surgical technique is the main factor that will affect the outcome. The use of anticoagulation to complement the anastomosis is a matter of personal choice and experience.

12.10   Complications

When considering at the success rate of free tissue transfer, it is not only flap survival that matters. It is important to look at the complications and assess the quality of life improvement. Complications in general can be divided into early and late in terms of timing. Another way to look at things is minor and major complications with respect to the overall outcome. In general, trauma patients have a higher rate of complications as compared to post-oncologic and congenital reconstructions [54].

12.10.1   Early Complications

Other than flap failure, early complications include partial flap loss, tip necrosis, hematomas, infection, and osteomyelitis. Partial flap loss and wound breakdown are often treated with debridement and local wound care. Wound infection is a common complication in this category of war trauma patients [65]. Whether soft tissue infection or osteomyelitis, early debridement, and coverage are critical for prevention. In case infection develops post-op, the initial treatment is aggressive antibiotic therapy [66]. Soft tissue reconstruction has a crucial role in the healing of the severely injured lower extremity. Even though initially it was thought that muscle flaps are more vascularized and so a wiser option for fighting infection, more recently it was shown that fasciocutaneous flaps have a similar efficacy [67].

12.10.2 Late Complications

Chronic osteomyelitis with sinus tract formation, bulky flaps, pressure ulcers, hypertrophic scarring, and limb length discrepancy are all late complications of free tissue transfer. In general flaps to the foot have a higher complication due to the inherent anatomic location [61]. The location of the foot puts it at increased pressure from both ambulation and weight bearing and from footwear, making it more prone to developing pressure ulcers [52].

Chronic osteomyelitis is a complex entity to treat. It happens to be common in post-traumatic injuries with reported rates between 4 and 64%. Even though a single-staged procedure is ideal, frequently multiple debridements, local and systemic antibiotic therapy, and dead space obliteration with vascularized tissue are the standard [68].

The need for flap debulking, in general, has decreased with the use of thin perforator flaps. Nevertheless, in areas where the native skin is thin such as the hand, foot, anterior leg, and the head and neck area flap debulking becomes essential. The two major methods for that are direct excision or liposuction, both of which if performed properly and at the correct timing, could be safe procedures [44].

Overall, late complications can be avoided with careful preoperative planning and attention to detail.

12.11 Special Consideration: Below the Age of 2 Years

Younger children below 2 years of age pose a special challenge. The decision to proceed to free tissue transfer in this population weighs heavily on both parents and surgeons. It is important before embarking on these procedures to speak to the parents and allow them to be part of the decision-making process because any failure of the flap will leave the child with a donor site defect that will be present for the rest of their lives.

There is a paucity of reports about free tissue transfer in children below the age of 2 years. In one series, it was reported that the vessels of these younger children are not more delicate than those of older children. The success rate was reported at 98% putting surgeons more at ease for performing these procedures [69]. Again, flap survival depends mostly on surgeon technique and skills rather than vessel size.

References

1. Patton GC, Coffey C, Sawyer SM, Viner RM, Haller DM, Bose K, et al. Global patterns of mortality in young people: a systematic analysis of population health data. Lancet. 2009;374(9693):881–92.
2. Carlson LC, Lafta R, Al-Shatari S, Stewart BT, Burnham G, Kushner AL. Pediatric injury during conflict and prolonged insecurity in Iraq from 2003–2014. Surgery. 2016;160(2):493–500.
3. Ursano RJ, Shaw JA. Children of war and opportunities for peace. JAMA. 2007;298(5):567–8.

4. Hargrave JM, Pearce P, Mayhew ER, Bull A, Taylor S. Blast injuries in children: a mixed-methods narrative review. BMJ paediatrics open. 2019;3(1).
5. Murray CK, Obremskey WT, Hsu JR, Andersen RC, Calhoun JH, Clasper JC, et al. Prevention of infections associated with combat-related extremity injuries. J Trauma Acute Care Surg. 2011;71(2):S235–S57.
6. Holcomb JB, Stansbury LG, Champion HR, Wade C, Bellamy RF. Understanding combat casualty care statistics. J Trauma Acute Care Surg. 2006;60(2):397–401.
7. Theodorakopoulou E, Mason KA, Pafitanis G, Ghanem AM, Myers S, Iwuagwu FC. Free-tissue transfer for the reconstruction of war-related extremity injuries: a systematic review of current practice. Mil Med. 2016;181(1):27–34.
8. Sabino JM, Slater J, Valerio IL. Plastic surgery challenges in war wounded I: flap-based extremity reconstruction. Adv Wound Care. 2016;5(9):403–11.
9. Tajsic NB, Husum H. Reconstructive surgery including free flap transfers can be performed in low-resource settings: experiences from a wartime scenario. J Trauma Acute Care Surg. 2008;65(6):1463–7.
10. Izadpanah A, Moran SL. Pediatric microsurgery: a global overview. Clin Plast Surg. 2017;44(2):313–24.
11. Devaraj V, Kay S, Batchelor A, Yates A. Microvascular surgery in children. J Plast Reconstr Aesthet Surg. 1991;44(4):276–80.
12. Quintana DA, Jordan FB, Tuggle DW, Mantor PC, Tunell WP. The spectrum of pediatric injuries after a bomb blast. J Pediatr Surg. 1997;32(2):307–11.
13. Ng ZY, Salgado CJ, Moran SL, Chim H. Soft tissue coverage of the mangled upper extremity. Seminars in plastic surgery. Thieme Medical Publishers; 2015.
14. Terzis JK, Kostopoulos VK. Free muscle transfer in posttraumatic plexopathies: part III. The hand. Plast Reconstr Surg. 2009;124(4):1225–36.
15. Terzis JK, Kostopoulos VK. Free muscle transfer in posttraumatic plexopathies part II: the elbow. Hand. 2010;5(2):160–70.
16. Laine JC, Cherkashin A, Samchukov M, Birch JG, Rathjen KE. The management of soft tissue and bone loss in type IIIB and IIIC pediatric open tibia fractures. J Pediatr Orthop. 2016;36(5):453–8.
17. Acar MA, Güleç A, Aydin BK, Erkoçak ÖF, Yilmaz G, Şenaran H. Reconstruction of foot and ankle defects with a free anterolateral thigh flap in pediatric patients. J Reconstr Microsurg. 2015;31(03):225–32.
18. Bibbo C, Ehrlich DA, Kovach SJ III. Reconstruction of the pediatric lateral malleolus and physis by free microvascular transfer of the proximal fibular physis. J Foot Ankle Surg. 2015;54(5):994–1000.
19. Yıldırım S, Calikapan GT, Akoz T. Reliable option for reconstruction of amputation stumps: the free anterolateral thigh flap. Microsurgery: Official Journal of the International Microsurgical Society and the European Federation of Societies for Microsurgery. 2006;26(5):386–90.
20. Upton J, Guo L. Pediatric free tissue transfer: a 29-year experience with 433 transfers. Plast Reconstr Surg. 2008;121(5):1725–37.
21. Seth AK, Friedstat JS, Orgill DP, Pribaz JJ, Halvorson EG. Microsurgical burn reconstruction. Clin Plast Surg. 2017;44(4):823–32.
22. Ibrahim A, Skoracki R, Goverman J, Sarhane K, Parham C, Abu-Sittah G. Microsurgery in the burn population–a review of the literature. Ann Burns Fire Disasters. 2015;28(1):39.
23. Losken A, Thourani V, Carlson G, Jones G, Culbertson J, Miller J, et al. A reconstructive algorithm for plastic surgery following extensive chest wall resection. Br J Plast Surg. 2004;57(4):295–302.
24. Netscher DT, Baumholtz MA. Chest reconstruction: I. Anterior and anterolateral chest wall and wounds affecting respiratory function. Plastic Reconstruct Surg. 2009;124(5):240e–52e.
25. Godina M. Early microsurgical reconstruction of complex trauma of the extremities. Orthopedic Trauma Directions. 2006;4(05):29–35.
26. Lee Z-H, Stranix JT, Rifkin WJ, Daar DA, Anzai L, Ceradini DJ, et al. Timing of microsurgical reconstruction in lower extremity trauma: an update of the Godina paradigm. Plast Reconstr Surg. 2019;144(3):759–67.

27. Colen DL, Colen LB, Levin LS, Kovach SJ. Godina's principles in the twenty-first century and the evolution of lower extremity trauma reconstruction. J Reconstr Microsurg. 2018;34(08):563–71.
28. Georgescu AV, Ivan O. Emergency free flaps. Microsurgery. 2003;23(3):206–16.
29. Rinker B, Valerio IL, Stewart DH, Pu LL, Vasconez HC. Microvascular free flap reconstruction in pediatric lower extremity trauma: a 10-year review. Plast Reconstr Surg. 2005;115(6):1618–24.
30. Lister G, Scheker L. Emergency free flaps to the upper extremity. J Hand Surg Am. 1988;13(1):22–8.
31. McCraw J, Vasconez L. Musculocutaneous flaps: principles. Clin Plast Surg. 1980;7(1):9–13.
32. Claes KE, Roche NA, Opsomer D, De Wolf EJ, Sommeling CE, Van Landuyt K. Free flaps for lower limb soft tissue reconstruction in children: systematic review. Reconstructive & Aesthetic Surgery: Journal of Plastic; 2019.
33. Banic A, Wulff K. Latissimus dorsi free flaps for total repair of extensive lower leg injuries in children. Plast Reconstr Surg. 1987;79(5):769–75.
34. Chiang Y-C, Jeng S-F, Yeh M-C, Liu Y-T, Chen H-T, Wei F-C. Free tissue transfer for leg reconstruction in children. Br J Plast Surg. 1997;50(5):335–42.
35. Momeni A, Lanni M, Levin LS, Kovach SJ. Microsurgical reconstruction of traumatic lower extremity defects in the pediatric population. Plast Reconstr Surg. 2017;139(4):998–1004.
36. F-c W, Jain V, Celik N, H-c C, Chuang D, Lin C-h. Have we found an ideal soft-tissue flap? An experience with 672 anterolateral thigh flaps. Plast Reconstr Surg. 2002;109(7):2219–26. discussion 27-30
37. Yildirim S, Gideroğlu K, Aköz T. Anterolateral thigh flap: ideal free flap choice for lower extremity soft-tissue reconstruction. J Reconstr Microsurg. 2003;19(04):225–34.
38. Saint-Cyr M, Wong C, Buchel EW, Colohan S, Pederson WC. Free tissue transfers and replantation. Plastic Reconstruct Surg. 2012;130(6):858e–78e.
39. Van Landuyt K, Hamdi M, Blondeel P, Tonnard P, Verpaele A, Monstrey S. Free perforator flaps in children. Plast Reconstr Surg. 2005;116(1):159–69.
40. Arnez ZM, Hanel DP. Free tissue transfer for reconstruction of traumatic limb injuries in children. Microsurgery. 1991;12(3):207–15.
41. Yazar S, Lin C-H, Wei F-C. One-stage reconstruction of composite bone and soft-tissue defects in traumatic lower extremities. Plast Reconstr Surg. 2004;114(6):1457–66.
42. Karami RA, Ghieh FM, Chalhoub RS, Saghieh SS, Lakkis SA, Ibrahim AE. Reconstruction of composite leg defects post-war injury. Int Orthop. 2019;43(12):2681–90.
43. Innocenti M, Delcroix L, Manfrini M, Ceruso M, Capanna R. Vascularized proximal fibular epiphyseal transfer for distal radial reconstruction. JBJS. 2004;86(7):1504–11.
44. Kim TG, Choi MK. Secondary contouring of flaps. Arch Plast Surg. 2018;45(4):319.
45. Chang EI, Chu CK, Chang EI. Advancements in imaging technology for microvascular free tissue transfer. J Surg Oncol. 2018;118(5):729–35.
46. Nahabedian MY, Patel KM. Maximizing the use of the handheld Doppler in autologous breast reconstruction. Clin Plast Surg. 2011;38(2):213–8.
47. Redmond JM, Levy BA, Dajani KA, Cass JR, Cole PA. Detecting vascular injury in lower-extremity orthopedic trauma: the role of CT angiography. Orthopedics. 2008;31(8)
48. Gilbert A. Reconstruction of congenital hand defects with microvascular toe transfers. Hand Clin. 1985;1(2):351–60.
49. Koshima I, Yamamoto T, Narushima M, Mihara M, Iida T. Perforator flaps and supermicrosurgery. Clin Plast Surg. 2010;37(4):683–9.
50. Srikanth R. Free tissue transfer in pediatric lower limb trauma. Indian J Plastic Surg. 2019;52(01):037–44.
51. Puckett CL, Winters RR, Geter RK, Goebel D. Studies of pathologic vasoconstriction (vasospasm) in microvascular surgery. J Hand Surg Am. 1985;10(3):343–9.
52. El-Gammal TA, El-Sayed A, Kotb MM, Saleh WR, Ragheb YF, El-Refai O, et al. Dorsal foot resurfacing using free anterolateral thigh (ALT) flap in children. Microsurgery. 2013;33(4):259–64.

53. Boyd L, Bond G, Jahromi AH, Kozusko S, Kokkalis Z, Konofaos P. Microvascular reconstruction of pediatric lower extremity trauma using free tissue transfer. Eur J Orthop Surg Traumatol. 2019;29(2):285–93.
54. Konttila E, Koljonen V, Kauhanen S, Kallio P, Tukiainen E. Microvascular reconstruction in children—a report of 46 cases. J Trauma Acute Care Surg. 2010;68(3):548–52.
55. Loos MS, Freeman BG, Lorenzetti A. Zone of injury: a critical review of the literature. Ann Plast Surg. 2010;65(6):573–7.
56. Çeliköz B, Şengezer M, Işik S, Türegün M, Deveci M, Duman H, et al. Subacute reconstruction of lower leg and foot defects due to high velocity-high energy injuries caused by gunshots, missiles, and land mines. Microsurgery. 2005;25(1):3–15.
57. Rappaport B, Mellon RD, Simone A, Woodcock J. Defining safe use of anesthesia in children. N Engl J Med. 2011;364(15):1387–90.
58. Cohen MM, Cameron CB, Duncan PG. Pediatric anesthesia morbidity and mortality in the perioperative period. Anesth Analg. 1990;70(2):160–7.
59. Bjorklund KA, Venkatramani H, Venkateshwaran G, Boopathi V, Sabapathy SR. Regional anesthesia alone for pediatric free flaps. J Plast Reconstr Aesthet Surg. 2015;68(5):705–8.
60. Inberg P, Kassila M, Vilkki S, Tarkkjla P, Neuvonen P. Anaesthesia for microvascular surgery in children. Acta Anaesthesiol Scand. 1995;39(4):518–22.
61. Jabir S, Sheikh F, Fitzgerald O'Connor E, Griffiths M, Niranjan N. A systematic review of the applications of free tissue transfer for paediatric lower limb salvage following trauma. J Plast Surg Hand Surg. 2015;49(5):251–9.
62. Askari M, Fisher C, Weniger FG, Bidic S, Lee WA. Anticoagulation therapy in microsurgery: a review. J Hand Surg Am. 2006;31(5):836–46.
63. Hanasono MM, Butler CE. Prevention and treatment of thrombosis in microvascular surgery. J Reconstr Microsurg. 2008;24(05):305–14.
64. Khouri RK, Sherman R, Buncke JH, Feller A-M, Hovius S, Benes CO, et al. A phase II trial of intraluminal irrigation with recombinant human tissue factor pathway inhibitor to prevent thrombosis in free flap surgery. Plast Reconstr Surg. 2001;107(2):408–15. discussion 16-8
65. Pollak AN, McCarthy ML, Burgess AR, Group LEAPS. Short-term wound complications after application of flaps for coverage of traumatic soft-tissue defects about the tibia. JBJS. 2000;82(12):1681.
66. Staruch RM, Hettiaratchy S. Warzone trauma and surgical infections. Surgery (Oxford). 2019;37(1):58–63.
67. Buono P, Castus P, Dubois-Ferrière V, Rüegg EM, Uçkay I, Assal M, et al. Muscular versus non-muscular free flaps for soft tissue coverage of chronic tibial osteomyelitis. World J Plastic Surg. 2018;7(3):294.
68. Pincher B, Fenton C, Jeyapalan R, Barlow G, Sharma HK. A systematic review of the single-stage treatment of chronic osteomyelitis. J Orthop Surg Res. 2019;14(1):393.
69. Pinder R, Hart R, Winterton R, Yates A, Kay S. Free tissue transfers in the first 2 years of life–a successful cost effective and humane option. J Plast Reconstr Aesthet Surg. 2010;63(4):616–22.

Management and Reconstruction of Long Bone Fractures

13

Said Sodki Saghieh, Serge Jean Sultanem, and Ahmad Salaheddine Naja

13.1 Introduction

13.1.1 Background

The battles of contemporary warfare have shifted tellingly from the classical battle-field to civilian areas, injuring more civilians [1, 2], which encompass around 35%–60% of all war casualties [3]. Approximately one in six children worldwide live in conflict zones [4]. These children are frequently exposed to high-order explosives including landmines and unexploded ordinance, shelling, and aerial bombardments or acts inflicted by non-state factors such as improvised explosive devices and suicide bombing [5]. In addition to the differences in anatomy and physiology inherent to the pediatric population, understanding the prevalence, nature, and sequence of events leading to these injuries is key to successful management.

13.1.2 Epidemiology

To date, literature about injury characteristics, including type and mechanism is limited in the pediatric population [5]. Although war brings firearms and penetrating wounds to the mind, studies have shown that the most common mechanism of injury is blunt trauma. However, the distribution of injury differs among the adult population. Head injury is more common in children, whereas abdominal and extremity injury rates were higher in adults. A study done by Helweg-Larsen et al. found that firearms and explosions were the leading mechanisms of injury in young patients and that the head was the most commonly injured area [6]. This finding might be related

S. S. Saghieh (✉) · S. J. Sultanem · A. S. Naja
Department of Surgery, Division of Orthopedic Surgery, American University of Beirut Medical Center, Beirut, Lebanon
e-mail: Ss15@aub.edu.lb; Ss199@aub.edu.lb; an85@aub.edu.lb

© Springer Nature Switzerland AG 2023
G. S. Abu-Sittah, J. J. Hoballah (eds.), *The War Injured Child*,
https://doi.org/10.1007/978-3-031-28613-1_13

to a higher risk of tertiary blast injury in the pediatric population attributed to lower weight and volume. A survey done by the red cross community through multiple conflict zones demonstrated that fragment mines and burns are the most frequent mechanism of injury in pediatric casualties compared to adults (gunshot wound). This is attributed to the lower tendency of children to participate actively in the conflict as well as the higher likelihood of children being the victims of landmines [7].

13.1.3 Mechanism

With the technological advances in weapons development witnessed since world war II, a shift has been noted in injury patterns. Thus, blast-related injuries have become the main contributor to civilian injuries, leading to physical and psychological disabilities [5]. From 1999 to 2006 this type of injury increased by eightfolds [8].

Blast injuries can be classified into primary, secondary, tertiary, and quaternary. Primary blast injury is mainly due to the overpressure that reaches the person and exerts its effect on the body, causing direct tissue damage affecting mainly the pulmonary, gastrointestinal, and auditory systems with a shock-like response lasting minutes to hours after the explosion exposure [9–12]. Secondary blast injury is created by the debris that is physically displaced by the overpressure winds leading to blunt and penetrating trauma [13–15]. Tertiary injury is derived from the physical displacement of a person from the peak overpressure leading to fractures, contusions, and head trauma [16]. Quaternary blast injuries termed miscellaneous include burns, toxic substances, asphyxiation, and psychological trauma [13, 17, 18]. Extremity and musculoskeletal injuries can be caused by primary, secondary, and tertiary forces, with children being particularly vulnerable to tertiary forces due to their lower body weight.

With modern warfare and the advancement of destructive weapons, gunshots have become less frequent contributors to injuries in the civilian population. Nevertheless, firearms still play a role in the clinical picture of emergency cases that present with orthopedic penetrating injuries [19–21]. Primary weapons of war are divided into explosive munitions like artillery, grenades, and small arms like pistols and machine guns [22]. The latter causes projectile injuries that create either permanent or temporary cavities. The permanent injury creates a localized area of necrosis symmetrical to the size of the projectile it passes. Whereas a temporary cavity creates a lateral displacement of tissue that might push the elastic tissue which can rebound and, fracture the inelastic tissue like bones.

13.2   Special Considerations in the Pediatric Population

Multiple aspects set aside the child from the adults when it comes to decision-making. Both physiologic and social differences should be taken into account when managing pediatric injuries. These include but are not limited to the active growth plate, the potential for remodeling, and caregiver influence.

13.2.1 Caregiver Influence

Children with severe trauma are commonly surgically treated with unnecessary aggressiveness. This goes back partially to the circumstances of the injury which are frequently emotive and associated with an emotional response from his/her surrounding support system [23]. However, the mortality rate has been shown to be higher in children with blast injuries compared to adults. Thus, a balance between a high index of suspicion and adequate management should be established to optimize patient care.

13.2.2 Growth

Longitudinal limb growth occurs interstitially through specialized cartilage of the growth plate [24]. Injury to the growth plate will result in growth arrest and subsequent limb length discrepancy or bone deformity. The severity of these deformities is predicted by the location of the injury, the skeletal maturity of the patient, and the extent of involvement of the growth plate. Identification and adequate assessment of the aforementioned factors are primordial to establishing individualized patient care.

Growth is dominated by genetic, intrinsic, and, extrinsic factors like weight bearing and muscle action. This dynamic regulation of growth exerted by the muscles should be taken into account when considering amputation since the loss of the distal attachment and the resulting variation in the tension of the remaining muscle fibers and forces exerted on the preserved proximal growth plate will interfere with its growth [25].

13.2.3 Remodeling and Regeneration

Two physiologic pediatric responses allow quicker regeneration and a faster healing process [26]: Rapid circulatory compensation of blood loss and tissue elasticity that has greater tolerance to muscle hypoxia and necrosis. This allows faster repair of bone defects compared to adults. Also, children's bone has higher collagen consistency with a thicker and more active periosteum. Thus, when the pediatric periosteum is intact, bone regeneration is steadily available even in cases of severe bone loss and open trauma. In addition, the higher collagen content increases bone elasticity allowing for plastic deformation and lowering the risk of fracture comminution.

Aside from the higher regenerative capacity of the pediatric bone, its remodeling potential makes conservative therapy acceptable in non-anatomical fractures compared to adults [27].

13.3 Management

Pediatric care in a conflict zone is often given by physicians for whom experience in dealing with pediatric blast injuries is minimal [28]. In addition, there is a lack of consensus as to whether evidence from the adult population can be applied to pediatric cohorts [29]. Directly applying adult trauma principles to the pediatric population might neglect social, anatomical, physiological, and psychological differences between adults and children affecting the outcome of these interventions [30].

13.3.1 Closed Fractures

The management of closed fractures in the war-injured child follows the same principles used for closed fractures in the general pediatric population. However, in view of the low socioeconomic status of most combat zones, treatment modalities might be scarce. One such example is the Camp Bastion military hospital established in 2006 in Afghanistan where casting remains the go-to, a most practical technique in the treatment of closed fractures. Traction and/or hip spicas require special equipment namely traction frames and spica table. The latter might not be available and as such using this treatment modality becomes more difficult. Pelvic fractures, although rarely seen, present another challenge since they might require stabilization using an external fixator. Stable pelvic fractures are treated conservatively with bed rest, DVT prophylaxis, and, gradual weight bearing as tolerated. Unstable fractures such as AP compression fractures with more than 2 cm diastasis, lateral compression, and, vertical shear fractures are treated with an external fixator. However, the only absolute indication for its use is hemodynamic instability [26].

13.3.2 Blast Injuries

Extremity injuries are one of the commonly discussed features following blast-related trauma. Its prevalence increases following blast injury within conflict zones [31]. An analysis study in children from Afghanistan and Iraq registries showed that in patients with blast injuries, 19% had an extremity/bony pelvis injury if they were younger than 7 years, 30% if they were between 8 and 14 years of age, and, 35% if they were 15–20 years old [32, 33]. In a study from Afghanistan by Bertani et al., blast injuries accounted for all traumatic amputations and 96% of bony injuries to the hand and foot [34]. Children are more prone to sustain upper limb injuries with a substantial increase in the percentage requiring amputation, especially at the level of the finger [35].

The rate of injury to the lower extremity due to blast injuries varies widely among different studies, ranging from 25 to 86%, with higher rates being associated with landmines [35]. Landmines drive debris, separating upward between planes of soft tissue and bone resulting in a degloving injury of the leg leading to serious complications and a higher rate of infection [36, 37]. These injuries leave the patient with a large bony defect of the lower limb which ought to be addressed by reconstruction with limited shortening [38]. This intervention is associated with a good prognosis, given that children have a significant capacity of the growth plate to remodel and compensate for bone loss [26, 34]. To note is that most growth occurs at the level of the distal femoral and proximal tibial growth plates which might be involved in the blast. However, up to 29% of pediatric landmine casualties end up with a transtibial amputation which has a major long-term influence on the physical, psychosocial, and financial burden.

Prevalence of pediatric upper extremity war injuries was eluded by a study done by Bertani et al. He discussed 89 cases of war-related extremity injuries that were managed in a combat support hospital in Afghanistan. He found that 3% had a soft tissue shoulder injury, and 9% had an arm soft tissue injury and fracture. Four patients had either elbow or forearm soft tissue injury and another four had either elbow or forearm fracture presenting 4% of all extremity injuries. Wrist injuries presented 2% of all extremity injuries. Hand injuries were the most common with 31%. Out of 19 patients with traumatic amputation 11 had upper extremity amputation. Most of the amputations were below the wrist.

13.3.3 Gunshot Injuries

In the pediatric population, children are victims of gunshot injuries resulting from wars, street fights, and accidents [39–41]. Most studies on pediatric gunshot injuries show a good prognosis with complete recovery [39, 41]. When deciding on the course of management for pediatric patients with gunshot injuries, acknowledging the type and velocity of the firearm is a must. Most low-velocity fractures in pediatric patients can be managed by external plaster immobilization whereas high-velocity fractures should be treated with external/internal fixators considering the large bone defects and comminution associated with this kind of injury [39, 41].

Arslan et al. investigated the clinical manifestations of gunshot wounds in children and their surgical management. High velocity, low velocity, and shotguns related fractures were managed by debridement with either early or late-stage surgical fixation [42]. Most fractures were displaced and/or comminuted with some having a large bone defect. The tibia was most commonly affected by high velocity and shotgun injuries while the femur was the most commonly injured bone, 4 out of 22 children had physeal injury, 2 patients had a hip joint injury with no major sequelae, and 1 elbow joint injury leading to decreased range of motion. Surgical management varied between cases ranging from conservative treatment in patients with a closed minimally displaced fracture to debridement and late surgical intervention like external fixation, decortication, and fibular or autologous bone graft in patients with infections, nonunion, and bone defects.

13.3.4 Salvage Procedures

The management of large bone defects in the pediatric population is challenging even in the highly advanced modern healthcare setting [43]. However, initially, same as any open wound fracture, explosive injuries resulting in complex open fractures should be managed following the fundamental principles of orthopedic trauma surgery. Urgent debridement procedures are usually the mainstay treatment with the removal of devitalized tissues and deep penetrating soil particles if any [44]. Then, restoration of length, alignment, and, rotation with the least available resources should be achieved [45]. Some of the treatment modalities include shortening followed by distraction osteogenesis, ipsilateral partial fibula transfer, free vascularized graft, and, allograft reconstruction [45, 46]. However, these surgical procedures require specialized centers, defined medical resources, and surgical expertise. In combat zones where the environment is austere medical resources are limited, hence amputation remains the last resort in large bone defects. But, due to several reasons including contralateral amputation, cultural beliefs, and patient preferences amputation is deferred.

Following multiple fingers amputation, a reconstructive option would be to lengthen the metacarpal using iliac bone improving the residual hand mechanics. It allows a partial restoration of thumb-to-finger grip facilitating fine motor motions. Another upper extremity salvage procedure that can improve function in patients with distal forearm amputation without resorting to a prosthetic implant is the Krukenberg procedure. This technique separates the radius and the ulna from each other, creating two movable fingers. The advantage of this technique over the prosthesis is the pinch movement which is basically the separation and approximation of the two bones achieving a closure movement that enables the patient to achieve basic hand dexterity helping in independence in activities of daily living [36].

13.3.5 Amputation

When contemplating lower extremity amputation in a pediatric patient, its effect on future growth should be taken into account.

In the femur, 75% of growth occurs at the distal physis, making its preservation vital at all possible costs otherwise a very short above-knee amputation will occur. In cases of inadequate soft tissue coverage preservation of distal physis can be executed through [36]:

1. Slightly shortening the femur at the level of the shaft and allowing soft tissue closure.
2. Keeping the skin open and using traction to stretch the soft tissue then performing secondary wound closure.
3. In contrast to adults, a split-thickness graft can be used to provide appropriate coverage in children and save limb length.

Moving down to the tibia, it is critical to preserve the physis of the proximal end. Again, attempting to do the amputation more proximally for wound closure will lead to excessively shortened residual limbs at maturity. In this case, the proper prosthetic fitting will become challenging at skeletal maturity. Thus, attempts to preserve the proximal tibial physis as much as possible are essential. Even a residual limb that is too short to fit a below-knee prosthesis at the time of amputation is worth retaining. The child might start with an above-knee amputation fit, then switch with time to a below-knee prosthesis as the stump grows.

These procedures are associated with a high rate of complications including varus bowing, heterotopic ossification, and osseous overgrowth requiring operative and prosthetic revision [47]. Overgrowth occurs particularly in patients below 12 years who undergo amputation mostly for the humerus, fibula, and, tibia [48] with 15% of them requiring revision surgery. It results from the excessive streaming of osteoblast from the periosteum leading to bony overgrowth around the stump. Terminal overgrowth is best addressed by performing amputations through the joint or by crowning the end of the transcortical bone piece of epiphyseal bone and overlying cartilage halting spicule formation. Another potential complication of both upper and lower extremity amputation is phantom limb syndrome which is reported in 50% of children following blast-related amputation [49–51].

13.3.6 Rehabilitation Management

Caring for landmine victims consists of emergency and medical care, hospital care, physical rehabilitation, and socioeconomic reintegration [52].

Physical rehabilitation involves prostheses fitting of absent limbs, assistive devices like crutches, and wheelchairs, and the occupational and physical therapy needed to get accommodated on the use of the above. Mine survivors with severe sequelae may require long-life rehabilitation protocol. However, in underdeveloped countries, appropriate management and support might become challenging [36]. Available rehabilitation centers are commonly unequally distributed between the capital and rural areas where most of the injuries occur. Even when accessible, the cost of these rehabilitation protocols makes them unavailable.

Prosthetic fitting of the upper extremity has amplified implications and struggles that make its optimization harder, especially in underdeveloped countries where most blast injuries occur. With the complexity of upper extremity/hand function and the need for the very sophisticated and advanced prosthesis to substitute partially the functions of native extremity, crude upper extremity prosthesis is technically non-useful.

A multidisciplinary approach is crucial in securing adequate rehabilitation services in patients with upper and lower extremity injuries. In addition to medical care, refurbishment to address limb amputations should address any concomitant sensory and/or cognitive deficits.

13.4 Conclusion

In conclusion, the management of bone injury in war-injured children remains a challenge. This is due both to the complexity of the injury resulting from high-energy devices as well as the scarceness of resources in such austere environments. A multidisciplinary approach remains essential for management in order to address all aspects of the injury be it bony, soft tissue, psychological, or rehabilitation. In addition, an intimate understanding of the mechanism of injury, pediatric physiology, and, available therapeutic options are needed to allow the surgeon to decide on the best course of action. Salvage should be attempted when possible but amputation is sometimes necessary. However, all efforts should be made to allow the patient to be autonomous and independent.

References

1. Coupland RM, Meddings DR. Mortality associated with use of weapons in armed conflicts, wartime atrocities, and civilian mass shootings: literature review. BMJ. 1999;319(7207):407–10.
2. Levy BS, Sidel VW. War and public health. Oxford University Press; 2008.
3. Meddings DR. Civilians and war: a review and historical overview of the involvement of non-combatant populations in conflict situations. Med Confl Surviv. 2001;17(1):6–16.
4. Frost A, et al. The effect of explosive remnants of war on global public health: a systematic mixed-studies review using narrative synthesis. Lancet Public Health. 2017;2(6):e286–96.
5. Wolf SJ, et al. Blast injuries. Lancet. 2009;374(9687):405–15.
6. Helweg-Larsen K, et al. Systematic medical data collection of intentional injuries during armed conflicts: a pilot study conducted in West Bank, Palestine. Scandinavian J Public Health. 2004;32(1):17–23.
7. Bitterman Y, et al. Role 1 pediatric trauma care on the Israeli–Syrian Border—First year of the humanitarian effort. Mil Med. 2016;181(8):849–53.
8. Incident, R.M. *RAND MIPT Terrorism Incident Database* [cited 2020 July 11 2020].
9. Sharpnack DD, Johnson AJ, Phillips Y. The pathology of primary blast injury. Conventional Warfare: Ballistic, Blast, and Burn Injuries. 1991:271–94.
10. Almogy G, Rivkind AI. Terror in the 21st century: milestones and prospects--part I. Curr Probl Surg. 2007;44(8):496.
11. Guy RJ, et al. Physiologic responses to primary blast. J Trauma Acute Care Surg. 1998;45(6):983–7.
12. Ohnishi M, et al. Reflex nature of the cardiorespiratory response to primary thoracic blast injury in the anaesthetised rat. Exp Physiol. 2001;86(3):357–64.
13. DePalma RG, et al. Blast injuries. N Engl J Med. 2005;352(13):1335–42.
14. Bellamy RF, Zajtchuk R, Grande C. Combat trauma overview. Textbook Military Med. 1995;4:1–42.
15. Schardin H. The physical principles of the effects of a detonation. German Aviation Medicine, World War. 1950;II(2):1207–24.
16. Arnold JL, et al. Mass casualty terrorist bombings: a comparison of outcomes by bombing type. Ann Emerg Med. 2004;43(2):263–73.
17. Severance HW. *Mass-casualty victim "surge" management.* Preparing for bombings and blast-related injuries with possibility of hazardous materials exposure. NCJM. 2002;63:242–6.
18. Yazbeck-Karam VG, et al. Methemoglobinemia after a blast injury. Anesthesiology: The Journal of the American Society of Anesthesiologists. 2004;100(2):448–9.
19. Barlow B, Niemirska M, Gandhi RP. Ten years' experience with pediatric gunshot wounds. J Pediatr Surg. 1982;17(6):927–32.
20. Hoffer M, Johnson B. Shrapnel wounds in children. JBJS. 1992;74(5):766–9.
21. Ordog GJ, et al. Infection in minor gunshot wounds. J Trauma. 1993;34(3):358–65.
22. Institute, B. Emergency war surgery 2013.
23. Aitken GT. Surgical amputation in children. JBJS. 1963;45(8):1735–41.
24. Chung R, Xian CJ. Recent research on the growth plate: mechanisms for growth plate injury repair and potential cell-based therapies for regeneration. J Mol Endocrinol. 2014;53(1):T45–61.
25. Brown KV, et al. Limb salvage of severely injured extremities after military wounds. BMJ Military Health. 2011;157(Suppl 3):S315–23.

26. Nordmann GR, et al. Paediatric trauma management on deployment. BMJ Military Health. 2011;157(Suppl 3):S334–43.
27. Wilkins KE. Principles of fracture remodeling in children. Injury. 2005;36:A3.
28. Harris C, McNicholas J. Paediatric intensive care in the field hospital. BMJ Military Health. 2009;155(2):157–9.
29. Bull A, et al. Paediatric blast injury: challenges and priorities. Lancet child and adolescent health, The. 2018;2(5):310–1.
30. Fendya DG, Snow SK, Weik TS. Using system change as a method of performance/quality improvement for emergency and trauma care of severely injured children: pediatric system performance improvement. J Trauma Nurs. 2010;17(1):28–33.
31. Inwald DP, et al. Management of children in the deployed intensive care unit at camp bastion, Afghanistan. BMJ Military Health. 2014;160(3):236–40.
32. Edwards MJ, et al. Blast injury in children: an analysis from Afghanistan and Iraq, 2002–2010. J Trauma Care Surg. 2012;73(5):1278–83.
33. Haverkamp FJ, et al. Global surgery for paediatric casualties in armed conflict. World J Emerg Surg. 2019;14(1):55.
34. Bertani A, et al. War-related extremity injuries in children: 89 cases managed in a combat support hospital in Afghanistan. Orthop Traumatol Surg Res. 2015;101(3):365–8.
35. Hargrave JM, et al. Blast injuries in children: a mixed-methods narrative review. BMJ Paediatr Open. 2019;3(1)
36. Watts HG. The consequences for children of explosive remnants of war: land mines, unexploded ordnance, improvised explosive devices, and cluster bombs. J Pediatr Rehabil Med. 2009;2(3):217–27.
37. Coupland RM, Korver A. Injuries from antipersonnel mines: the experience of the International Committee of the red Cross. Br Med J. 1991;303(6816):1509–12.
38. Franke A, et al. Management of soft-tissue and bone defects in a local population: plastic and reconstructive surgery in a deployed military setting. Mil Med. 2017;182(11–12):e2010–20.
39. Stucky W, Loder RT. Extremity gunshot wounds in children. J Pediatr Orthop. 1991;11(1):64–71.
40. Valentine J, Blocker S, Chang J-H. Gunshot injuries in children. J Trauma. 1984;24(11):952–6.
41. Washington E, Lee WA, Ross W Jr. Gunshot wounds to the extremities in children and adolescents. Orthop Clin North Am. 1995;26(1):19.
42. Arslan H, et al. Problem fractures associated with gunshot wounds in children. Injury. 2002;33(9):743–9.
43. Keenan AJ, et al. Ipsilateral fibular transfer as a salvage procedure for large traumatic tibial defects in children in an austere environment. BMJ Military Health. 2016;162(6):476–8.
44. Mathieu L, et al. Wartime paediatric extremity injuries: experience from the Kabul international airport combat support hospital. J Pediatr Orthopaedics B. 2015;24(3):238–45.
45. Covey DC. Blast and fragment injuries of the musculoskeletal system. JBJS. 2002;84(7):1221–34.
46. Edwards MJ, et al. Surgical interventions for pediatric blast injury: an analysis from Afghanistan and Iraq 2002 to 2010. J Trauma Acute Care Surg. 2014;76(3):854–8.
47. Eichelberger MR. Pediatric surgery and medicine for hostile environments. J Pediatr Surg. 2011;46(8):1683.
48. Pellicore RJ, et al. Incidence of bone overgrowth in juvenile amputee population. Inter-Clinic Information Bulletin. 1974;13(5):1–8.
49. Ketz AK. The experience of phantom limb pain in patients with combat-related traumatic amputations. Arch Phys Med Rehabil. 2008;89(6):1127–32.
50. Jaffe DH, Peleg K, I.T. Group. Terror explosive injuries: a comparison of children, adolescents, and adults. Ann Surg. 2010;251(1):138–43.
51. Kauvar DS, et al. Burns sustained in combat explosions in operations Iraqi and enduring freedom (OIF/OEF explosion burns). Burns. 2006;32(7):853–7.
52. Forsythe DP. The humanitarians: the international committee of the red cross. Cambridge University Press; 2005.

Reconstruction of Pediatric Craniomaxillofacial Injuries

14

Rawad Chalhoub and Ghassan Soleiman Abu-Sittah

14.1 Introduction

Millions of children have been injured and many more will suffer in the numerous wars and armed conflicts, which we have witnessed throughout history. Some of the most debilitating injuries are craniofacial injuries that are challenging to treat and often leave long-term sequelae. Children are logically more prone to devastating injuries from armed conflicts and explosions due to their smaller bodies and closer anatomic regions such as the head and chest to the explosion center. Pediatric craniofacial trauma secondary to armed conflicts was caused mostly by blast and/or penetrating trauma [1]. The pattern of pediatric maxillofacial trauma depends on the size of the explosive, the distance from the child, and the child's body mass; also the position of the body and angle of the body with respect to blast cone will impact the outcome.

14.2 Mechanisms of Injury

Blasts result in what is known as a shock front, which propagates rapidly in all directions from the epicenter of the explosion. The effects of this shock front cause body tissue devastation due to the shrapnel/fragments and ground particles that propagate toward the body. Explosions also cause devastation by propelling the body against walls, vehicles, and other objects, which may manifest as blunt trauma or crush injuries [2]. Shock waves moving from a high-density to a lower-density medium create fragmentations or spalling at the interface of two different media.

R. Chalhoub · G. S. Abu-Sittah (✉)
Conflict Medicine Program, Global Health Institute, American University of Beirut, Beirut, Lebanon
e-mail: rc58@aub.edu.lb; ga60@aub.edu.lb

© Springer Nature Switzerland AG 2023
G. S. Abu-Sittah, J. J. Hoballah (eds.), *The War Injured Child*,
https://doi.org/10.1007/978-3-031-28613-1_14

Facial soft tissue directly in line with the front wave will experience sudden loading and when the tension exceeds the tensile strength of soft tissue, collagen fibers, and bones these will fracture and shatter. These will result in ragged facial skin, widespread contusions, and multiple puncture wounds [3].

14.3   Comparative and Developmental Anatomy in the Pediatric Patient

An appreciation of facial development is imperative in understanding the differences between adult and pediatric injuries and having a better understanding of therapeutic and reconstructive approaches. Several differences between adult and pediatric maxillofacial injuries make facial fractures more common in the adult population. First, children's bones are less calcified than adults, which make "greenstick" flexing of the bone more common than a fracture upon subjection to a force. Second, pneumatized sinuses are not developed in the pediatric age group until adolescence. The pneumatized sinuses would act as a cushion in adults and hence protects the brain whereas in children any impact force would be transmitted to the brain leading to a traumatic brain injury rather than fractures in the facial skeleton [4]. Third, the cranial to facial volume decreases with age, which explains why adults exhibit more facial injuries than intracranial injuries [5]. Fourth, children have more fat pads than adults, especially around the mandible and the maxilla that allow cushioning against external forces and reduce the rate of fractures. Moreover, the retruded position of the face in children less than 5 years of age protects against midfacial and mandibular fractures [6]. Another factor that is unique to the pediatric population is incomplete dentition, which increases the stability of the mandible and is protective against fractures. All these unique features in pediatric patients act to protect from significant bony and soft tissue injuries, nevertheless; potential growth disturbances must be considered when planning treatment. On the other hand, due to the unpredictability of conflict-related injuries, planning treatment for such maxillofacial defects could be challenging.

14.4   Injury Site

For children below the age of 2 years, the most common maxillofacial injury is to the frontal region. The most commonly injured bone is the frontal bone, especially when pneumatization occurs later on during puberty. However, it is important to keep in mind that frontal bone injuries are frequently associated with other intracranial injuries. Moreover, as in adults, the nasal bones are the least resistant to the facial skeleton.

Mandibular fractures on the other hand are the fractures that most commonly require hospitalization. The condylar region is the most frequently fractured segment and due to its high vascularity in pediatric patients, most of these fractures are intracapsular rather than extracapsular.

In the midface, other than the nasal bone and maxilla, zygomatic fractures are also common. Le Fort fractures are rarely seen in children below the age of 2 years and as the child grows and the eruption of permanent teeth takes place along with the expansion of the maxillary sinuses the incidence of midfacial fractures also increase.

Most orbital injuries occur as a result of force transmission directly from the orbital rim to the thin orbital walls indirectly through the hydraulic pressure effect. Another theory that describes orbital fracture is the bone conduction theory the energy absorbed by the orbital rim results in buckling of the floor at the thinnest point. As seen previously, sinus development also plays a role in injury type and location as the child grows. Orbital roof fractures are more common prior to maxillary sinus development and as the sinus grows beyond the equator of the globe, orbital floor fractures become more common.

14.5   Emergency Management

As in any type of trauma, pediatric maxillofacial trauma requires strict adherence to the basic principles of trauma management. The primary survey should clear the child's airway, breathing, and circulation.

Depending on the type of injury, several airway interventions are available. When an injury is only isolated to the face, adequate positioning of the head is usually sufficient to maintain the airway, along with suctioning any blood and removing any intraoral debris. Orotracheal intubation becomes a necessity if there's concomitant bleeding associated with midfacial fractures, intracranial injuries, orotracheal obstruction, or posterior protrusion of the mandible.

An extensively injured and fractured face in a child could result in significant blood loss causing hypovolemic shock. Hence, volume expansion with crystalloid solution is necessary via two peripheral large bore IVs and eventually, a blood transfusion may be required. Secondary surveys of maxillofacial injuries should proceed in an orderly fashion, with neurological assessment done first including evaluation of the eyes, otoscopy, rhinoscopy as well as cranial nerve testing.

14.6   Physical Examination

The examination should begin with inspection and followed by palpation. Signs to look out for are facial asymmetry, ecchymosis, trismus, malocclusion, and periorbital swelling. Palpation of the orbital margins may reveal step-offs, which indicate a point of fracture. Enophthalmos or inferior displacement of the globe usually indicates orbital floor fracture. The bimanual examination goes over all the bony prominences of the face to reveal any crepitus, step-offs, or tenderness. The stability of the maxilla is assessed by placing one hand on the cranium and the other hand on the premaxilla while testing for mobility. Intra-orally, the palate should be examined to rule out any lacerations or fractures while also paying close attention to the gingiva for any bruising and ecchymosis. The mandibular examination proceeds from the temporomandibular joint and progresses until reaching the symphysis. Moreover, any injury to the nasal complex should include an endonasal examination to rule out a septal hematoma.

14.7   Imaging Evaluation

Computed tomography (CT) is the gold standard for viewing craniofacial fractures. An axial CT is indicated for orbital and maxillary fractures to assess changes in facial width and orbital volume. Coronal cuts are useful for complex nasoethmoid fractures and orbital fractures. Moreover, reformatting images into 3D reconstruction and important perspectives for preoperative planning.

Although mandibular fractures can be assessed via a CT, panoramic radiographs are more useful as it displays the anatomy of the condyles as well as the upper and lower teeth; however, this might not be too feasible in an injured child as they are rarely cooperative in such situations.

14.8   Pediatric Facial Fracture Management

Principles of pediatric facial fractures differ from the management of fractures in adults and these should be adhered to. In pediatrics, a more conservative approach is usually advocated. Large and bulky fixations are not recommended as they might interfere with tooth development. In case fixation was absolutely needed 1.5 or 2.0 millimeters plates and monocortical screws are used. Removing of fixation is not usually recommended in children unless these become symptomatic.

14.8.1 Frontal Bone Injury

All non-displaced frontal bone fractures do not require any surgical intervention. On the other hand, displaced fractures and fractures with nasofrontal duct injuries should be explored and reduced. Moreover, cerebrospinal fluid leak is also common after frontal bone fracture occurring in around 18%–36% of the cases.

The goals of frontal fracture repair include protection of the neurocapsule, management of CSF leaks, prevention of infection, and esthetic craniofacial contours. The best surgical access to the frontal bone is via a coronal approach and fixation is usually achieved with microplate fixation. Any subdural hematomas should be evacuated and dural lacerations repaired. Traumatic disruption of the frontal sinus usually prompts sinus destruction with mucosal ablation and nasofrontal duct obliteration to ensure complete separation of the nose from the intracranial cavity, this is done by using vascularized tissue such as a pericranial flap. In patients older than 5 years of age any involvement of the posterior table of the frontal sinus mandates a multidisciplinary approach from the maxillofacial and neurosurgeons.

14.8.2   Orbital Fractures

Pediatric orbital fractures are distinct from adult fractures. Supraorbital fractures are classified as skull base fractures because they include the frontal bones prior to sinus pneumatization. The neurocranium in children is relatively larger than in adults, which increases the susceptibility to neurological injuries as a result of orbital fractures. It is critical to examine the extraocular muscle movement to rule out any underlying entrapment. Symptoms of entrapment include nausea, vomiting, diplopia, and an oculocardiac reflex. Forced duction testing performed under anesthesia is useful to distinguish between diplopia of entrapment and pseudoentrapment from a nerve injury due to swelling. Meanwhile, superior orbital fissure syndrome should be treated as an emergency; this includes internal and external ophthalmoplegia, proptosis, and CN VI paresthesia.

In the absence of any entrapment or acute globe malposition, management is often conservative. Moreover, the goals of orbital fracture treatment are the restoration of globe position, correction of diplopia, and release of entrapment. Several surgical approaches are described when the need for open reduction internal fixation (ORIF) arises. Most commonly the transconjunctival approach is used, as it is associated with the least risk of ectropion. Subciliary or midlid incisions with lateral extensions could afford more exposure without the need for lateral cantholysis, which would otherwise be used in transconjunctival approach. Any herniated tissue in the sinuses should be reduced and debris from the fractures cleaned and irrigated. Finally, fixation is done after identifying stable bony edges for anchoring either with bone grafts or plates. Commonly used bone grafts include split calvarial bone grafts, rib grafts, and iliac bone grafts.

14.8.3   Nasal and Nasoethmoid Fractures

Isolated nasal injuries as a result of war are very rare and due to the high energy trauma usually from blasts and weapons, complex naso-orbital ethmoidal (NOE) is more often seen. Patterns of these fractures differ considerably from adults this is mainly due to proportional differences in midface to neurocranium and lack of pneumatization of the frontal sinus. In the pediatric population, these fractures are characterized by posterior and lateral displacement of nasal bones and medial orbital walls, including the ethmoid. Any injury to the medial orbital wall could lead to traumatic telecanthus due to the disruption of the medial canthus; however, this might become apparent 10 days after the injury when the edema subsides.

Although less common in combat injuries, non-displaced nasal fractures can be managed with an external splint. It is important to remember that the septum is important for midfacial growth in the developing child; therefore any definitive open management for displaced facial fractures is postponed until skeletal maturity unless the fractures are so severe that the airway is significantly compromised. Nevertheless, such fractures do need closed reduction under general anesthesia.

Pediatric NOE fractures with traumatic telecanthus require restoration of the intercanthal distance. Reducing the medial orbital rims and reattachment of the medial canthal tendons with transnasal wires reduces the intercanthal distance. It is important to attach the transnasal wires superiorly and posteriorly to the lacrimal crest. Occasionally, the anterior skull base is also involved in these fractures and a subcranial approach could be used just like in adults.

14.8.4 Midface and Zygomticomaxillary Complex Fractures

Zygomaticomaxillary complex (ZMC) fractures refer to the dislocation of the malar eminence from the temporal bone, frontal bone, and maxilla. As mentioned previously these fractures are rare in children especially the classic Le Fort types of fractures. This is due to the underdeveloped sinus system, undeveloped buttress system, and unerupted tooth buds. ZMC fractures usually present with malar flattening, enophthalmos, and lateral canthal dystopia.

The goals of treating midfacial fractures are obtaining stable bony fixation to allow proper healing and eventual undisturbed growth. They may require closed reduction or ORIF with mandibulomaxillary fixation (MMF). The duration of fixation to allow bone healing is usually less than in adults but special care must be taken to avoid disruption of the erupting tooth buds. For ZMC fractures, it is important to correct malocclusion if present and restoration of the malar contour and prominence. The surgical approach for these fractures involves either a brow incision or an upper lid blepharoplasty incision and usually, a 3-point fixation is required for zygomaticofrontal suture, inferior orbital rim, and zygomaticomaxillary buttress.

14.8.5 Mandible

Traumatic mandibular fractures usually present with a risk of airway compromise. Therefore, the first step is to secure the airway with endotracheal intubation or even a surgical airway if needed. Ecchymosis, intraoral lacerations, mucosal bruising, and edema may represent underlying mandibular fractures. Paresthesia over the area innervated by the inferior alveolar nerve may occur in displaced fractures. Drooling and trismus are also alarming signs. Trismus in children can present with malocclusion without bony displacement. Palpation of the temporomandibular joint (TMJ) at the external auditory canal during jaw movement may demonstrate crepitation and or a displaced mandibular head.

Treatment goals include achieving normal occlusion and bony union without disruption of facial growth. Nevertheless, in a developing mandible, minor occlusal discrepancies are allowed and are corrected in the future by orthodontics. Conservative management is also indicated with minimally displaced mandibular fractures usually with jaw rest and immobilization with a compressive jaw wrap or cervical collar as well as a liquid diet. Dentoalveolar fractures can be managed with occlusive splinting, arch bars, and/or bonded wires. MMF fixation in children is challenging, especially during primary and mixed dentition but can be safely performed.

Mandibular condyles are growth centers and are very sensitive to blood flow disruptions from fractures. Intracapsular fractures, high condylar neck fractures, and coronoid fractures should be managed conservatively to avoid such blood flow disruptions. Moreover, early range-of-motion exercises should be commenced early on after injury, usually within 5 days. Blast or bullet injuries usually contaminate the TMJ with foreign material hence an open approach is advocated in these cases usually through the preexisting lacerations.

Body and angle fractures are managed through the standard anterior sulcus incision while taking care to leave a small cuff of mentalis muscle attached to the upper edge to prevent the witch's chin deformity.

14.9 Soft Tissue Injuries

In the growing face, it is important to minimize scar tissue as this places constraints on proper growth. In general, soft tissue defects in children are repaired primarily without using rotational flaps initially. This is especially accurate in combat areas during mass casualty cases and primary care centers with inadequate personnel and equipment. These defects should be revisited after allowing healing and full scar maturation, taking into account the exquisite healing capabilities of the pediatric population. Specialized structures such as the facial nerve, lacrimal ducts, and salivary ducts may require microsurgical reconstruction.

14.10 Complications

In general, postoperative complications following facial fracture repair are uncommon in children. This is due to the higher osteogenic potential, faster healing response, and less frequent need for open reduction and rigid fixation. Nevertheless, due to the highly contaminating nature of combat injuries, infections, and malunion rates become similar to that in adults. Long-term complications such as growth disturbance are unique to that population.

Malocclusion is always a risk when treating maxillary and mandibular fractures. Also, any malposition of facial skeletal bones during the repair could result in facial deformities. Such as malpositioning of medial canthal tendons will result in an unsightly telecanthus that will be evident weeks after surgical repair.

14.11 Long-Term Follow-Up

Long-term follow-up is recommended in children until they reach skeletal maturity since skeletal growth could be affected. Moreover, psychological counseling is usually required for patients and families sustaining these injuries because of the initial trauma and the disfiguring nature of these injuries.

References

1. McGuigan R, et al. Pediatric trauma: experience of a combat support hospital in Iraq. J Pediatr Surg. 2007;42(1):207–10.
2. Shuker ST. Effect of biomechanism mine explosion on children: craniofacial injuries and management. J Craniofac Surg. 2013;24(4):1132–6.
3. Shuker ST. Facial skin-mucosal biodynamic blast injuries and management. J Oral Maxillofac Surg. 2010;68(8):1818–25.
4. Haug RH, Foss J. Maxillofacial injuries in the pediatric patient. Oral Surg Oral Med Oral Pathol Oral Radiol Endod. 2000;90(2):126–34.
5. Hatef DA, Cole PD, Hollier LH Jr. Contemporary management of pediatric facial trauma. Curr Opin Otolaryngol Head Neck Surg. 2009;17(4):308–14.
6. Morris C, Kushner GM, Tiwana PS. Facial skeletal trauma in the growing patient. Oral Maxillofac Surg Clin North Am. 2012;24(3):351–64.

War-Related Amputations and Prostheses in the Pediatric Population

15

Paul Beaineh, Seif Emseih,
and Ghassan Soleiman Abu-Sittah

15.1 Introduction

Despite violating international laws and norms, children continue today to bear the brunt of war and armed conflicts. The United Nations designated 2018 as the most violent year for children in terms of the record-high number of killings and maiming since the establishment of a mechanism on surveilling and reporting war-related violations against children in 2005 [1]. The UN Security Council also recognizes the killing and maiming of children during conflict as one of six grave violations [2]. With no sign of violence calming down and the continued presence of armed conflicts throughout the different quarters of the world, this brings to the forefront the need to address the impact of armed conflict on children's health and how permanent disability resulting from such conflicts, namely amputations, could be targeted. This is especially important considering the paucity of epidemiological data on pediatric healthcare in combat zones.

P. Beaineh
Department of Surgery, American University of Beirut Medical Center, Beirut, Lebanon

S. Emseih
Department of Surgery, Division of Plastic and Reconstructive Surgery, American University of Beirut Medical Center, Beirut, Lebanon

G. S. Abu-Sittah (✉)
Conflict Medicine Program, Global Health Institute, American University of Beirut, Beirut, Lebanon
e-mail: ga60@aub.edu.lb

© Springer Nature Switzerland AG 2023
G. S. Abu-Sittah, J. J. Hoballah (eds.), *The War Injured Child*,
https://doi.org/10.1007/978-3-031-28613-1_15

15.2 Epidemiology

Limbs are frequently the most common site of combat injury in pediatric patients across different conflict zones. This can be attributed to the direct morbidity of war on children resulting from bombs, missiles, burns, and bullet injuries that could be experienced either through the recruitment of children into combat or through the targeting of schools, hospitals, and civilian populations [3].

For example, children accounted for 28% of all civilian casualties in Afghanistan in 2018, with 2135 cases of maiming reported as a result of improvised explosive devices (IEDs) and aerial operations. In fact, IEDs accounted for around 4 in every 5 pediatric extremity injuries in Afghanistan, with a reported one-fifth of pediatric war-related extremity injuries requiring treatment by amputation [4]. In the Gaza Strip, one out of every 5 patients who required a war-related traumatic extremity amputation in 2018 was a child [5]. In Iraq, 84 children were maimed as a result of explosive remnants left behind by ISIS. In Syria, there were 784 cases of limb disability reported in 2018, where 70% of attacks on schools and hospitals were the result of air strikes, shelling, and IEDs [1], and 38% of children experienced traumatic limb injuries [6]. The list of countries with armed conflicts where children bear the brunt of war goes on and on and also includes Somalia, South Sudan, Yemen, Pakistan, and many others.

15.3 History

With advancements in healthcare, this means that fewer people die as a result of war injuries, whereas more and more survive and have to live with these injuries. Of course, with severe limb injuries comes the dilemma of whether to amputate primarily or attempt to salvage the damaged limb and with amputations comes the need for prostheses to enable children to maintain mechanics of movement that are as close to normal as possible.

While the most rudimentary prostheses from the first World War took the form of a split tree trunk attached to the limb by means of a leather strap, there have so far been monumental advancements in the designs of these prostheses. They trace their roots back to their mass production at a time when amputations were carried out as a necessity in the pre-antibiotic era as a result of gangrene and infections [7]. Later came prostheses with hinged designs that would mimic joints and others equipped with suspension systems, thereby better-suiting individuals with amputations occurring proximal to joints such as above-knee amputations and allowing for better shock absorption [8]. More advanced and lighter-weight materials such as aluminum and carbon fiber also replaced wood to allow for greater versatility and ease of use. Then in 1960 came the birth of myoelectric prostheses, ushered in by Alexander Kobrinski, allowing the amputee to stimulate the movement of the prosthetic [9], and 2004 saw the idea of a revolutionary surgical technique to reroute spare nerves from the amputated part to specific muscle groups, dubbed "targeted motor reinnervation [10]." However, a major rate-limiting factor for prostheses continues to be their financial cost despite all these advancements [11].

15.4 Primary Amputation Versus Limb Salvage

15.4.1 Objective Scoring Systems

A number of scoring systems have been devised to eliminate the subjectivity of the decision of whether to amputate or salvage the limb and to help guide decision-making based on objective criteria. The most commonly used and best-studied system is the Mangled Extremity Severity Score (MESS), where a score of 7 and above can be used as an indication to go for early amputation (Table 15.1). However, there is no consensus in the literature on the reliability of each of these systems to predict functional outcomes and the need for secondary amputation in cases where salvage fails [12]. With regard to the pediatric age group, the controversy surrounding these scores is also present, with some authors believing they are more sensitive in children compared to adults and others advocating against their use [13] [14] [15]. What is certain is that data on their use in the pediatric age group is limited, and surgeons should be cautious about being too overzealous in relying on these scores in general and in children in particular. Failed efforts to salvage a limb would lead to the need for secondary amputation with its resulting physical, psychological, social, and financial impacts on the child and their families [16].

15.4.2 Functional Outcomes

To assess the differences in functional outcomes between patients with mangled extremities undergoing primary amputation versus limb salvage, a large multicenter

Table 15.1 Variables considered in the different scoring systems for primary amputation vs. limb salvage

	MESS	LSI	PSI	NISSSA
Age	X			X
Shock	X			X
Warm ischemia time	X	X	X	X
Bone injury		X	X	
Muscle injury		X	X	
Skin injury		X		
Nerve injury		X		X
Deep vein injury		X		
Skeletal/soft tissue injury	X			X
Contamination				X
Time to treatment		X		
Comorbid conditions				

MESS Mangled Extremity Severity Score, *LSI* Limb Salvage Index, *PSI* Predictive Salvage Index, *NISSSA* Nerve injury, Ischemia, Soft-tissue injury, Skeletal injury, Shock, and Age of patient [12].

prospective observational study dubbed the Lower Extremity Assessment Project (LEAP) was carried out. While targeted toward trauma in the civilian rather than the military setting, this study followed patients with trauma-related lower extremity injuries who were treated with either primary amputation or limb salvage and assessed their functional outcomes at 2 and 7 years post-operatively [17]. It concluded that there was actually no difference between the two groups, albeit both experienced substandard physical and psychosocial outcomes. However, it showed that outcomes and quality of life are influenced by the patient's pre-existing economic, social, and personal factors, regardless of the initial treatment [18].

While functional outcomes related to the treatment of severe upper extremity injuries have not been as thoroughly addressed as their lower extremity counterpart, similar results have been noted in the Military Extremity Trauma Amputation/Limb Salvage (METALS) study, whereby long-term functional outcomes are similar for both amputation and limb salvage groups. [19] However, this study similarly demonstrates the persistence of overall disability in this population regardless of what type of treatment is pursued.

15.5 Level of Amputation

In some scenarios, limb salvage may fail due to local factors such as wound infections, complete damage to bones or soft tissues, or systemic factors affecting wound healing such as smoking, diabetes, peripheral artery disease, and neuropathy, in which cases amputation should be considered [20]. When taking this path, it is important to prepare a functional and painless residual limb for ambulation and activity [21]. Early counseling for patients and their families play a pivotal role in expected outcomes from such procedures [21]. It is also of uttermost importance to determine the level of amputation that gives the patient the best results in terms of activity, motility, and preservation of joint functions. The location of the most severe injury sustained by the traumatized limb is usually the main determinant of the level of amputation [21].

Table 15.2 shows that function and length are generally directly correlated, whereas energy consumption and length are inversely related.

Recent studies suggested that patients with below-knee amputation have a significantly better outcome than those who underwent above-knee amputation [21, 23]. It is also worth mentioning that patients with knee disarticulation have a better

Table 15.2 Energy expenditure as a function of lower extremity amputation level [22]

Amputation level	Energy above baseline, %	Speed, m/min	Oxygen cost, mL/kg/min
Long transtibial	10	70	0.17
Average transtibial	25	60	0.20
Short transtibial	40	50	0.20
Bilateral transtibial	41	50	0.20
Transfemoral	65	40	0.28
Wheelchair	0–8	70	0.16

quality of life than those with above-knee amputation [23]. Therefore, it is important to maintain the maximal length of the stump during surgery. In brief, the most used lower extremity amputation levels in order of length preference are trans metatarsal, Lis franc, Chopart, Syme, transtibial or below-knee amputation (BKA), knee disarticulation, transfemoral or above-knee amputation (AKA), hip disarticulation, and hemipelvectomy [21, 24].

15.6   Transtibial Amputation

From clinical experience in the current conflicts, this level represents the workhorse of amputations performed on the leg and below [25]. Taking into consideration that the knee joint will be preserved, this will allow the amputee to have a near normal gait with less energy required for ambulation [21, 26]. Patient who underwent below-knee amputation have a high rate of prosthetic use and are usually active [26]. At present, most BKAs are performed using a long posterior myocutaneous flap that is based on the blood supply from the gastrocnemius muscle [21]. This technique first described and popularized by Burgess in 1969 is based on the fact that the poorly vascularized anterior skin flap is compensated by the highly vascularized posterior flap [27, 28]. Later on, different techniques have been proposed for below-knee amputation that differ based on the soft tissue coverage used. In 1982, Robinson described the skewed flap based on the observations that thermographic mapping of the leg shows a higher temperature profile on the anteromedial as well as the posterolateral aspect this finding indicates a better blood flow, or say better nutrition, of the anteromedial as well as the posterolateral areas below the knee joint [29]. A recent meta-analysis showed the choice of amputation skin flap, including skew flaps and sagittal flaps, has not improved outcomes when compared with the posterior myocutaneous flap [21, 30]. No difference was also found in terms of wound healing, stump infection, and re-amputation rate [23]. The standard below-knee amputation techniques may not always be always used in war-related injuries due to the highly damaged soft tissues, therefore the surgeons may use local "flaps of opportunity" to cover the defect [21].

15.7   Surgical Technique

In terms of surgery, the main steps remain the same regardless of the level of amputation. The gold standard in war-related amputations is the aggressive removal of all necrotic and dead tissues [21]. The essential principles of amputation surgery at any level include removal of diseased tissue, providing a residual limb that allows for prosthetic fitting, tapering the ends of the bone to avoid sharp edges, providing a conical-shaped limb to allow better prosthetic fitting, controlling post-surgical edema, avoiding hematoma formation, allowing for nerve retraction, preservation of length, and optimized post-operative pain control [22, 31]. It is also important to minimize operation time and reduce blood loss; therefore, the use of a tourniquet is usually recommended [21, 27]. Copious irrigation with normal saline is advised with low-pressure irrigation preferred over high-pressure jet lavage [27]. The viability of the tissues must be assessed in the operating room based on the 4 Cs: color, consistency, contractility, and capillary bleeding when cut [32]. As mentioned above, the cornerstone of war surgery is to remove all non-viable tissue, fat, fascia, and muscle. At a later stage, the bone should be tackled with adequate length preservation; removal of small bone fragments and foreign bodies is essential to reduce infection rates. However, it is also of uttermost importance to preserve viable tissue and to preserve function.

Since injuries sustained in battle are usually contaminated, amputations are left open in either a guillotine fashion or with retaining muscle and skin flaps that could be used later in closure. To reduce infection rates, the use of subatmospheric wound dressings is becoming more popular for large wounds and cavitary defects [33]. Usually, serial irrigation and debridement will follow the primary surgery and are usually spaced for 48 hours. Once the wound is adequately debrided, stump closure should be performed [21, 27].

15.8   Anatomic and Physiologic Considerations in the Pediatric Patient

15.8.1 Bone Growth

The pediatric patient is a growing patient, whereby the physis plays a pivotal role in the growing extremity. As such, maximal effort must be exerted to preserve the physis, as this will have great implications later down the line when it comes to rehabilitation and prosthetic fitting [34]. However, when removal of one of the growth plates of a long bone is warranted, as happens in most through-bone amputations, growth is inhibited at the remaining growth plate on the proximal end of that bone. Therefore, the longitudinal growth of the remaining bone stump is generally stunted, resulting in a remnant that is shorter than would be expected as the child grows [35]. However, the child will require frequent prosthesis modifications, with socket revisions or replacement, as the residual limb does continue to grow, even if at a below-ideal rate [36].

15.8.2 Stump Length

While resection of devitalized soft tissue or bone is needed following severe extremity injury, pediatric patients generally have a superior healing capacity compared to adults, and damaged and infected tissues may respond more readily to medical resuscitation [21, 37]. This enables a more conservative approach to debridement, whereby it could be enough to simply debride non-viable tissue that is encountered during the first surgical intervention [37], with secondary revisions warranted in the days thereafter to assess the viability of tissues and whether an amputation would be needed.

Taking into account the aforementioned idea that growth of the amputated long bone is stunted, recognizing the importance of an adequate stump length following an amputation is vital so as to achieve good functional skeletal length at maturity. As such, all efforts should be exerted by the surgeon to maintain as much bone and soft tissues as possible without, however, compromising the adequacy of the debridement process so as to achieve an acceptable stump [38]. Negative pressure wound therapy (NPWT), or vacuum-assisted closure (VAC), has become a useful temporary adjunct once the wound has been adequately debrided and has become stable, as a plan for final bony level and soft tissue coverage is being formulated [39] [40].

15.8.3 Tissue Coverage

A number of reconstructive options are available to ensure soft tissue coverage of the stump should primary skin apposition not be attainable. Options include local flaps, free flaps, or tissue expansion so as to create an expandable flap. Soft tissue coverage of the distal end of an amputated extremity is important so as to control bony overgrowth with its associated complications [41]. Moreover, owing to its higher elasticity, the skin of a child can be stretched to cover the end of the residual limb, and skin grafts in the pediatric patient could better tolerate weight bearing and the shear forces experienced in the socket of the prosthesis [42].

15.8.4 Stump Overgrowth

Following an amputation performed through a bone, a common complication experienced by pediatric patients is appositional or intramembranous ossification at the transected end of the bone. This osseous overgrowth, or exostosis, can be problematic in several ways: compromising the adequacy of prosthetic fitting and injuring the surrounding soft tissues in the stump, leading to the development of pressure injuries or perforation through the skin [43]. This often necessities either prosthetic modifications or secondary surgical procedures to revise these overgrowths when the former fails [44]. It is important to recognize that the problem of stump overgrowth is not encountered with joint disarticulation but is only faced in the setting of through-bone amputations. Other events that can complicate post-op recovery include neuroma formation and phantom limb sensation.

15.9   Prostheses

An important consideration for children is that they are growing entities both physically and socially, and a child who experiences an acquired limb loss will have a sense of incompleteness and will undergo a period of readjustment, the success of which greatly depends on how well the child accepts the replacement prosthetic limb. While a prosthesis will never truly replace the missing limb, it will be needed to regain functionality as much as possible so that the child can continue to proceed through their developmental milestones [45].

Both upper and lower extremity prostheses share similar overall structures and are composed of: a socket, suspension system, pylon, and terminal section. Additionally, it is important to note that the prosthesis can also include an elbow or knee section that would mimic the lost joint in above-elbow and above-knee amputations.

15.9.1 The Socket

The socket is the weight-bearing part of the prosthesis that establishes contact with the stump of the residual limb and, as such, has to be custom-designed to fit a given amputation stump. While sockets have been historically designed so that weight bearing is mainly concentrated at the tip of the stump, newer sockets are total surface bearing and are designed to distribute the weight equally throughout the stump, thereby minimizing complications [46]. A comfortable fit is essential for the child to accept the prosthesis [41].

15.9.2 The Suspension System

This is the means by which the prosthesis is held in its proper position during different types of movements of the given extremity so as to prevent displacement of the socket out of its fit with the amputation stump. In other words, the suspension system ensures that the socket and the amputation stump are completely adherent to one another at all times and during different types of movements of the limb so as to prevent displacement of the stump within the socket and to minimize pain and gait instability [47]. This suspension system can take the form of a belt that anchors the stump and the socket to one another. Alternatively, internal suspension systems have replaced their more cumbersome and bulky external counterparts, and these include atmospheric/suction systems and pin-lock systems, among others [48]. It is not uncommon for more than one suspension system to be used at a given time [23].

15.9.3 The Pylon

This is the structure that lies between the socket and the terminal section. In other words, it is the arm/forearm section in an upper extremity prosthesis and the thigh/leg section in a lower extremity prosthesis. The pylon can either be rigid or flexible, and the latter is particularly important for lower extremity prostheses so as to allow shock absorption during running and walking activities and is referred to as a shock-absorbing pylon (SAP) [27, 49].

15.9.4 The Terminal Section

This is either the hand in an upper extremity prosthesis or the foot in a lower extremity prosthesis.

15.9.5 The Hand

While the hand was originally designed as a rigid unit, advancements today have allowed the construction of an artificial hand with moveable, articulated fingers given the importance of dexterity that is attributed to the hand. The most common configuration is that whereby the first three digits can be operated, whereas the fourth and fifth digits are composed of a flexible material that conforms to the shape of the object that is being held in the hand [45]. A number of terminal devices can be attached to the end of the hand prosthesis to enable performing particular functions by the amputee, one example of which could be a hook [45].

15.9.6 The Foot

The ankle and foot assembly in a lower extremity prosthesis exists in articulated and non-articulated forms. In the former, the ankle and the foot are a single rigid entity, and there is no separation between the two. In the latter, the foot and the ankle are separate entities, thereby enabling movements such as plantarflexion-dorsiflexion and/or inversion-eversion of the foot [50].

15.9.7 Power Source

A major distinguishing feature between upper extremity prostheses is the energy source used to power their movements. The prosthesis could be body-powered, whereby movements of the more proximal parts of the body such as the shoulder or the stump allow the motion of more distal parts of the prosthesis due to changes in tension being applied to a cable system that runs along the length of the prosthesis. The prosthesis could alternatively be electric-powered by a chargeable battery that operates an electric motor in the pylon, and this motor could be switched on or off by movements of the stump [47].

More recent is the advent of the myoelectric prosthesis, or the bionic hand, whereby the amputee is able to stimulate its movement by simply thinking about making an effort to open or close the fingers. Sensors present in the socket are able to pick up the electric potentials being transmitted through the stump as the amputee makes a conscious effort to move the hand or fingers, and these signals are transmitted to a motor unit in the hand or wrist section to obtain the desired movement.

In contrast to the upper extremity prosthesis, dexterity, and manipulation of objects are not required from the lower extremity counterpart. However, it is primarily needed to generate propulsive power to achieve motion of the body as a whole by walking or running, and an external energy source is often not needed. However, the effort is currently in place to produce myoelectric ankle/foot prostheses similar to the bionic hand so as to trigger movements of the ankle by means of neural signals [51, 52]. It is also worth noting that electric-powered knee units are available but have not been successful owing to poor battery life, noise, and weight [21].

References

1. UN Security Council. Children and armed conflict: Report of the Secretary-General. 2019. Report No.: S/2019/509.
2. UN Security Council Resolution 1261, S/RES/1261 (1999).
3. Pearn J. Children and war. J Paediatr Child Health. 2003;39(3):166–72.
4. Bertani A, Mathieu L, Dahan JL, Launay F, Rongieras F, Rigal S. War-related extremity injuries in children: 89 cases managed in a combat support hospital in Afghanistan. Orthop Traumatol Surg Res. 2015;101(3):365–8.
5. Heszlein-Lossius HE, Al-Borno Y, Shaqqoura S, Skaik N, Giil LM, Gilbert M. Life after conflict-related amputation trauma: a clinical study from the Gaza strip. BMC Int Health Hum Rights. 2018;18(1):34.
6. Naaman O, Yulevich A, Sweed Y. Syria civil war pediatric casualties treated at a single medical center. J Pediatr Surg. 2019;
7. A century of advances in prostheses. Nat Mater. 2018;17(11):945.
8. Fleigel O, Feuer SG. Historical development of lower-extremity prostheses. Archives of Medicine and Rehabilitation. 1966;47:275–85.
9. Sherman ED. A Russian bioelectric-controlled prosthesis: report of a research team from the rehabilitation institute of Montreal. Can Med Assoc J. 1964;91:1268–70.
10. Kuiken TA, Dumanian GA, Lipschutz RD, Miller LA, Stubblefield KA. The use of targeted muscle reinnervation for improved myoelectric prosthesis control in a bilateral shoulder disarticulation amputee. Prosthetics Orthot Int. 2004;28(3):245–53.
11. MacKenzie EJ, Jones AS, Bosse MJ, Castillo RC, Pollak AN, Webb LX, et al. Health-care costs associated with amputation or reconstruction of a limb-threatening injury. J Bone Joint Surg Am. 2007;89(8):1685–92.
12. Schiro GR, Sessa S, Piccioli A, Maccauro G. Primary amputation vs limb salvage in mangled extremity: a systematic review of the current scoring system. BMC Musculoskelet Disord. 2015;16:372.
13. Mommsen P, Zeckey C, Hildebrand F, Frink M, Khaladj N, Lange N, et al. Traumatic extremity arterial injury in children: epidemiology, diagnostics, treatment and prognostic value of mangled extremity severity score. J Orthop Surg Res. 2010;5:25.
14. Stewart DA, Coombs CJ, Graham HK. Application of lower extremity injury severity scores in children. J Child Orthop. 2012;6(5):427–31.
15. Fagelman MF, Epps HR, Rang M. Mangled extremity severity score in children. J Pediatr Orthop. 2002;22(2):182–4.
16. Prasarn ML, Helfet DL, Kloen P. Management of the mangled extremity. Strategies Trauma Limb Reconstr. 2012;7(2):57–66.
17. Higgins TF, Klatt JB, Beals TC. Lower Extremity Assessment Project (LEAP)--the best available evidence on limb-threatening lower extremity trauma. Orthop Clin North Am. 2010;41(2):233–9.

18. MacKenzie EJ, Bosse MJ. Factors influencing outcome following limb-threatening lower limb trauma: lessons learned from the lower extremity assessment project (LEAP). J Am Acad Orthop Surg. 2006;14(10):S205–10.
19. Mitchell SL, Hayda R, Chen AT, Carlini AR, Ficke JR, MacKenzie EJ, et al. The military extremity trauma amputation/limb salvage (METALS) study: outcomes of amputation compared with limb salvage following major upper-extremity trauma. J Bone Joint Surg Am. 2019;101(16):1470–8.
20. Molina CS, Faulk J. Lower extremity amputation. StatPearls Publishing.
21. Fergason J, Keeling JJ, Bluman EM. Recent advances in lower extremity amputations and prosthetics for the combat injured patient. Foot Ankle Clin. 2010;15(1):151–74.
22. Waters RL, Perry J, Antonelli DA, Hislop H. Energy cost of walking of amputees: the influence of level of amputation. J Bone Joint Surg Am. 1976;58(1):42–6.
23. Guerra-Farfán E, Nuñez JH, Sanchez-Raya J, Crespo-Fresno A, Anglés F, Minguell J. Prosthetic limb options for below and above knee amputations: making the correct choice for the right patient. Current Trauma Reports. 2018;4(4):247–55.
24. Meier RH, Melton D. Ideal functional outcomes for amputation levels. Phys Med Rehabil Clin. 2014;25(1):199–212.
25. Peterson LT. Administrative considerations in the amputation program. Orthopedic surgery in the zone of interior. Washington, DC: Office of the Surgeon General, Department of the Army; 1970. p. 865–912.
26. Purry NA, Hannon MA. How successful is below-knee amputation for injury? Injury. 1989;20(1):32–6.
27. Karami R, Hoballah JJ. Amputations and prostheses. In: Reconstructing the war injured patient. Cham: Springer; 2017. p. 165–80.
28. Burgess EM. The below-knee amputation Bull Prosthet Res. 1968;5:19–25.
29. Jain SK. Skew flap technique in trans-tibial amputation. Prosthetics Orthot Int. 2005;29(3):283–90.
30. Tisi PV, Callam MJ. Type of incision for below knee amputation (Cochrane review). The Cochrane. Library. 2004;1
31. Schnur D, Meier RH. Amputation surgery. Physical Medicine and Rehabilitation Clinics. 2014;25(1):35–43.
32. Bowyer G. Debridement of extremity war wounds. JAAOS-Journal of the American Academy of Orthopaedic Surgeons 2006 Oc;14(10):S52–S56.
33. Bluman EM, Hills C, Keeling JJ, Hsu JR. Augmented subatmospheric wound dressings (SAWDA): technique tip. Foot Ankle Int. 2009 Jan;30(1):62–4.
34. Khan MA, Javed AA, Rao DJ, Corner JA, Rosenfeld P. Pediatric traumatic limb amputation: the principles of management and optimal residual limb lengths. World J Plast Surg. 2016;5(1):7–14.
35. Brown KV, Henman P, Stapley S, Clasper JC. Limb salvage of severely injured extremities after military wounds. J R Army Med Corps. 2011;157(3 Suppl 1):S315–23.
36. Lambert CN. Amputation surgery in the child. Orthop Clin North Am. 1972;3(2):473–82.
37. Stewart DG Jr, Kay RM, Skaggs DL. Open fractures in children. Principles of evaluation and management. J Bone Joint Surg Am. 2005;87(12):2784–98.
38. Homann HH, Lehnhardt M, Langer S, Steinau HU. Stump retention and extension on the lower extremity. Chirurg. 2007;78(4):308–15.
39. Kneser U, Leffler M, Bach AD, Kopp J, Horch RE. Vacuum assisted closure (V.a.C.) therapy is an essential tool for treatment of complex defect injuries of the upper extremity. Zentralbl Chir. 2006;131(Suppl 1):S7–12.
40. Harrison DK, Hawthorn IE. Amputation level viability in critical limb ischaemia: setting new standards. Adv Exp Med Biol. 2005;566:325–31.
41. Davids JR, Meyer LC, Blackhurst DW. Operative treatment of bone overgrowth in children who have an acquired or congenital amputation. J Bone Joint Surg Am. 1995;77(10):1490–7.

42. Kent T, Yi C, Livermore M, Stahel PF. Skin grafts provide durable end-bearing coverage for lower-extremity amputations with critical soft tissue loss. Orthopedics. 2013;36(2):132–5.
43. Vocke AK, Schmid A. Osseous overgrowth after post-traumatic amputation of the lower extremity in childhood. Arch Orthop Trauma Surg. 2000;120(7–8):452–4.
44. Potter BK, Burns TC, Lacap AP, Granville RR, Gajewski DA. Heterotopic ossification following traumatic and combat-related amputations. Prevalence, risk factors, and preliminary results of excision. J Bone Joint Surg Am. 2007;89(3):476–86.
45. Bowker H, Michael J. Atlas of limb prosthetics: surgical, prosthetic, and rehabilitation principles. 2nd ed. American Academy of Orthopedic Surgeons; 1992.
46. Sewell P, Noroozi S, Vinney J, Andrews S. Developments in the trans-tibial prosthetic socket fitting process: a review of past and present research. Prosthetics Orthot Int. 2000;24(2):97–107.
47. Agarwal AK. Chapter 8: upper limb prosthesis. In: Essentials of prosthetics and orthotics. Jaypee Brothers Medical Publishers; 2013.
48. Gholizadeh H, Abu Osman NA, Eshraghi A, Ali S, Razak NA. Transtibial prosthesis suspension systems: systematic review of literature. Clin Biomech (Bristol, Avon). 2014;29(1):87–97.
49. Berge JS, Czerniecki JM, Klute GK. Efficacy of shock-absorbing versus rigid pylons for impact reduction in transtibial amputees based on laboratory, field, and outcome metrics. J Rehabil Res Dev. 2005;42(6):795–808.
50. Agarwal AK. Chapter 6: lower limb prosthesis. In: Essentials of prosthetics and orthotics. Jaypee Brothers Medical Publishers; 2013.
51. Au S, Berniker M, Herr H. Powered ankle-foot prosthesis to assist level-ground and stair-descent gaits. Neural Netw. 2008;21(4):654–66.
52. Sawicki GS, Ferris DP. Powered ankle exoskeletons reveal the metabolic cost of plantar flexor mechanical work during walking with longer steps at constant step frequency. J Exp Biol. 2009;212(Pt 1):21–31.

Rehabilitation of the War Injured Child

16

Natasha Habr and Ghassan Soleiman Abu-Sittah

16.1 Chapter Text

Injuries in children caused by firearms were often found to lead to considerable functional limitations. In addition, the psychological and social disruptions, which are present in a state of war, could influence children's recovery.

16.2 Outcomes After War-Related Trauma to Children

Jandric looked at 193 children aged 1–16 years to see if the grade of functional status differed considerably depending on the severity of the damage (firearms, other mechanisms of injury). The most common injuries were musculoskeletal and brain injuries. The extremities were the most commonly injured areas. Many badly injured children were shown to have long-term physical limitations. They were frequently discovered unable to walk without assistance and required the assistance of another person, a walker, or a prosthetic. Despite the suppleness, children who experienced significant trauma suffered long-term repercussions. Only 35.6% of children who had severe trauma and roughly 10% of children who were injured by firearms recovered fully functionally [1–4].

N. Habr
Department of Plastic and Reconstructive Surgery, American University of Beirut Medical Center, Beirut, Lebanon
e-mail: Nh117@aub.edu.lb

G. S. Abu-Sittah (✉)
Conflict Medicine Program, Global Health Institute, American University of Beirut, Beirut, Lebanon
e-mail: ga60@aub.edu.lb

© Springer Nature Switzerland AG 2023
G. S. Abu-Sittah, J. J. Hoballah (eds.), *The War Injured Child*,
https://doi.org/10.1007/978-3-031-28613-1_16

16.3   Medical Therapy

Increased protein breakdown is accompanied by insufficient synthesis in the post-injury hypermetabolic reaction. This causes a loss of lean body mass and, as a result, muscle weakening. However, the catabolic consequences are not restricted to muscle, as bone mineral content (BMC) and fat mass are also reduced. To enhance anabolism in trauma patients, strong nutritional support is required both during acute hospitalization and after discharge. These steps, however, have not proven to be sufficient. Several therapy options have been looked upon. Insulin, growth hormone, insulin growth factor I, oxandrolone, and testosterone are examples of anabolic hormones that have been utilized with varying degrees of success. Insulin has been found to be the most efficient in increasing net protein synthesis.

In badly burned children, oxandrolone 0.1 mg/kg/day has been proven to greatly speed healing. It has been shown to greatly boost muscular anabolism. Patients on oxandrolone had greater insulin growth factor-1 secretion, lean body mass, and muscle strength after a year of follow-up. In severely burned individuals, oxandrolone given over a shorter length of time paired with a 12-week exercise regimen produces much better outcomes than either alone. It has been shown that a dose of 0.1 mg/kg twice daily for up to a year is relatively safe. Patients should, however, be constantly monitored for potential side effects such as hepatotoxicity, testicular shrinkage, hirsutism, or behavioral abnormalities.

Endogenous catecholamines are important regulators of the hypermetabolic response in the aftermath of significant trauma. They increase myocardial contractility, myocardial oxygen consumption, and local myocardial hypoxia, resulting in tachycardia. Catecholamine concentrations in plasma increase tenfold almost immediately after injury and stay high for 2 years. Cardiotoxicity has been linked to high doses. The use of propranolol (a nonselective beta-antagonist) to block beta-adrenergic receptors in seriously injured patients can reduce hypermetabolic adrenergic effects and reduce catecholamine-induced muscle catabolism and lipolysis. It reduces oxygen consumption, mandatory thermogenesis, cardiac effort, heart rate, and cardiac oxygen consumption. It also improves immunological response and reduces infectious consequences by correcting any catecholamine-mediated impairment in lymphocyte activation. Beta-blockers may also reduce the inflammatory response by lowering the levels of IL-6 and MCP-1.

Propranolol medication for 12 months is safe in children with burns covering more than 30% of their entire body surface area. In children with minimal bouts of bradycardia and hypoglycemia, a daily dose of 4 mg/kg is well tolerated [5, 6].

16.4   Physical Therapy

Patients require considerable physical therapy in addition to medical treatment. Physical weakness is frequently linked to impaired osteogenesis, discomfort, and psychosocial stress in those who have suffered severe burns. Scars and contractures, which can be socially and physically debilitating, can worsen these issues. Because scars do not expand at the same pace as normal skin, burn scar contractures are a primary cause of late morbidity, especially in children who are still growing. Splinting and positioning are considered necessary to restrict and avoid the development of contractures, however, they might be difficult in the pediatric population.

Physical therapy can help counteract decreasing range of motion and avoid severe contractures in the extremities and fingers if started early. During outpatient rehabilitation, supervised resistance training and aerobic exercise regimens have been demonstrated to provide significant advantages. Cardiopulmonary capacity, the muscular mass, and pulmonary function improve 6 months after a burn when an organized program is undertaken. Strengthening occurs in severely burned youngsters as a result of greater muscle and neurological adaptations. It could be linked to an increase in endogenous anabolic hormones like growth hormone (GH) and testosterone secretion.

Improved physical exercise can help the patient ambulate more comfortably and execute things on their own. This alone would boost a child's emotional and physical self-esteem, resulting in a better quality of life.

16.5   Pain Management

The stages that follow an injury are marked by a lot of pain and concern. Patients should be given adequate pain control during the rehabilitation process in order to maintain their psychological and physical well-being. Procedural pain and physical therapy discomfort can have a substantial impact on a patient's willingness to participate in rehabilitation therapy. If the child has had a bad first experience, he or she is more likely to endure increasing discomfort and anxiety during subsequent sessions.

Understanding and addressing the requirements of individual patients is critical, and standardized processes must be reassessed on a regular basis. Because sedation is used during the treatment, a variety of analgesic, amnesic, and anxiolytic regimens can be used. When compared to the use of opioids alone, which has been proven to cause a drop in SaO_2 of more than 90%, this is favorable. In burned children, non-pharmacological cognitive (distraction tactics), behavioral (conditioning/relaxation techniques), and learning techniques have helped manage procedural pain. In therapy, the utilization of purposeful playing activity can produce excellent outcomes. Their focus is directed away from the discomfort, making the encounter less painful.

Multimodal distraction creates a subjective illusion in a child's mind based on sensory inputs from a virtual reality that successfully captivated the attention from feelings of pain and anxiety. A statistically significant reduction in pain-related brain stimuli was recorded in patients who underwent virtual reality [7].

16.6   Scar Management

Hypertrophic scarring is defined by chronic inflammation and proliferation of dermal tissue, as well as excessive deposition of fibroblast-derived extracellular matrix proteins, primarily collagen, in children who have been exposed to trauma causing extensive burns. Scar prevention and management is one of the most essential rehabilitation challenges for trauma sufferers. Early and vigorous interventions are the cornerstones of successful management. However, there is no consensus in the research on how to avoid and cure these scars. Surgical excision and grafting, occlusive dressings, topical or intralesional steroids, cryotherapy, laser therapy, radiation, pressure therapy, silicone gel sheeting and creams, and a range of other topical extracts have all been recommended.

Pressure therapy is designed to prevent the formation of hypertrophic scars and should be used as soon as the wound is closed. Recommendations for the amount of pressure and length of therapy are based on observational studies and are not conclusive. To overcome capillary pressure, it is recommended that the pressure be provided at roughly 24 mm Hg for 23 h per day. Maceration and paresthesia can occur when pressures exceed 40 mm Hg. Although the specific mechanism of action is uncertain, it has been associated with a reduction in scar blood flow and the stimulation of structured collagen deposition. Unfortunately, sticking to the prescribed routine can be challenging, especially during the summer.

The pressure garments can be utilized with gel sheeting, either hydrogel or silicone sheeting. They frequently soften scars by keeping them hydrated and reducing tension. They appear to promote scar maturation while reducing scar enlargement. Skin maceration, recurrent pruritus, skin rash, bad odor, and poor long-term compliance are all commonly reported adverse effects. In rehabilitation institutes that specialize in scar treatments, massage therapy, whether manual or mechanical (compressed air, threadlike showers, and vacuotherapy) is commonly used. Although different approaches can be used, none of them have been proven to be effective [8–11].

16.7 Transition to Outpatient Rehabilitation

Transitioning from intensive care and inpatient wards to outpatient care might raise the chance of misunderstanding and miscommunication, resulting in a lack of necessary care and increased stress. It is critical to recognize and address the challenges that families will experience once the child is brought home. The method for providing an efficient and effective changeover procedure is still unknown. Unmet needs are typical in children who have had brain damage, particularly in the first few months after the accident. It was discovered that post-discharge phone calls from an experienced rehabilitation nurse were able to clear up any misunderstandings and aid families with the difficult transition.

References

1. Kirk S, Fallon D, Fraser C, Robinson G, Vassallo G. Supporting parents following childhood traumatic brain injury: a qualitative study to examine information and emotional support needs across key care transitions. Child Care Health Dev. 2015;41:303–13.
2. Dudas V, Bookwalter T, Kerr KM, Pantilat SZ. The impact of follow-up telephone calls to patients after hospitalization. Am J Med. 2001;111:26S–30S.

3. Dossa A, Bokhour B, Hoenig H. Care transitions from the hospital to home for patients with mobility impairments: patient and family caregiver experiences. Rehabil Nurs. 2012;37:277–85.
4. Snow V, Beck D, Budnitz T, Miller DC, Potter J, Wears RL, et al. Transitions of care consensus policy statement: American College of Physicians, Society of General Internal Medicine, Society of Hospital Medicine, American Geriatrics Society, American College of Emergency Physicians, and Society for Academic Emergency Medicine. J Hosp Med. 2009;4:364–70.
5. Atiyeh BS, Gunn SWA, Dibo SA. Nutritional and pharmacological modulation of the metabolic response of severely burned patients: review of the literature (part 2). Ann Burns Fire Disasters. 2008;21:119–23.
6. Atiyeh BS, Gunn SWA, Dibo SA. Metabolic implications of severe burn injuries and their management: a systematic review of the literature. World J Surg. 2008;32:1857–69.
7. Perry S, Heidrich G, Ramos E. Assessment of pain by burn patients. J Burn Care Rehabil. 1981;2:322–7.
8. Carr-Collins JA. Pressure techniques for the prevention of hyper trophic scar. Clin Plast Surg. 1992;19:733–43.
9. Patiño O, Novick C, Merlo A, et al. Massage in hypertrophic scars. J Burn Care Rehabil. 1999;20:268–71.
10. Atiyeh B, El-Khatib A, Dibo SA. Pressure garment therapy (PGT) of burn scars: evidence-based efficacy. Ann Burns Fire Disasters. 2013;26:205–12.
11. Atiyeh BS, Esselman PC, Thumbs BD, Magyar-Russell G. Non-surgical management of hypertrophic scars (HSS): evidence based therapy, standard practices and emerging modalities. Aesthetic Plast Surg. 2007;31:468–92.

The Microbiology of War Wounds

17

Fadi M. Ghieh, Ismail Soboh, and Abdul Rahman Bizri

17.1 Introduction

Children living in conflict zones are nothing but victims of the actions of adults. Civilian casualties, including those in children, are part of the collateral damage resulting from modern war [1]. Children's injuries result from various scenarios including direct and indirect trauma, imprisonment, and recruitment of minors in combat. No matter the cause, the resultant injuries to children bring about both physical and psychological trauma, with the latter being more severe in some cases. Part of the suffering of injured children is the wounds they acquire, complicated by infections leading to amputations and disability.

In fact, all war-related wounds are grossly contaminated by various types and forms of bacteria [2]. Contaminated wounds caused by blasts and gunshots increase the risk of wound infection. Throughout history, several epidemics and pandemics from smallpox to cholera were responsible for greater morbidity and mortality than those caused by the injury sustained during wartime. However, upgrading the health care systems and the sanitation infrastructure were key elements in decreasing some of the morbidities and mortality rates related to these infections [3].

F. M. Ghieh
Division of Plastic and Reconstructive Surgery, American University of Beirut Medical Center, Beirut, Lebanon

I. Soboh
Department of Surgery, American University of Beirut Medical Center, Beirut, Lebanon

A. R. Bizri (✉)
Division of Infectious Diseases, American University of Beirut Medical Center, Beirut, Lebanon
e-mail: ab00@aub.edu.lb

© Springer Nature Switzerland AG 2023
G. S. Abu-Sittah, J. J. Hoballah (eds.), *The War Injured Child*,
https://doi.org/10.1007/978-3-031-28613-1_17

Improving the survival rates among injured patients during wars has increased the risk of acquiring wound infections and their subsequent complications including multi-drug-resistant organisms and sepsis [3]. On the other hand, early surgical interventions with aggressive surgical debridement and delayed primary closure were all part of a better treatment regimen leading to superior outcomes in terms of lower complications and mortality rates.

War injuries, whether due to trauma or post-operative complications, as in surgical site infections, pose a great burden not only on the patient but also on the treating physician and healthcare system [4].

17.2 Pediatric Pathophysiology of Wound Infection

There is no doubt that skin plays a significant role in preventing the bacterial flora living on its surface from invading and infecting the tissues and structures underneath [5]. Aside from the complexity and integrity of the skin, several other important factors determine the risk of developing a wound infection. These include the type of wound, depth, site of injury, and the host immune response to contaminants [6]. However, the anatomical and physiological responses to wounds differ between children and adults, and among children themselves according to age group. Younger children have thinner skin, a smaller body surface area, a smaller intravascular volume, less capable of preventing and fighting wound infections [7–9].

There are multiple sources through which bacteria responsible for wound infection can penetrate:

- Environmental Contamination is one of the major sources at the time of injury referring to contaminated clothes, shrapnel, bullets, and dirt associated with explosives [6].
- Skin-associated normal flora including *Staphylococcus epidermidis*, Propionibacteria, Micrococci, and skin diptheroids [5].
- The bacterial flora colonizing the internal organs mainly genitourinary, oropharyngeal, and gastrointestinal mucosa [10]. Multiple studies done on patients with wound infections have shown a close correlation between the bacterial contaminants found on wound culture and those present in the gut or oral cavity [11–13].

The resultant tissue hypoxia from wound injuries leads to cellular death and tissue necrosis. This creates a perfect environment for fastidious anaerobes to grow and proliferate consuming the local residual oxygen; this process was first described by Alexander Fleming during World War I [14].

Furthermore, tissue hypoxia is known to impair the local immune response, especially against invading microorganisms. The Antimicrobial burst of polymorphonuclear cells and its activity is impaired when reaching levels lower than 30 mmHg of PO2 [15]. Consequently, impaired tissue perfusion increases the risk of wound infection when compared to well-perfused tissue [16].

17.3 Diagnosis of Infection

The multiplicity of wound presentation in combat injuries makes it a laborious task to culture all wounds effectively. This may be due to numerous reasons such as a superficial or fluid swab culture taken for a wound that has a deeper infection brewing or a deep tissue culture taken while an osteomyelitic bone infection is lying underneath. Such examples lead to the initiation of inappropriate treatment for combat wound infections resulting in long and arduous ineffective treatment regimens. The complexity of combat wounds should be always taken into consideration when diagnosing wound infections and initiating treatment. Computed tomography imaging to diagnose deeper collections and magnetic resonance imaging or bone scans when available to rule out osteomyelitis should be ordered when needed and clinically suspected. However, this does not negate the need for proper testing and avoiding unnecessary cultures when the clinical scenario does not require. Over-testing is as bad as under-testing when trying to culture the microorganisms from war injuries. Another major requirement is early testing for suspected wound infections, which helps in avoiding further complications such as delayed wound healing, prolonged hospital stay, deeper infections, and systemic infections [5].

17.4 Bacterial Contaminants of Pediatric War Wounds

Searching through the literature, there is a severe dearth of studies on the microbiology involved in war injuries targeting the pediatric population. Most studies citing microbiology of war injury include very few if any pediatric patients in their sample. In a study comparing infantile to the adult cutaneous microbiome, a close similarity was observed between the two groups, and hence part of the conclusions in this article were based on adult findings to account for the scarcity of pediatric microbiology studies [17].

The microbiology of war injuries in adults has involved both Gram-positive and Gram-negative bacteria. Among Gram-positive bacteria, *Staphylococcus aureus* has been the most commonly involved pathogen [18]. Regarding Gram-negative bacteria, *Pseudomonas* spp. and *Acinetobacter baumannii* were the most commonly isolated [19, 20]. An interesting finding in war-associated osteomyelitic infections is the predominance of Gram-negative cultures in the early phases of infection and the predominance of Gram-positive cultures in the later phases [21, 22]. This finding can be attributed to several reasons, including nosocomial infections and inappropriate antibiotic usage.

It is clearly evident that pediatric physiology, along with the pathophysiology of wound infection, differs significantly from adults. This is mainly related to the fact that both skin and the intravascular volume are much greater in adults compared to the pediatric population and thus the reaction to traumatic events differs too [23, 24]. However, there is not enough data stating the differences in bacterial contaminants among the pediatric age groups susceptible to wound infections.

Nonetheless, certain constants remain regarding the common pathogens present in war wound infections whether in pediatrics or in adults [25, 26]. Several pathogens are commonly present and identified in wounds causing infection:

– Gram-positive cocci: *S. aureus* and beta-hemolytic streptococci are part of the normal human skin flora [1]. Recently, the presence of methicillin resistant *S. aureus* (MRSA) has increased the burden of treatment in many conflict countries [27, 28].
– Gram-positive bacilli: including the *Clostridia* species are widely spread in the environment and might cause gas gangrene and tetanus infections [2, 29].
– Gram-negative bacilli: Enterobacteriaceae such as *Escherichia coli*, Proteus and Klebsiella spp., *Pseudomonas aeruginosa*, and Bacteroides are found in the gastrointestinal tract with *Acinetobacter baumannii* being one of the major pathogens recently associated with nosocomial infections [30, 31].

Since World War I, studies done by Alexander Fleming have shown that the bacteriological nature of wound infections has evolved over time [32]. In other words, the development of wound infection and the microbiological etiology can evolve from the instant of wounding, self-contamination, and might end up with hospital-acquired nosocomial bacteria stepping in [2]. This highlights the importance of proper surgical debridement and wound hygiene as well as the need for proper antibiotics whether prophylactically or postoperatively to prevent evolvement of infection. Negative pressure wound therapy has an important role as bridging therapy, especially in contaminated wounds or those not ready for definite coverage. It has also been proven to help reduce the number of major soft tissue coverage procedures such as local muscle flaps and free tissue transfer [33].

17.5   Antimicrobial Resistance

Wars have been a notorious source of multi-drug-resistant (MDR) bacteria. These drug-resistant strains have been a problem for both military and civilian patients alike. The transfer of military personnel back to their home country and civilians to regional care centers has contributed to the widespread and dissemination of MDR organisms. Nosocomial transmission in sub-optimally equipped care centers has also played a role in spreading drug-resistant bacteria.

To begin with, refugees from war-torn countries such as Syria have been known to have high rates of MDR bacteria, due to several reasons such as non-prescription antibiotic sale [34–36]. MDR pathogens are present in as much as 83% of pediatric infections, with 58% of those infections having MDR bacteria similar to those present during the initial screening cultures [37].

Extended spectrum beta-lactamase producing *E. coli* and *Klebsiella pneumoniae*, are the most commonly isolated MDR pathogens followed by Acinetobacter *baumannii*, carbapenem resistant Enterobacteriaceae (CRE), MRSA, and vancomycin resistant Enterococci [37].

MDR bacterial infections have been linked with higher rates of failure of limb salvage, operative take-backs, and late amputations [38]. Furthermore, they have been associated to lower functional outcomes from limb injuries [38].

Consequently, firm infection control measures should be taken to impede the nosocomial transmission of MDR bacteria. They include early contact precautions, early culturing when needed, and hand hygiene. Appropriate antibiotic regimens should be initiated when required, with reservation of empiric broad-spectrum antibiotics for more severe and critical infections.

17.6   Antibiotic Prophylaxis and Management of War-Related Injuries

Prophylactic antibiotics in war injuries are commonly prescribed, regardless of the wound contamination status and mechanism of injury [39, 40]. Using targeted antibiotics with a narrower spectrum and for appropriate courses decreases the complications of wound infections and the incidence of MDR bacteria [41].

Wound care in combat-related injuries begins with copious irrigation of the affected wound, especially if the status of the wound is contaminated. Irrigation and removal of debris is followed by proper debridement procedures, as frequent and numerous as needed until healthy viable tissue is obtained. When required in contaminated wounds, antimicrobials should be given within 3 h preferably, along with the tetanus toxoid or immune globulin when indicated as per the guidelines of the Infectious Diseases Society of America and the Surgical Infection Society [41]. The latter measures help prevent sepsis and wound-associated complications. Targeted antimicrobial therapy depends on the area of the body affected; cefazolin is used for extremity, central nervous system, and thoracic injuries; metronidazole is added to cefazolin for penetrating abdominal injuries and thoracic injuries with esophageal perforation. Topical antimicrobials, such as silver sulfadiazine and mafenide acetate, are reserved for burn injuries where systemic antibiotics are not needed. As the aforementioned recommendations are for adults, several modifications apply to pediatric patients. Mafenide acetate is to be avoided in neonatal patients as it may cause kernicterus. Doses in pediatric patients less than 40 kg should be adjusted based on weight. Cefazolin and metronidazole doses should be based on patient's weight and divided into several doses [41]. Ertapenem, with usual dosing of once daily in adults, should be divided into two doses daily in children up to 12 years [41]. An alternative for abdominal penetrating injuries is ciprofloxacin or levofloxacin combined with metronidazole. Vancomycin can be added in cases of central nervous system trauma when needed. In septic patients, empiric antibiotics such as meropenem and amikacin are indicated [37]. Severe sepsis or CRE/ MDR *Acinetobacter baumannii* presence requires the addition of colistin [37]. Fluoroquinolones, tetracycline, and chloramphenicol should be avoided in children depending on age [42, 43].

17.7   Major Clinical War Wound Infections in Pediatrics

The polymicrobial nature of wound contamination might lead to various forms of infection [2]. Multiple fatal infections are ubiquitous in war wounds, mainly those which are neglected or mismanaged without proper excision and debridement [2, 44, 45]. The spectrum through which wound infection runs ranges from the minor superficial surgical site or wound infection to a more severe organ or surgical space infection to sepsis and septicemia [2, 46]. War wounds are frequently grossly contaminated with foreign materials and dirt [47]. They might initially start as cellulitis with/without local abscess formation through which the bacteria begin to spread from areas that are contiguous to the wound [48]. Cellulitis represents acute infection of the skin involving the dermis and subcutaneous tissues with the predominating microorganisms being Gram-positive cocci such as *Streptococcus* spp. and *Staphylococcus aureus* [49, 50]. The clinical picture in pediatric patients does not differ from that of the adult including pain, heat, erythema, and swelling, with skin penetration being the major risk factor [49].

Myositis and deep tissue infections result from further bacterial spread into the muscles and tissues underneath [2]. Systemic symptoms such as fever and tachycardia are more pronounced in this case and can dominate the clinical picture [2, 51].

Before the era of penicillin, deep tissue infections were usually caused by Clostridia and invasive beta-hemolytic Streptococci for the profound amount of tissue damage and the most severe systemic signs and symptoms [2, 52, 53]. The clinical picture since the presence of penicillin has significantly changed [54].

However, multiple invasive deep tissue infections in war-injured children have been observed in the literature including gas gangrene in mismanaged and neglected wounds, tetanus due to the disruption of immunizations and poverty in conflict and combat areas, invasive streptococcal infection, bone infection, necrotizing fasciitis, and pyogenic deep tissue infections [2, 55, 56].

17.8   Complications of Wound Infections

A variety of complications result from wound infections, whether correctly managed or not. Rates of complications have been reported to be higher than 25% in evacuated patients [38]. Incorrect and ineffective treatment, along with delay in initiation of treatment, results in a higher frequency and severity of wound infection complications. Deep wound infections and osteomyelitis can result as sequelae from more superficial infections. Further infectious complications include the emergence of MDR bacteria [38].

17.9   Conclusion

Prevention is key in war injuries; it should begin when injury occurs including copious irrigation, proper surgical debridement, adequate wound care, fracture fixation, and antibiotic prophylaxis when indicated [38]. Strict infection control measures should be applied when possible. Major obstacles remain in the way such as the severe environments of battle and gross contamination of wounds, improperly equipped medical health facilities in conflict zones, and the lack of availability of appropriate treatment at some centers.

References

1. Bertani A, Mathieu L, Dahan J-L, Launay F, Rongiéras F, Rigal S. War-related extremity injuries in children: 89 cases managed in a combat support hospital in Afghanistan. Orthop Traumatol Surg Res. 2015;101(3):365–8.
2. Giannou C, Baldan M, Molde Å. War surgery. Working with limited resources in armed conflict and other situations of violence. 2010;1:225.
3. Murray CK, Horvath LL, Ericsson CD, Hatz C. An approach to prevention of infectious diseases during military deployments. Clin Infect Dis. 2007;44(3):424–30.
4. Horwitz JR, Chwals WJ, Doski JJ, Suescun EA, Cheu HW, Lally KP. Pediatric wound infections: a prospective multicenter study. Ann Surg. 1998;227(4):553.
5. Bowler P, Duerden B, Armstrong DG. Wound microbiology and associated approaches to wound management. Clin Microbiol Rev. 2001;14(2):244–69.
6. Abu-Sittah GS, Hoballah JJ, Bakhach J. Reconstructing the war injured. Patient: Springer; 2017.
7. Fluhr J, Pfisterer S, Gloor M. Direct comparison of skin physiology in children and adults with bioengineering methods. Pediatr Dermatol. 2000;17(6):436–9.
8. Kong F, Galzote C, Duan Y. Change in skin properties over the first 10 years of life: a cross-sectional study. Arch Dermatol Res. 2017;309(8):653–8.
9. Özçelik S, Kulaç İ, Yazıcı M, Öcal E. Distribution of childhood skin diseases according to age and gender, a single institution experience. Turkish Archives of Pediatrics/Türk Pediatri Arşivi. 2018;53(2):105.
10. Duerden BI. Virulence factors in anaerobes. Clin Infect Dis. 1994;18(Supplement_4):S253–S9.
11. Brook I, Randolph JG. Aerobic and anaerobic bacterial flora of burns in children. J Trauma. 1981;21(4):313–8.
12. Brook I, Frazier EH. Aerobic and anaerobic microbiology of infection after trauma. Am J Emerg Med. 1998;16(6):585–91.
13. Muchuweti D, Jönsson KU. Abdominal surgical site infections: a prospective study of determinant factors in Harare, Zimbabwe. International wound journal. 2015;12(5):517–22.
14. Diggins FW. The true history of the discovery of penicillin, with refutation of the misinformation in the literature. Br J Biomed Sci. 1999;56(2):83.
15. Mukaida T, Takahashi K, Yamauchi Y, Horiuchi T. The effect of O2 tension on the blastocyst (BL) development of mouse embryos in vitro. Fertil Steril. 2000;74(3):S195–S6.
16. Davidson JD, Mustoe TA. Oxygen in wound healing: more than a nutrient. Wound Repair Regen. 2001;9(3).175–7.
17. Schoch JJ, Monir RL, Satcher KG, Harris J, Triplett E, Neu J. The infantile cutaneous microbiome: a review. Pediatr Dermatol. 2019;36(5):574–80.
18. Murphy RA, Ronat J-B, Fakhri RM, Herard P, Blackwell N, Abgrall S, et al. Multidrug-resistant chronic osteomyelitis complicating war injury in Iraqi civilians. J Trauma Acute Care Surg. 2011;71(1):252–4.
19. Teicher CL, Ronat J-B, Fakhri RM, Basel M, Labar AS, Herard P, et al. Antimicrobial drug–resistant bacteria isolated from Syrian war–injured patients, august 2011–March 2013. Emerg Infect Dis. 2014;20(11):1949.
20. Petersen K, Riddle MS, Danko JR, Blazes DL, Hayden R, Tasker SA, et al. Trauma-related infections in battlefield casualties from Iraq. Ann Surg. 2007;245(5):803.
21. Brown KV, Murray CK, Clasper JC. Infectious complications of combat-related mangled extremity injuries in the British military. J Trauma Acute Care Surg. 2010;69(1):S109–S15.
22. Johnson EN, Burns TC, Hayda RA, Hospenthal DR, Murray CK. Infectious complications of open type III tibial fractures among combat casualties. Clin Infect Dis. 2007;45(4):409–15.

23. Wheeler DS, Wong HR, Zingarelli B. Pediatric sepsis–part I:"children are not small adults!". Open Inflamm J. 2011;4:4.

24. Pickering LK, Dajani AS. Pediatric. Infections: WB Saunders; 1992.

25. Eardley W, Brown K, Bonner T, Green A, Clasper J. Infection in conflict wounded. Philosophical Transactions of the Royal Society B: Biological Sciences. 2011;366(1562):204–18.

26. PULVERTAFT RJ. Bacteriology of war wounds. Lancet. 1943;242:1–2.

27. Vento TJ, Calvano TP, Cole DW, Mende K, Rini EA, Tully CC, et al. Staphylococcus aureus colonization of healthy military service members in the United States and Afghanistan. BMC Infect Dis. 2013;13(1):325.

28. Falagas ME, Karageorgopoulos DE, Leptidis J, Korbila IP. MRSA in Africa: filling the global map of antimicrobial resistance. PLoS One. 2013;8(7):e68024.

29. Walker B. Gas Gangrene. The Lancet. 1939;233(6021):150.

30. Wassilew S. Infections of the skin caused by gram-negative pathogens. Foot infections--wound infections--folliculitis. Zeitschrift fur Hautkrankheiten. 1989;64(1):17–20.

31. Pondei K, Fente BG, Oladapo O. Current microbial isolates from wound swabs, their culture and sensitivity pattern at The Niger delta university teaching hospital, Okolobiri, Nigeria. Tropical medicine and health. 2013;41(2):49–53.

32. Fleming A. On the bacteriology of septic wounds. Lancet. 1915;186(4803):638–43.

33. Dedmond BT, Kortesis B, Punger K, Simpson J, Argenta J, Kulp B, et al. Subatmospheric pressure dressings in the temporary treatment of soft tissue injuries associated with type III open tibial shaft fractures in children. J Pediatr Orthop. 2006;26(6):728–32.

34. Al-Assil B, Mahfoud M, Hamzeh AR. Resistance trends and risk factors of extended spectrum β-lactamases in Escherichia coli infections in Aleppo, Syria. Am J Infect Control. 2013;41(7):597–600.

35. Al-Faham Z, Habboub G, Takriti F. The sale of antibiotics without prescription in pharmacies in Damascus, Syria. The Journal of Infection in Developing Countries. 2011;5(05):396–9.

36. Heudorf U, Krackhardt B, Karathana M, Kleinkauf N, Zinn C. Multidrug-resistant bacteria in unaccompanied refugee minors arriving in Frankfurt am Main, Germany, October to November 2015. Eurosurveillance. 2016;21(2)

37. Kassem DF, Hoffmann Y, Shahar N, Ocampo S, Salomon L, Zonis Z, et al. Multidrug-resistant pathogens in hospitalized Syrian children. Emerg Infect Dis. 2017;23(1):166.

38. Yun HC, Murray CK, Nelson KJ, Bosse MJ. Infection after orthopaedic trauma: prevention and treatment. J Orthop Trauma. 2016;30:S21–S6.

39. Velmahos GC, Jindal A, Chan L, Kritikos E, Vassiliu P, Berne TV, et al. Prophylactic antibiotics after severe trauma: more is not better. Int Surg. 2001;86(3):176–83.

40. Velmahos GC, Toutouzas KG, Sarkisyan G, Chan LS, Jindal A, Karaiskakis M, et al. Severe trauma is not an excuse for prolonged antibiotic prophylaxis. Arch Surg. 2002;137(5):537–42.

41. Hospenthal DR, Murray CK, Andersen RC, Bell RB, Calhoun JH, Cancio LC, et al. Guidelines for the prevention of infections associated with combat-related injuries: 2011 update: endorsed by the Infectious Diseases Society of America and the surgical infection society. J Trauma Acute Care Surg. 2011;71(2):S210–S34.

42. Sharland M, Rodvold KA, Tucker HR, Baillon-Plot N, Tawadrous M, Hickman MA, et al. Safety and efficacy of tigecycline to treat multidrug-resistant infections in pediatrics: an evidence synthesis. Pediatr Infect Dis J. 2019;38(7):710–5.

43. Jackson MA, Schutze GE, CoI D. The use of systemic and topical fluoroquinolones. Pediatrics. 2016;138(5):e20162706.

44. Negut I, Grumezescu V, Grumezescu A. Treatment strategies for infected wounds. Molecules [Internet] MDPI AG. 2018;23(9):2392.

45. Kalbitz M, von Baum H. Frühe postoperative Wundinfektionen. Orthopädie und Unfallchirurgie up2date. 2009;4(01):49–62.

46. Percival S, Cutting K. Microbiology of wounds. CRC Press; 2010.

47. Onyekwelu I, Yakkanti R, Protzer L, Pinkston CM, Tucker C, Seligson D. Surgical wound classification and surgical site infections in the orthopaedic patient. J Am Acad Orthopaedic Surg Global Res Rev. 2017;1(3)

48. Rubin RH. Surgical wound infection: epidemiology, pathogenesis, diagnosis and management. BMC Infect Dis. 2006;6(1):171.
49. Phoenix G, Das S, Joshi M. Diagnosis and management of cellulitis. BMJ. 2012;345:e4955.
50. Yarbrough PM, Kukhareva PV, Spivak ES, Hopkins C, Kawamoto K. Evidence-based care pathway for cellulitis improves process, clinical, and cost outcomes. J Hosp Med. 2015;10(12):780–6.
51. Jung N, Eckmann C. Essentials in the management of necrotizing soft-tissue infections. Infection. 2019;47(4):677–9.
52. Ki V, Rotstein C. Bacterial skin and soft tissue infections in adults: a review of their epidemiology, pathogenesis, diagnosis, treatment and site of care. Canadian J Infect Dis Med Microbiol. 2008;19(2):173–84.
53. Ramakrishnan K, Salinas RC, Higuita NIA. Skin and soft tissue infections. Am Fam Physician. 2015;92(6):474–83.
54. Polhemus ME, Kester KE. Infections. Combat Medicine: Springer; 2003. p. 149–73.
55. Nnadi C, Etsano A, Uba B, Ohuabunwo C, Melton M, Wa Nganda G, et al. Approaches to vaccination among populations in areas of conflict. J Infect Dis. 2017;216(suppl_1):S368–S72.
56. Strain RE. Gas Gangrene. Indian Medical Gazette. 1943;78(6):275.

The Invisible Wounds: Mental Health Support for the War Injured Children

18

Evelyne Baroud and Leila Akoury Dirani

18.1 Background and Epidemiology

In the world of today, there has been a shift in the type of armed conflict and war, from well-defined battlefields to civilian and community targeting [1]; conflicts have also become more stretched out and prolonged with a tendency to wax and wane [2]. Over the last few decades, there has been a consistent and steady rise in the number of children living in conflict areas [3]. In 2017, an estimated 1.8 billion children live in areas or countries torn apart by armed conflict [3]. In terms of the total number of children living in such areas, Asia has the highest figures; yet this must be taken in the context of the overall population size [3]. It is in fact the Middle East—with an approximate 40%, or 2 out of 5 children living in conflict regions—which has the highest portion of children affected by conflict; relative to its overall population [3]. The numbers for Africa, Asia, the Americas, and Europe, are as follows: 26%, 16%, 11%, and 5%, respectively [3]. Quite alarmingly, more than 420 million children live less than 50 km away from actual fighting zones [3]. In 2017, approximately a third (33.7%) of the world's children in conflict areas were reported to live in "high intensity" conflict regions where the census for battle-associated deaths exceeds 1000 children in a year's time [3]. There is a wide array of harms that befall children and adolescents during the conflict, these include but are not limited to death, physical injury, disfigurement, disease [3, 4] the failure of structures that deliver preventive, curative, and ameliorative care [4], as well as the hindrance of proper humanitarian help such as medical care, which according to United Nation reports, has become more widespread in recent years [3]. Deeper wounds that involve the mental health and psychological well-being of these children have also been well-documented in the literature [5–7]. The aims of the present chapter are to (1) provide an overview of the impact of war on children's mental health; (2)

E. Baroud · L. A. Dirani (✉)
Department of Psychiatry, American University of Beirut, Beirut, Lebanon
e-mail: eb22@aub.edu.lb; la55@aub.edu.lb

© Springer Nature Switzerland AG 2023
G. S. Abu-Sittah, J. J. Hoballah (eds.), *The War Injured Child*,
https://doi.org/10.1007/978-3-031-28613-1_18

explore some of the moderating factors in this complex relationship; (3) provide an overview of the assessment of children and adolescents exposed to war trauma; and (4) briefly review the evidence-based interventions and treatments that may help this vulnerable population.

18.2 Impact of War on Children's Mental Health

18.2.1 Stressors and Resilience

Stressors that may lead to acute and chronic stress responses in children may be classified into primary and secondary [8]. Primary stressors relate to the direct experience of harm or danger of harm, while secondary stressors encompass the repercussions of the disaster (i.e., adversities such as loss of home and injury). In many cases, if given appropriate support, children recover from acute stress responses over the course of time [8]. The American Psychological Association defines resilience as "the process of adapting well in the face of adversity, trauma, tragedy, threats or even significant sources of stress" [9]. Though resilience is an intricate concept and has been defined in many different ways; it generally refers to the capacity of a dynamic system to effectively adjust to disruptions that pose a danger to its viability; and an individual's ability to achieve a stable course of healthy function following an adverse experience [10]. For children in particular; there is an added layer of complexity to the concept of resilience; as a number of factors including parents or caretakers, family, and community/social come into play and are necessary for resilience to develop in children [11]. In trying to understand what adds to the resilience of children who experience war, factors are conceptualized on three levels [12–14]. The first level pertains to the children themselves and their individual characteristics; this includes their coping styles whereby resilient children characteristically evaluate traumatic incidents as less devastating and are able not only to appreciate the existing social resources but also to use relevant cognitive-emotional means that are appropriate to the stresses of the particular traumatic incident [12, 15]. Family is at the second level, as it is the main contributor to the healthy development of a child, especially after exposure to trauma [16]. The existing literature documents the buffering effect that a protective family environment can have. A study by Barber in 2001 showed that better parental education, integration in the family, and good parenting safeguarded the mental health of Palestinian children exposed to military violence. Specifically, the development of antisocial behavior among adolescents was precluded if they had elevated levels of parental acceptance and support [17]. In another study among Palestinians, supportive parenting styles were related to creativity and cognitive capacity in children, which in turn, added to psychological adjustment despite heavy war trauma experiences [18]. What is more, constructive relationships with siblings and connectedness with peers can dampen the mental health effects of war trauma particularly when It comes to symptoms of anxiety and depression [19, 20]. Having explored this, it is worthwhile to be aware that there are a number of other

Table 18.1 Factors that moderate the detrimental effects of war on children [21]

Solid bond between the primary caregiver and the child
Maternal mental health
Presence of additional caregivers
Social support from persons in the community who have been exposed to the same suffering
Shared sense of values
Religious beliefs that find meaning in suffering
Assuming responsibility for the protection and well-being of others
Having an internal locus of control
Using humor and altruism as defense mechanisms

factors that moderate the detrimental effects of war on children [21]. Table 18.1 lists the factors that were found to moderate the negative repercussions of war on children in the literature.

18.2.2 War and Psychopathology in Children and Adolescents

According to some researchers, traumatic experiences represent a continuum and it is the magnitude of the stress or the effect of moderating factors rather than the nature of the stress itself that is more important in determining aftermaths. According to this perspective, traumatic events may result in a wide variety of and are a risk for a number of different psychopathologies; and the particular psychiatric outcome may be related to characteristics of the child him/herself rather than the traumatic exposure [22]. On the other hand, other research explores that different types of stress may be specifically associated with different types of psychopathologies. For example, dangerous experiences usually generate distinctive signs of fear in a child, while losing essential relationships (for example, death of a loved one) may result in dysphoria [23]. It is important to keep in mind that during war times, multiple traumatic exposures are the rule rather than the exception; and that cumulative experiences are associated with greater symptomatology [24, 25]. Exposure to war results in a myriad of behavioral, emotional, and mental problems in children and adolescents; and the number of conflict-related traumatic occurrences is positively correlated with the prevalence of these problems[7]. The severity of traumatic experience is also a robust predictor of outcome, but other factors such as children's individual characteristics as well as elements related to their environment are also involved [26]. This range of exposure- and child-related influences entails that there are a number of possible targets for interventions intended to promote resilience in children [27]. In general, the more common diagnoses encountered in children exposed to war trauma are Post-Traumatic Stress Disorder (PTSD), depressive disorders, and anxiety disorders; and these may be comorbid [28]. A 2009 systematic review by Attanayake et al. of 17 studies included approximately 8000 children between the ages of 5 and 17 years, who have been exposed to wars in several regions including Central America, Bosnia, Cambodia, Rwanda, and the Middle East indicates that PTSD is the main sequel, with a prevalence of 47%, followed by depression (43%), and anxiety (27%) [6]. In the middle east, the prevalence of PTSD among children and adolescents in war zones is approximately 5–8% in Israel; it ranges between 23 and 70% in Palestine and between 10 and 30% in Iraq. As for Lebanon, litte is know about the prevalence of PTSD, althought the country faces major challenges. These numbers are similar to those in other war-burdened regions, namely 70% in Kuwait following the Iraqi invasion [29]; 52% in Bosnia-Herzegovina [30], and 50% among Cambodian children after war trauma [31]. Studies led after the War on Gaza (2008–2009) showed that more than half of children [32, 33], exhibited clinically significant post-traumatic stress symptoms, and a third endorsed symptoms of depression [33].

18.2.3 A complex Interplay of Factors That Perpetuate Psychological Suffering

Children and adolescents in war-afflicted regions are at risk of physical injury, torture, and witnessing or participating themselves in combat; they are at subsequent risk for several forms of violence including abuse and neglect [34–38]. There are also exposures to community and school-level violence [39] as well as domestic violence [35, 36]. Caregivers who have themselves endured armed conflict are in fact more likely to engage in child neglect and abuse, and there are higher rates of both child- and caregiver-reported child abuse in caregivers who suffer mental health illness or stress associated with their experience of armed conflict [34–36]. Conflict also precludes children from attending school and lowers their overall educational achievement [40, 41]. Economic sequelae of war also influence psychopathology, as rates of anxiety, post-traumatic stress disorder and depression in children and adolescents are higher in families who have lower income [42–44], perhaps because those with higher income are able to provide basic necessities during times of war[42]. Children may also take on adult responsibilities and obligations prematurely; this involves becoming providers for their families and delivering care for ill or disabled parents [45–47]. During war conflicts children may experience, be a witness to, and perpetrate acts of sexual violence and sexual exploitation [48, 49]. The sequelae of sexual violence are broad and far-reaching. A recent systematic review has categorized them into physical aftermaths such as pregnancy, sexual dysfunction, sexually transmitted illnesses, and traumatic genital injuries; and mental health consequences which include post-traumatic stress disorder, depression, and anxiety; as well as social outcomes such as rejection[50]. Conflicts also drive children and families to abandon their homes and flee within national or across international borders[48]; a journey during which they are vulnerable to illness, psychological trauma as well as exploitation and during which they may be separated from their families [51, 52]. Even in cases of re-settlement in a foreign country; post-migration socioeconomic factors influence the risk of developing depression, post-traumatic stress disorder, and anxiety [53].

18.3 Special Considerations in the Assessment of Children and Adolescents Exposed to War Trauma.

The assessment of children exposed to war trauma is different from adults. A key point is that a child's clinical presentation depends on his or her developmental level [8], and the reactions to trauma can be most understood from the perspective of the children's social, emotional, and cognitive development [54]. For example, younger children may show regressive behaviors while school-aged children may struggle at school, and older children or adolescents may engage in substance misuse [55]. Depression may be more common among older children as well [56]. Specific features of the stressor and the exposure to it, as well as individual-level factors such as age, developmental level, gender, previous history of psychiatric illness, and other larger-scale factors such as family characteristics and social environment all, play a role in the response to trauma and influence the recovery trajectory of the child/ adolescent [57]. The extent of exposure to acutely dangerous experiences appears to predict a greater risk for the development of subsequent psychiatric symptoms [22, 58]. A number of children will show non-specific behavioral and emotional symptoms, such as new-onset fears; clinging, and over-reliance on caregivers; they may also exhibit low frustration tolerance, aggressive behaviors, and changes in their eating patterns [1].

While assessing the sense of safety in children, one should consider the following. Infants and very young children rely on their parents or caregivers to estimate the actual degree of danger while preschoolers start to consciously incorporate the safety and protection of their parents as well as their own in their representations of danger [59]. By school age, children begin to grasp the complexity of dangerous situations and start to visualize self-efficacy as they become more and more involved in the safety and protection of themselves and others [59]. By mid-adolescence, they rely on themselves and on peers to evaluate threats and protection [59].

To assess the impact of the traumatic or stressful events, one should assess what is spoken by the child as much as the behavioral and somatic manifestations, particularly in young children and in children with limited cognitive and verbal abilities. Magical thinking, confusion, and self-accusation are developmentally related examples of early childhood thinking and emotional processing after a traumatic experience [54]. In the very young age group ranging from infancy to 6 years old, the following are some of the manifestations of distress: fear, increased startling, seeking attention from caregivers, temper tantrums, crying spells, and sleep interruptions along with trouble sleeping [1]. These young children are also more prone to experience somatic symptoms, such as gastrointestinal pains and changes in bowel movements [1]. They also show alterations in their play, which may change to more aggressive or on the contrary more inhibited [1]. Play is an important area of focus, as children tend to reflect on their traumatic experiences in the content of play; such as re-enacting the trauma, repetitive play, fantasy devoid play as well as macabre themes in the play. Their play is also less rich in social interactions and with a predominance of negative affect [60–62]. Young children may exhibit sleep-related difficulties such as refusing to sleep alone, instance on sleeping with their parents; experiencing nightmares, and repeated awakenings[63–67]. On the other hand, while separation anxiety is a usual normative occurrence in younger children; it may become apparent in school-aged children as a manifestation of their distress[1]. In general, boys have more exposure to severe traumatic events than girls [42, 68]; and though both genders suffer from anxiety and depression symptoms; girls report considerably more symptoms of depression than boys [43]. After exposure to war trauma, adolescents experience elevated levels of intrusion, avoidance, and depression symptoms; with the female gender being a significant risk factor for depression[44]. What is more, adolescents who have increased exposure to war events and those who suffer from PTSD as a result, have greater rates of substance abuse and are more likely to be involved in violence within schools [69].

The following are some of the signs of distress in children exposed to war trauma across age groups: physical symptoms such as headaches and abdominal pain with no apparent physical origin; crying spells, sadness, or irritability; difficulties sustaining attention and focus; fear and anxiety; insomnia or hypersomnia; nightmares; recurrent thoughts about the traumatic event or avoiding discussion the event and avoiding reminders of the event; being distressed by reminders of the traumatic event; difficulties managing behavior or emotions; flashbacks; not engaging with others in play or in activities that were enjoyable and hopelessness [70].

As previously mentioned, signs of distress in children may vary according to age categories and developmental level. Below are some examples of distress stratified by age groups [70, 71]:

1. **Preschool Children**: Preschool children may experience a regression to younger behaviors which may include bed-wetting, thumb-sucking, and mutism. They may have unexplained physical symptoms as well as trouble separating from their parents or caregivers. They may also throw temper tantrums or have aggressive behaviors such as throwing kicking, biting, or hitting. They may be reluctant to engage in play or engage in a repetitive re-enactment of the traumatic event during their play.

2. **Elementary School Children:** These children may experience difficulties with concentration, memory, and attention, causing them to struggle in school. They may also have peer problems and aggression toward others. They may present with new-onset fears such as fear of separation from parents or caregivers and fear of something bad happening. They may isolate themselves from others; and may experience anger and irritability as well as feelings of sadness, self-blame, and guilt.

3. **Middle and High school children and Adolescents:** This category of children/adolescents may experience more complex emotions, such as a sense of guilt or responsibility for bad things that have happened; feelings of shame or embarrassment, and helplessness. They may have difficulties in interpersonal relationships with their parents, teachers, friends, and family. They may have changes in

their perception of the world or experience a loss of faith. Alternatively, they may have conduct problems or engage in substance use or misuse.

Because children are embedded within families, and because it is the parents who usually are the closest and most impactful people in a child's development, particularly during the early years[72], it is crucial to incorporate parental mental health in the overall evaluation of a war-affected child. Indeed, children in families where a parent has suffered from war trauma may experience secondary traumatization and may suffer from the repeated use of ineffective coping skills by the distressed parent, generally the mother [73]. Furthermore, the psychological distress of parents mediates and moderates the connection between war trauma and developmental consequences in children including behavioral and emotional problems [72]. In particular, parental distress after exposure to war trauma may present a specific risk for depressive symptoms in the child [74]. In young children, the effect of the parents' responses may have an equal or bigger impact than that of the actual traumatic experience [75]. Not only is there a correlation between parental and children's psychopathology but the family environment and parental functioning moderate the relationship between exposure to trauma and outcome for children [1].

18.4   The Interplay Between Direct Physical Injuries, Pain, and Mental Health

There is a wide array of possible physical harms affecting all organ systems that may befall children as a result of penetrating injuries, burns, crush injuries, and blunt trauma [48]. Chronic physical illness places children at a higher risk of behavioral and emotional problems as well as at an increased risk of developing psychiatric disorders [76]. Between a quarter to a third of children who suffer from burns display some PTSD symptoms [77, 78], they may also suffer from anxiety and mood symptoms, sleep problems, as well as conduct, learning, and attention problems [79]. Interestingly, pathways leading to the development of PTSD in children with burns are mediated by separation anxiety and dissociative responses, with trauma magnitude being a mediator of both pathways, and pain having an influence on the development of PTSD indirectly through separation anxiety; thereby highlighting the complex and dynamic interaction between pain, family effects and the development of PTSD [80]. During the acute phase of burn injuries, for example, children experience a psychological reaction to the trauma of the burn injury itself and to its subsequent treatment [81]. Anxiety, fear, and pain frequently have comparable symptoms, particularly in younger children who may experience dread, tremulousness, restlessness, muscle tension, tachycardia, dizziness, sweating, dyspnea, cold hands and feet, excessive worries; nightmares as well as difficulties falling asleep [81]. Therefore, the child and adolescent psychiatrist, psychologist, or clinician assesses injury severity to plan interventions that can alleviate pain and reinforce coping strategies to manage the risk of death, disability, and effects on body image [82]. Later on, in the recovery process, children may show aggression, disruptive behaviors, mood symptoms, learned helplessness, enuresis and encopresis, food refusal as well as sleep and attention difficulties [82]. Some suggested methods for the psychiatric care of the injured child include pain management, brief consultation, and crisis intervention followed by brief psychotherapeutic techniques [82]. As a first step, explaining and clarifying what is going on and what is going to happen, as well as giving the children reasonable choices about how a procedure can be performed boosts their sense of control, and can help diminish their sense of being a victim. For example, during dressing changes, a child may gain a sense of control by aiding in the removal of the dressing and will trust this will cause him or her less distress [83]. Particular attention should be paid to pain. While pharmacological interventions remain the core of pain treatment, it is important to be mindful of the large number of psychological factors that accompany pain and that may contribute to the sensation of pain [83]. These include emotional distress, stressful memories, anticipatory apprehension about both the treatment of the injury itself and the recovery period, as well as being restricted in a new and possibly frightening hospital environment. These factors are the target of psychotherapeutic interventions [83, 84]. Specific intervention approaches include cognitive behavioral therapy, hypnosis, relaxation training, guided imagery, art, music, and play therapies as well as biofeedback and distraction therapy [85–88]. In biofeedback, patients learn through self-regulation to voluntarily control body processes [89]. Common methods of distraction [81, 90] that help in alleviating pain in burned children are playing, reading a story, watching television, and listening to music [91]. Other techniques include biofeedback, massage [92], and even virtual reality [93]. The two principal psychotherapeutic methods used to treat an injured child are psychodynamic psychotherapy and cognitive behavioral therapy, and they are generally used together and explicitly oriented to the pain [94], the injury itself, coping with surgery, and other needed medical care, as well as addressing responses to disfigurement or disability and grieving losses [28]. Cognitive restructuring, management of anxiety, strategies to cope with anger, and exposure-based interventions are the main features of cognitive behavioral therapy in injured children who suffer from PTSD [95] and in those with facial deformities [96]. Table 18.2 lists some strategies to help children cope

Table 18.2 Techniques to help children coping with anger

Immediate reaction to anger outbursts from the caregiver	
Do not yell	Use a neutral tone of voice
Do not scold	Encourage the child, or take him to a quiet place (remove him or her from the heat of the situation)
After the anger outburst	
Do not blame	Partner with the child in defining the problem that led to anger
	Find several alternative solutions
Do not shame	Encourage emotional expression
	Encourage peaceful conflict resolution
Continuous preventive measures and coping techniques to adopt with the child	
Identifying the bodily sensations as signs of emergent anger outburst	
Use relaxation techniques (breathing, distraction, humor)	
Step out of the "circle of anger"	
Promise to get back to problem solving after the anger is tamed	

with anger. Further on in the recovery process, clinicians should be mindful that burn disfigurement impacts children's self-confidence, affects their social interactions, and marks their identity [97]. These children are more likely to be bullied [98]. In adolescents, predictors of positive body image and improved self-esteem are linked to perceived social support [99]. This applies to all other types of acquired disabilities.

18.5 Interventions for Recovery from War Trauma Among Children and Adolescents

Research in the field of the resilience of war-exposed children and their growth post-trauma has recognized potentially changeable protective processes that may become the focus of interventions [21, 100]. Once the armed conflict is over; essential needs such as primary health care, limiting the spread of infectious diseases, access to clean water, food, shelter, and sanitation must be met; and educational activities should be started or reinstated as soon as possible [100]. Indeed, a large number of children may improve when access to water, food, shelter, health care, and security is restored [71]. Other children and adolescents will need dedicated support, with particular consideration for the child, family, and group. This psychological first aid should be delivered by health workers [71]. Lastly, children who suffer from exceptionally stressful reactions may require focused support for months; this may encompass counseling by social workers, teachers, and health care workers as well as broader social and cultural activities with Non-Governmental Organizations or groups within the community [71]. In general, the principles of management in line with those of Psychological First Aid include the following: (1) Creating a sense of safety, (2) instilling calm and lessening physiologic arousal, (3) reinstating a sense of personal efficacy, (4) re-establishing a sense of connectedness to others, and (5) imparting hope [101]. For those who will be working on the front line with traumatized children, it is important to keep in mind that the goal of Psychological First Aid for children is to provide relief from distress, help their current needs, and to foster adaptive functioning, and does not aim to gather details of painful experiences and loss [71].

18.5.1 Encounter with the Trauma-Affected Child or Adolescent

In general, the evaluation of the child begins with extracting the storyline of the trauma, preferably from the child himself or herself [28]. Children as young as ages 2–12 years can remember details of stressful incidents after injury [102]. Throughout the child's narrative, it is important to be mindful of his or her account of related memories, thoughts, and feelings, the occurrence of alterations, and potential recurrent themes [103]. Afterward, in addition to assessing existing symptoms, it is important to look into the child's developmental history and the presence of previous psychopathology [28]. This information may be obtained from the parent or caretaker whenever possible. Before beginning the assessment of traumatized child or adolescent, patience is of the utmost importance. The interviewer should not take for granted that children or their parents/caregivers will respond positively straightaway [71]. The interviewer must remain sensible, sensitive, and attentive and must follow the pace of the child, all the while providing support for difficult emotions [71]. Accepting that the child may be experiencing difficult emotions such as anger, guilt and grief is paramount, and this involves avoiding telling the child or adolescent how he or she should feel, and rather mirroring the feelings of sadness; and acknowledging the overwhelming nature of these emotions [71]. Equally imperative is to offer hope to the child without dismissing or minimizing the reality of the situation [71]. Figure 18.1 provides general instructions when performing an interview with a child/adolescent following a traumatic experience. Specifically, the use of active listening helps to reinforce cooperation and nurtures understanding between the interviewer and the child/adolescent [71]. Active listening is a communication technique based on the work of psychologist Carl Rogers, which involves providing full attention to the speaker; and encompasses both verbal and non-verbal communication approaches [104]. There are five elements to active listening: (1)attentive focus, (2) paraphrasing, (3)

Fig. 18.1 General considerations in the interview of a child/adolescent following a traumatic experience

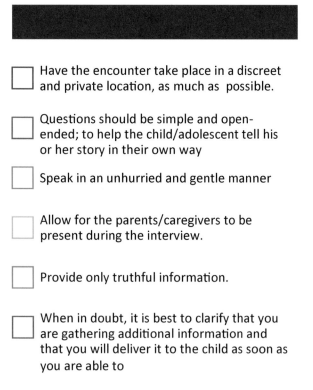

Have the encounter take place in a discreet and private location, as much as possible.

Questions should be simple and open-ended; to help the child/adolescent tell his or her story in their own way

Speak in an unhurried and gentle manner

Allow for the parents/caregivers to be present during the interview.

Provide only truthful information.

When in doubt, it is best to clarify that you are gathering additional information and that you will deliver it to the child as soon as you are able to encouragement, (4) questioning/clarifying, and (5) summarizing [71]. In attentive focus, the emphasis is on listening while avoiding interruptions, regardless of what the child is saying; and on being aware of one's own body language [71]. In paraphrasing the interviewer may restate important words spoken by the child/adolescent, and may reprise what was heard in a descriptive rather than an interpretative way; for example, by using statements such as "I understand what you are saying"; "Did I understand correctly?"; and "It sounds like this experience made you feel scared; is that so? [71]. Depending on the context of the assessment, and the level of acuity of the situation, the interviewer may be faced with an emotionally overwhelmed and very distressed child or adolescent. Stabilization of this state of hypervigilance and hyperarousal may be achieved through the use of some relaxation and grounding techniques [71], examples of which are shown in Figure 18.2. As previously mentioned, it is imperative to involve the parents/caregivers in the evaluation of traumatized children and adolescents. Priority should be given to educating the parents/caregivers about the wide range of signs and symptoms and possible reactions of their child's distress depending on the child's age and development level [71], keeping in mind that parents are themselves traumatized or at least heavily affected by the situation which means that they are also in need of active listening and support.

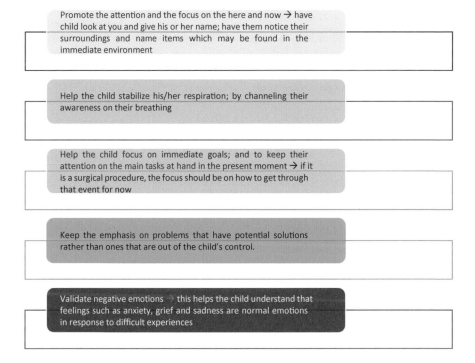

Fig. 18.2 Examples of relaxation and grounding techniques

18.5.2 Evidence-Based Approaches for Treating War-Affected Children and Adolescents

There is increasing awareness and emphasis on incorporating the mental health and psychosocial support needs of people who experience humanitarian crises into humanitarian aid responses [105]. Mental health and psychosocial support programs are defined as any local or external support that purposes to safeguard or promote psychosocial well-being [106] or to prevent or treat mental health problems [107]. This definition is used broadly in the area of humanitarian emergencies to describe strategies devised to tackle the mental health and psychosocial difficulties of people in disaster and conflict situations [108]. There are numerous challenges to implementing proper evidence-based interventions in low and middle-income countries following trauma. These include the paucity of mental health services, insufficiently qualified clinicians, and barriers to modifying established interventions to the needs of contexts that are specific to low and middle-income countries [109]. The more common mental health and psychosocial support interventions relate to community-based social support, structured social activities, providing information and counseling, psychoeducation, and fostering awareness [110].

Randomized trials in conflict-affected areas propose that brief and structured intervention may improve outcomes in traumatized children and adolescents when carefully applied [111, 112]. A 2011 meta-analysis that comprised four randomized controlled trials in children and adolescents who experienced mass traumatic events showed that school-based interventions did not improve symptoms of post-traumatic stress disorder per se, but that psychosocial interventions (group interpersonal psychotherapy, group meetings with parents, and school-based interventions) were beneficial for internalizing symptoms (anxiety or depression) [110]. However, there is much heterogeneity in the literature, and the effects of various programs may depend on the initial intervention objectives [113], the characteristics of the program itself, as well as its quality and delivery [107, 114]. The specifics of the target population also play a role, including the type of trauma exposure, gender, level of social support, and context-related considerations such as degree of insecurity [115]. It is therefore important to identify common practice features of interventions that are successful at inducing targeted change [114]. It is equally important to describe different effects for dissimilar subgroups of participants [116] with regard to age, gender, socioeconomic level, geographic location, and trauma exposure [117]. A 2017 systematic review evaluated the effectiveness of mental health and psychosocial support programs in areas affected by humanitarian crises, though these were not limited to war-ridden areas [107]. The programs were likely to use cognitive behavioral techniques or other psychotherapy modalities including interpersonal grief-focused therapy and narrative exposure and were typically given in school-based environments, for the longest duration of 3 months [107]. The following evidence emerged:

1. Strong evidence is that the programs reduce functional impairment but have little impact on anxiety.

2. Moderate evidence that the programs marginally improve symptoms of post-traumatic stress disorder conduct problems, and psychological distress; and that they may have no effect on depression or prosocial behaviors.
3. Moderate evidence that Trauma-focused cognitive behavioral therapy is helpful in effectively ameliorating post-traumatic stress disorder symptoms as well as emotional and conduct problems.
4. Moderate evidence is that classroom and school-based interventions do not help reduce anxiety.
5. Moderate evidence that Narrative Exposure Therapy helps functional impairment but has little effect on post-traumatic stress symptoms.

18.6 Conclusion

War-related consequences are common worldwide and relate not only to the direct impact of war on the children themselves but also to major societal breakdowns, leading to consequential psychiatric morbidity [118–121]. War consequences such as death, injury, illness, disability, child soldiers, sexual violence as well as social and cultural losses [122] to name a few perpetuate psychological suffering in children exposed to war. Post-traumatic stress disorder, depression, and anxiety are among the most common disorders after traumatic events, including physical injuries; but other problems include sleep and elimination difficulties, conduct, learning, and attention problems as well as longer terms effects on body image and self-esteem may become apparent. The clinical presentation of distress in a child is developmentally dependent and must be grasped from the perspective of the child's social, emotional, and cognitive development. The elaboration of clear, consistent, and effective interventions for managing war-related traumatic experiences can only be done through a better understanding of conflicts and the multitude of mental health problems that result from them[123]. It is imperative to keep in mind the importance of social resources in trauma—particularly the role of family—and their potential to shield children from the detrimental effects of war, as well as their contribution to the resilience of children [124, 125]. Cognitive behavioral therapy and trauma focused cognitive behavioral therapy, remain validated therapeutic approaches for children and adolescents who suffer from trauma-related symptoms. The potential for children to recover is inherently related to resilience, which in turn depends on broader systems of care. Residual symptoms in children who have experienced war may be considered normal reactions to very abnormal situations; therefore there is a need for longer-term follow-up of these children, to better understand which symptom dimensions remain as psychopathology; and which fade away when a normal life balance is restored. Lastly, when trauma exposure becomes chronic and danger is ongoing, strong reactions may become a mechanism for survival, rather than a manifestation of psychopathology. More research is needed into what strategies work best to foster resilience in war-exposed children and to help them overcome, step by step, the difficulties they may face in the long road to recovery.

These children without a childhood
Without youth and without joy
Who shivered helplessly
With sorrow and cold
Who defied suffering
And silenced their turmoil
But lived in hope
Are like you and me
Charles Aznavour

References

1. Slone M, Mann S. Effects of War, Terrorism and Armed Conflict on Young Children: A Systematic Review. Child Psychiatry Hum Dev. 2016;47:950–65.
2. Austin A, MRN FM. Trends and causes of armed conflict. In: Transform. New York: Ethnopolitical Confl. Berghof Handb. VS Verlag für Sozialwissenschaften; 2004. p. 111–27.
3. Østby G, Aas Rustad S, Forø Tollefsen A. Children Affected by Armed Conflict, 1990–2017. Oslo; 2018.
4. Devakumar D, Birch M, Osrin D, Sondorp E, Wells JC. The intergenerational effects of war on the health of children. BMC Med. 2014;12:57.
5. Shaar KH. Post-traumatic stress disorder in adolescents in Lebanon as wars gained in ferocity: a systematic review. J Public health Res. 2013;2:e17.
6. Attanayake V, McKay R, Joffres M, Singh S, Burkle F, Mills E. Prevalence of mental disorders among children exposed to war: a systematic review of 7,920 children. Med Confl Surviv. 25:4–19.
7. Dimitry L. A systematic review on the mental health of children and adolescents in areas of armed conflict in the Middle East. Child Care Health Dev. 2012;38:153–61.
8. Chrisman AK, Dougherty JG. Mass Trauma. Child Adolesc Psychiatr Clin N Am. 2014;23:257–79.
9. American Psychological Association. The Road to Resilience. Washington DC: American Psychological Association. 2014. http://www.apa.org/helpcenter/road-resilience.aspx.
10. Southwick SM, Bonanno GA, Masten AS, Panter-Brick C, Yehuda R. Resilience definitions, theory, and challenges: interdisciplinary perspectives. Eur J Psychotraumatol. 2014;5:25338.
11. Pine DS, Cohen JA. Trauma in children and adolescents: risk and treatment of psychiatric sequelae. Biol Psychiatry. 2002;51:519–31.
12. Betancourt TS, Meyers-Ohki SE, Charrow AP, Tol WA. Interventions for Children Affected by War. Harv Rev Psychiatry. 2013;21:70–91.
13. Dubow EF, Huesmann LR, Boxer P. A social-cognitive-ecological framework for understanding the impact of exposure to persistent ethnic–political violence on children's psychosocial adjustment. Clin Child Fam Psychol Rev. 2009;12:113–26.
14. Ungar M. Resilience, Trauma, Context, and Culture. Trauma, Violence, Abus. 2013;14:255–66.
15. Tol WA, Song S, Jordans MJD. Annual Research Review: Resilience and mental health in children and adolescents living in areas of armed conflict - a systematic review of findings in low- and middle-income countries. J Child Psychol Psychiatry. 2013;54:445–60.
16. Bowlby J. Attachment and loss: Retrospect and prospect. Am J Orthopsychiatry. 1982;52:664–78.
17. Barber BK. Political violence, social integration, and youth functioning: Palestinian youth from the Intifada. J Community Psychol. 2001;29:259–80.
18. Punamaki R-L, Qouta S, El SE. Models of traumatic experiences and children's psychological adjustment: the roles of perceived parenting and the children's own resources and activity. Child Dev. 1997;68:718.

19. Peltonen K, Qouta S, El Sarraj E, Punamäki R-L. Military trauma and social development: The moderating and mediating roles of peer and sibling relations in mental health. Int J Behav Dev. 2010;34:554–63.
20. Betancourt TS, Salhi C, Buka S, Leaning J, Dunn G, Earls F. Connectedness, social support and internalising emotional and behavioural problems in adolescents displaced by the Chechen conflict. Disasters. 2012;36:635–55.
21. Werner EE. Children and war: Risk, resilience, and recovery. Dev Psychopathol. 2012;24:553–8.
22. Steinberg L, Avenevoli S. The role of context in the development of psychopathology: a conceptual framework and some speculative propositions. Child Dev. 71:66–74.
23. Eley TC, Stevenson J. Specific life events and chronic experiences differentially associated with depression and anxiety in young twins. J Abnorm Child Psychol. 2000;28:383–94.
24. Hubbard J, Realmuto GM, Northwood AK, Masten AS. Comorbidity of psychiatric diagnoses with posttraumatic stress disorder in survivors of childhood trauma. J Am Acad Child Adolesc Psychiatry. 1995;34:1167–73.
25. Wright MO, Master A, Northwood J, Hubbard J. The effects of trauma on the developmental process. In: Cicchetti D, Toth L, editors. Rochester Symp. Dev. Psychopathol. Rochester: University of Rochester Press; 1997. p. 181–225.
26. Masten AS, Coatsworth JD. The development of competence in favorable and unfavorable environments: Lessons from research on successful children. Am Psychol. 1998;53:205–20.
27. Pine DS, Costello J, Masten A. Trauma, proximity, and developmental psychopathology: the effects of war and terrorism on children. Neuropsychopharmacology. 2005;30:1781–92.
28. Caffo E, Belaise C. Psychological aspects of traumatic injury in children and adolescents. Child Adolesc Psychiatr Clin N Am. 2003;12:493–535.
29. Nader KO, Pynoos RS, Fairbanks LA, Al-Ajeel M, Al-Asfour A. A preliminary study of PTSD and grief among the children of Kuwait following the Gulf crisis. Br J Clin Psychol. 1993;32:407–16.
30. Smith P, Perrin S, Yule W, Hacam B, Stuvland R. War exposure among children from Bosnia-Hercegovina: psychological adjustment in a community sample. J Trauma Stress. 2002;15:147–56.
31. Kinzie JD, Sack WH, Angell RH, Manson S, Rath B. The psychiatric effects of massive trauma on cambodian children: I. the children. J Am Acad Child Psychiatry. 1986;25:370–6.
32. Thabet AA, Ibraheem AN, Shivram R, Winter EA, Vostanis P. Parenting support and PTSD in children of a war zone. Int J Soc Psychiatry. 2009;55:226–37.
33. Qouta SR, Palosaari E, Diab M, Punamäki R-L. Intervention effectiveness among war-affected children: a cluster randomized controlled trial on improving mental health. J Trauma Stress. 2012;25:288–98.
34. Reese Masterson A, Usta J, Gupta J, Ettinger AS. Assessment of reproductive health and violence against women among displaced Syrians in Lebanon. BMC Womens Health. 2014;14:25.
35. Rees S, Silove D, Verdial T, et al. Intermittent explosive disorder amongst women in conflict affected Timor-Leste: associations with human rights trauma, ongoing violence, poverty, and injustice. PLoS One. 2013;8:e69207.
36. Saile R, Ertl V, Neuner F, Catani C. Does war contribute to family violence against children? Findings from a two-generational multi-informant study in Northern Uganda. Child Abuse Negl. 2014;38:135–46.
37. Rabenhorst MM, McCarthy RJ, Thomsen CJ, Milner JS, Travis WJ, Colasanti MP. Child maltreatment among U.S. Air Force parents deployed in support of Operation Iraqi Freedom/Operation Enduring Freedom. Child Maltreat. 2015;20:61–71.
38. Rentz ED, Marshall SW, Loomis D, Casteel C, Martin SL, Gibbs DA. Effect of deployment on the occurrence of child maltreatment in military and nonmilitary families. Am J Epidemiol. 2007;165:1199–206.

39. Sullivan K, Capp G, Gilreath TD, Benbenishty R, Roziner I, Astor RA. Substance abuse and other adverse outcomes for military-connected youth in california: results from a large-scale normative population survey. JAMA Pediatr. 2015;169:922–8.

40. Poirier T. The effects of armed conflict on schooling in Sub-Saharan Africa. Int J Educ Dev. 2012;32:341–51.

41. Di Maio M, Nandi TK. The effect of the Israeli–Palestinian conflict on child labor and school attendance in the West Bank. J Dev Econ. 2013;100:107–16.

42. Qeshta HA, AL Hawajri AM, Thabet AM (2019) The Relationship between War Trauma, PTSD, Anxiety and Depression among Adolescents in the Gaza Strip. Heal Sci J. https://doi.org/10.21767/1791-809X.1000621\

43. Dawwas MK, Thabet AAM. The Relationship between Traumatic Experience, Posttraumatic Stress Disorder, Resilience and Posttraumatic Growth among Adolescents in Gaza Strip. Glob J Intellect Dev Disabil. 2017;3(3):73–82.

44. Kolltveit S, Lange-Nielsen II, Thabet AAM, Dyregrov A, Pallesen S, Johnsen TB, Laberg JC. Risk factors for PTSD, anxiety, and depression among adolescents in gaza. J Trauma Stress. 2012;25:164–70.

45. Mann G. 'Finding a Life' Among Undocumented Congolese Refugee Children in Tanzania. Child Soc. 2010;24:261–70.

46. Erjavec K, Volčič Z. Living with the sins of their fathers: an analysis of self-representation of adolescents born of war rape. J Adolesc Res. 2010;25:359–86.

47. Dickson-Gomez J. Growing Up in Guerrilla Camp: the long-term impact of being a child soldier in El Salvador's civil war. Ethos J Soc Psychol Anthropol. 2002;30:327–56.

48. Kadir A, Shenoda S, Goldhagen J. Effects of armed conflict on child health and development: a systematic review. PLoS One. 2019;14:e0210071.

49. Betancourt TS, Borisova II, de la Soudière M, Williamson J. Sierra Leone's child soldiers: war exposures and mental health problems by gender. J Adolesc Health. 2011;49:21–8.

50. Ba I, Bhopal RS. Physical, mental and social consequences in civilians who have experienced war-related sexual violence: a systematic review (1981-2014). Public Health. 2017;142:121–35.

51. ISSOP Migration Working Group. ISSOP position statement on migrant child health. Child Care Health Dev. 2018;44:161–70.

52. Marquardt L, Krämer A, Fischer F, Prüfer-Krämer L. Health status and disease burden of unaccompanied asylum-seeking adolescents in Bielefeld, Germany: cross-sectional pilot study. Trop Med Int Health. 2016;21:210–8.

53. Bogic M, Njoku A, Priebe S. Long-term mental health of war-refugees: a systematic literature review. BMC Int Health Hum Rights. 2015;15:29.

54. Joshi PT, O'Donnell DA. Consequences of child exposure to war and terrorism. Clin Child Fam Psychol Rev. 2003;6:275–92.

55. Dyregrov A, Salloum A, Kristensen P, Dyregrov K. Grief and traumatic grief in children in the context of mass trauma. Curr Psychiatry Rep. 2015;17:48.

56. Papageorgiou V, Frangou-Garunovic A, Iordanidou R, Yule W, Smith P, Vostanis P. War trauma and psychopathology in Bosnian refugee children. Eur Child Adolesc Psychiatry. 2000;9:84–90.

57. Pfefferbaum B. Posttraumatic stress disorder in children: a review of the past 10 years. J Am Acad Child Adolesc Psychiatry. 1997;36:1503–11.

58. Smith P, Perrin S, Yule W, Rabe-Hesketh S. War exposure and maternal reactions in the psychological adjustment of children from Bosnia-Hercegovina. J Child Psychol Psychiatry. 2001;42:395–404.

59. Pynoos RS, Steinberg AM, Piacentini JC. A developmental psychopathology model of childhood traumatic stress and intersection with anxiety disorders. Biol Psychiatry. 1999;46:1542–54.

60. Almqvist K, Brandell-Forsberg M. Refugee children in Sweden: post-traumatic stress disorder in Iranian preschool children exposed to organized violence. Child Abuse Negl. 1997;21:351–66.

61. Cohen E, Chazan S, Lerner M, Maimon E. Posttraumatic play in young children exposed to terrorism: an empirical study. Infant Ment Health J. 2010;31:159–81.
62. Smith E. The play behaviors of young children exposed to a traumatic event. Columbia University; 2011.
63. Zahr LK. Effects of war on the behavior of Lebanese preschool children: Influence of home environment and family functioning. Am J Orthopsychiatry. 1996;66:401–8.
64. Pat-Horenczyk R, Achituv M, Rubenstein AK, Khodabakhsh A, Brom D, Chemtob C. Growing up under fire: building resilience in young children and parents exposed to ongoing missile attacks. J Child Adolesc Trauma. 2012;5:303–14.
65. Thabet AAM, Karim K, Vostanis P. Trauma exposure in pre-school children in a war zone. Br J Psychiatry. 2006;188:154–8.
66. Klein TP, Devoe ER, Miranda-Julian C, Linas K. Young children's responses to September 11th: The New York City experience. Infant Ment Health J. 2009;30:1–22.
67. Chemtob CM, Nomura Y, Abramovitz RA. Impact of conjoined exposure to the World Trade Center attacks and to other traumatic events on the behavioral problems of preschool children. Arch Pediatr Adolesc Med. 2008;162:126–33.
68. Thabet AA, Abu Tawahina A, El Sarraj E, Vostanis P. Exposure to war trauma and PTSD among parents and children in the Gaza strip. Eur Child Adolesc Psychiatry. 2008;17:191–9.
69. Schiff M, Pat-Horenczyk R, Benbenishty R, Brom D, Baum N, Astor RA. High school students' posttraumatic symptoms, substance abuse and involvement in violence in the aftermath of war. Soc Sci Med. 2012;75:1321–8.
70. The National Child Traumatic Stress Network. https://www.nctsn.org/what-is-child-trauma/trauma-types/refugee-trauma/effects.
71. Save The Children (2017) Psychological First Aid for Children: Training manual.
72. Khamis V. Does parent's psychological distress mediate the relationship between war trauma and psychosocial adjustment in children? J Health Psychol. 2016;21:1361–70.
73. Khamis V. Long-term psychological effects of the last Israeli offensive on Gaza on Palestinian children and parents. In: Gaza strip: Gaza community mental health programme; 2013.
74. Lai BS, Hadi F, Llabre MM. Parent and child distress after war exposure. Br J Clin Psychol. 2014;53:333–47.
75. Green BL, Korol M, Grace MC, Vary MG, Leonard AC, Gleser GC, Smitson-Cohen S. Children and disaster: Age, gender, and parental effects on PTSD symptoms. J Am Acad Child Adolesc Psychiatry. 1991;30:945–51.
76. Hysing M, Elgen I, Gillberg C, Lie SA, Lundervold AJ. Chronic physical illness and mental health in children. Results from a large-scale population study. J Child Psychol Psychiatry. 2007;48:785–92.
77. Stoddard FJ, Norman DK, Murphy JM. A diagnostic outcome study of children and adolescents with severe burns. J Trauma. 1989;29:471–7.
78. Stoddart F. Care of infants. children and adolescents with burn injuries. In: Lewis M, editor. Child Adolesc. psychiatry a Compr. Textb. Williams & Wilkins; 1996. p. 1016–37
79. Tarnowski K, Rasnake L. In: Tarnowski K, editor. Behavioral aspects of pediatric burns. New York; 1994. p. 81–118.
80. Saxe GN, Stoddard F, Hall E, Chawla N, Lopez C, Sheridan R, King D, King L, Yehuda R. Pathways to PTSD, part I: children with burns. Am J Psychiatry. 2005;162:1299–304.
81. Arceneaux LL, Meyer WJ. Treatments for common psychiatric conditions among children and adolescents during acute rehabilitation and reintegration phases of burn injury. Int Rev Psychiatry. 2009;21:549–58.
82. Stoddard FJ, Saxe G. Ten-year research review of physical injuries. J Am Acad Child Adolesc Psychiatry. 2001;40:1128–45.
83. Stoddard FJ, Sheridan RL, Saxe GN, King BS, King BH, Chedekel DS, Schnitzer JJ, Martyn JAJ. Treatment of pain in acutely burned children. J Burn Care Rehabil. 23:135–56.
84. Latarjet J, Choinère M. Pain in burn patients. Burns. 1995;21:344–8.
85. Henry DB, Foster RL. Burn pain management in children. Pediatr Clin North Am. 2000;47(681–98):ix–x.

86. Miller AC, Hickman LC, Lemasters GK. A distraction technique for control of burn pain. J Burn Care Rehabil. 13:576–80.
87. Pal SK, Cortiella J, Herndon D. Adjunctive methods of pain control in burns. Burns. 1997;23:404–12.
88. Patterson DR. Practical applications of psychological techniques in controlling burn pain. J Burn Care Rehabil. 13:13–8.
89. Frank DL, Khorshid L, Kiffer JF, Moravec CS, McKee MG. Biofeedback in medicine: who, when, why and how? Ment Health Fam Med. 2010;7:85–91.
90. Stoddard FJ. Psychiatric management of the burned patient. In: Martyn J, editor. Acute Manag. Burn. patient; 1990. p. 256–72.
91. Prensner JD, Yowler CJ, Smith LF, Steele AL, Fratianne RB. Music therapy for assistance with pain and anxiety management in burn treatment. J Burn Care Rehabil. 22:83–8. discussion 82-3
92. Hernandez-Reif M, Field T, Largie S, Hart S, Redzepi M, Nierenberg B, Peck TM Childrens' distress during burn treatment is reduced by massage therapy. J Burn Care Rehabil 22:191–5.; discussion 190
93. Hoffman HG, Doctor JN, Patterson DR, Carrougher GJ, Furness TA. Virtual reality as an adjunctive pain control during burn wound care in adolescent patients. Pain. 2000;85:305–9.
94. Berde C, B M (1999) Pain in children. In: Wall P, Melzack R (eds) Textb. pain, 4th ed. London, pp 1463–1478
95. March JS, Amaya-Jackson L, Murray MC, Schulte A. Cognitive-behavioral psychotherapy for children and adolescents with posttraumatic stress disorder after a single-incident stressor. J Am Acad Child Adolesc Psychiatry. 1998;37:585–93.
96. Robinson E, Rumsey N, Partridge J. An evaluation of the impact of social interaction skills training for facially disfigured people. Br J Plast Surg. 1996;49:281–9.
97. Tarnowski K, Brown R. Pediatric Burns. In: Roberts M, editor. Handb. Pediatr. Psychol; 2003. p. 451–61.
98. Rimmer RB, Foster KN, Bay CR, Floros J, Rutter C, Bosch J, Wadsworth MM, Caruso DM. The reported effects of bullying on burn-surviving children. J Burn Care Res. 28:484–9.
99. Fauerbach JA, Heinberg LJ, Lawrence JW, Bryant AG, Richter L, Spence RJ. Coping with body image changes following a disfiguring burn injury. Health Psychol. 2002;21:115–21.
100. Barenbaum J, Ruchkin V, Schwab-Stone M. The psychosocial aspects of children exposed to war: practice and policy initiatives. J Child Psychol Psychiatry. 2004;45:41–62.
101. Hobfoll SE, Watson P, Bell CC, et al. Five essential elements of immediate and mid-term mass trauma intervention: empirical evidence. Psychiatry. 2007;70:283–315. discussion 316-69
102. Peterson C, Bell M. Children's memory for traumatic injury. Child Dev. 1996;67:3045–70.
103. Terr LC. Childhood traumas: an outline and overview. Am J Psychiatry. 1991;148:10–20.
104. Robertson K. Active listening: more than just paying attention. Aust Fam Physician. 2005;34:1053–5.
105. Sarah M, Mary-Beth M. Mental health and psychosocial support in humanitarian settings: reflections on a review of UNHCR's approach and activities. Intervention. 2013;13:235–47.
106. IASC Guidelines for mental health and psychosocial support in emergency settings- WHO 7 February 2007.
107. Bangpan M, Dickson K, Felix L (2017) The impact of mental health and psychosocial support interventions on people affected by humanitarian emergencies: A systematic review.
108. Mayer S. UNHCR's Mental Heatlh and Psychosocial Support in Emergency Settings. Geneva; 2013.
109. Morina N, Rushiti F, Salihu M, Ford JD. Psychopathology and well-being in civilian survivors of war seeking treatment: a follow-up study. Clin Psychol Psychother. 17:79–86.
110. Tol WA, Barbui C, Galappatti A, Silove D, Betancourt TS, Souza R, Golaz A, van Ommeren M. Mental health and psychosocial support in humanitarian settings: linking practice and research. Lancet (London, England). 2011;378:1581–91.
111. Betancourt TS, McBain R, Newnham EA, Akinsulure-Smith AM, Brennan RT, Weisz JR, Hansen NB. A behavioral intervention for war-affected youth in Sierra Leone: a randomized controlled trial. J Am Acad Child Adolesc Psychiatry. 2014;53:1288–97.

112. Jordans MJD, Komproe IH, Tol WA, Kohrt BA, Luitel NP, Macy RD, de Jong JTVM. Evaluation of a classroom-based psychosocial intervention in conflict-affected Nepal: a cluster randomized controlled trial. J Child Psychol Psychiatry. 2010;51:818–26.

113. Bolton P, Bass J, Betancourt T, Speelman L, Onyango G, Clougherty KF, Neugebauer R, Murray L, Verdeli H. Interventions for depression symptoms among adolescent survivors of war and displacement in northern Uganda: a randomized controlled trial. JAMA. 2007;298:519–27.

114. Brown FL, de Graaff AM, Annan J, Betancourt TS. Annual Research Review: Breaking cycles of violence - a systematic review and common practice elements analysis of psychosocial interventions for children and youth affected by armed conflict. J Child Psychol Psychiatry. 2017;58:507–24.

115. Ziadni M, Hammoudeh W, Rmeileh NMEA, Hogan D, Shannon H, Giacaman R. Sources of human insecurity in post-war situations: the case of gaza. J Hum Secur. 2011; https://doi.org/10.3316/JHS0703023.

116. Das JK, Salam RA, Lassi ZS, Khan MN, Mahmood W, Patel V, Bhutta ZA. Interventions for adolescent mental health: an overview of systematic reviews. J Adolesc Health. 2016;59:S49–60.

117. Panter-Brick C, Dajani R, Eggerman M, Hermosilla S, Sancilio A, Ager A. Insecurity, distress and mental health: experimental and randomized controlled trials of a psychosocial intervention for youth affected by the Syrian crisis. J Child Psychol Psychiatry. 2018;59:523–41.

118. Toole MJ, Galson S, Brady W. Are war and public health compatible? Lancet (London, England). 1993;341:1193–6.

119. Ladd GW, Cairns E. Children: ethnic and political violence. Child Dev. 1996;67:14–8.

120. Laor N, Wolmer L, Cohen DJ. Mothers' Functioning and Children's Symptoms 5 Years After a SCUD Missile Attack. Am J Psychiatry. 2001;158:1020–6.

121. Aboutanos MB, Baker SP. Wartime civilian injuries: epidemiology and intervention strategies. J Trauma. 1997;43:719–26.

122. Santa Barbara J. Impact of war on children and imperative to end war. Croat Med J. 2006;47:891–4.

123. Murthy RS, Lakshminarayana R. Mental health consequences of war: a brief review of research findings. World Psychiatry. 2006;5:25–30.

124. Cohen E, Dekel R, Solomon Z. Long-term adjustment and the role of attachment among Holocaust child survivors. Pers Individ Dif. 2002;33:299–310.

125. Mikulincer M, Shaver PR, Horesh N. Attachment Bases of Emotion Regulation and Posttraumatic Adjustment. In: Emot. Regul. couples Fam. Pathways to Dysfunct. Heal. Washington: American Psychological Association. p. 77–99.

Index

© Springer Nature Switzerland AG 2023
G. S. Abu-Sittah, J. J. Hoballah (eds.), *The War Injured Child*,
https://doi.org/10.1007/978-3-031-28613-1

Printed by Printforce, the Netherlands